ON CALL
PRINCIPLES AND PROTOCOLS

ON CALL
PRINCIPLES AND PROTOCOLS

Second Edition

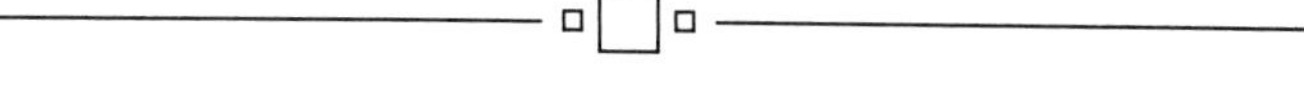

SHANE A. MARSHALL, M.D., F.R.C.P.C.

Director, Cardiac Ultrasound Laboratory
King Edward VIIth Memorial Hospital
Paget, Bermuda

Formerly Chief Resident, Internal Medicine
St. Paul's Hospital
University of British Columbia
Vancouver, British Columbia, Canada

JOHN RUEDY, M.D., F.R.C.P.C.

Dean, Faculty of Medicine
Dalhousie University
Halifax, Nova Scotia, Canada

Formerly Head, Department of Medicine
St. Paul's Hospital
University of British Columbia
Vancouver, British Columbia, Canada

W.B. SAUNDERS COMPANY
A Division of Harcourt Brace & Company
Philadelphia London Toronto Montreal Sydney Tokyo

W.B. SAUNDERS COMPANY
A Division of
Harcourt Brace & Company

The Curtis Center
Independence Square West
Philadelphia, Pennsylvania 19106

Cover illustration is a reproduction of *Speed* by Virgil Cantini, porcelain enamel on steel.

Library of Congress Cataloging-in-Publication Data

Marshall, Shane A.
   On call : principles and protocols / Shane A. Marshall, John Ruedy.—2nd ed.
         p.   cm.
   Rev. ed. of: On Call : principles and protocols / Jean H. Gillies, Shane A. Marshall, John Ruedy.   1989.
   Includes bibliographical references and index.
   ISBN 0-7216-3982-8
   1.   Medical emergencies.   2.   Hospitals—Medical staff.   I.   Ruedy, John.   II.   Gillies, Jean H. On call.   III.   Title.
      [DNLM: 1.   Emergencies—handbooks.   2.   Emergency Medicine—handbooks.   WB29 M369o]
   RC86.7.G55   1993
   616.02'5—dc20
   DNLM/DLC   92-49077

ON CALL: Principles and Protocols   ISBN 0-7216-3982-8

                                                          International Edition
                                                          ISBN   0–7216–4801–0

Printed in United States of America

Last digit is the print
number: 9   8   7   6   5   4   3   2

To our families
in Bermuda and Canada

❑ ❑ ❑

PREFACE

The responsibility for calls at night is one of the traditional duties of medical students and residents in teaching hospitals. *On Call: Principles and Protocols* is designed to facilitate the transition of medical students and residents from the classroom to the hospital setting. We believe that the initiation of the medical student to hospital practice need not be one of trial and error and need not be recalled as a year of stress and uncertainty.

On Call emphasizes the assessment and management of the common problems for which medical students and residents are called at night. The second edition provides more comprehensive assessment and management strategies for the elderly and those with acquired immunodeficiency syndrome, two groups whose numbers comprise increasingly larger segments of the hospitalized population. The second edition of *On Call* includes the On Call Formulary, a quick reference of commonly prescribed medications. We have been careful to maintain an approach that provides both instruction and reference while emphasizing the rational thought processes required for optimal patient care in specific clinical situations. It is our belief that this structured approach deserves greater emphasis in the undergraduate years, and we are hopeful that it will help in the introduction of students to clinical medicine.

Shane A. Marshall
John Ruedy

ACKNOWLEDGMENTS

We are grateful to the many physicians from St. Paul's Hospital in Vancouver, British Columbia, who provided helpful and detailed comments on individual chapters: Drs. B. Chan, S. Clarke, A. Dodek, L. Halperin, S.A. Kline, L. Lawson, A. Levin, I. MacDonald, J. Martini, W.A. McLeod, J. Onrot, P.T. Phang, J. Russell, H. Stein, C. Thompson, H. Tildesley, and J. Ward. We would also like to thank Dr. J. Gillies for her major contribution to the first edition of *On Call*, and to Mr. John Dyson for his patience and encouragement during the preparation of the first and second editions of this book.

DOSAGE NOTICE

Extraordinary efforts have been made by the authors and the publisher of this book to ensure that dosage recommendations are precise and in agreement with the highest standards of practice. [The drug dosage recommendations are those for adults.]

Dosage schedules are changed from time to time in the light of accumulating clinical experience and continuing laboratory studies. These changes are most likely to occur in the case of recently introduced products.

We urge, therefore, that you check the package information data for the manufacturer's recommended dosage. In addition, there are some quite serious situations, each encountered only rarely, in which drug therapy must be individualized, and expert judgment advises the use of a higher dosage or administration by a different route than is included in the manufacturer's recommendations.

STRUCTURE OF THE BOOK

The book is divided into three main sections.

Section I covers introductory material in four chapters: (1) Approach to the Diagnosis and Management of On-Call Problems, (2) Documentation of On-Call Problems, (3) Assessment and Management of Volume Status, and (4) AIDS and the House Officer. Volume status is discussed in the introductory section as its assessment is essential in the proper management of many problems in hospitalized patients. A statement on AIDS is included because of the small but real risk that caring for HIV patients poses to the health care worker.

Section II contains the common calls associated with patient-related problems. Each problem is approached from its inception, beginning with the relevant questions that should be asked over the phone, the temporary orders that should be given, and the major life-threatening problems to be considered as one approaches the bedside:

PHONE CALLS

Questions

Pertinent questions to assess the urgency of the situation.

Orders

Urgent orders to be carried out before the housestaff arrives at the bedside.

Inform the RN

RN to be informed of the time the housestaff anticipates arrival at the bedside.

ELEVATOR THOUGHTS

The differential diagnosis to be considered by the housestaff while they are on their way to assess the patient (i.e., while they are in the elevator).

MAJOR THREAT TO LIFE

Identification of the major threat to life is essential in providing focus for the subsequent effective management of the patient.

BEDSIDE
Quick Look Test

The quick look test is a rapid visual assessment to place the patient into one of three categories: well, sick, or critical. This helps determine the necessity of immediate intervention.

Vital Signs
Selective History
Selective Physical Examination
Management

Section III contains the common calls associated with laboratory-related problems.

The appendix consists of reference items that we have found useful in managing calls.

The On Call Formulary is a compendium of commonly used medications that are likely to be prescribed by the student or resident on call. The formulary serves as a quick, alphabetically arranged reference for indications, drug dosages, routes of administration, side effects, contraindications, and modes of action.

COMMONLY USED ABBREVIATIONS

ABD	Abdomen
ABG	Arterial blood gas
AC	Before meals
ACTH	Adrenocorticotropic hormone
AIDS	Acquired immunodeficiency syndrome
ANA	Antinuclear antibody
A/P	Anteroposterior
aPTT	Activated partial thromboplastin time
ARDS	Adult respiratory distress syndrome
ASD	Atrial septal defect
AV	Atrioventricular
BID	Two times a day
BP	Blood pressure
BPH	Benign prostatic hypertrophy
Ca	Cancer
CBC	Complete blood count
CCU	Coronary care unit
CGL	Chronic granulocytic leukemia
CHF	Congestive heart failure
CLL	Chronic lymphocytic leukemia
CMV	Cytomegalovirus
CNS	Central nervous system
CO	Cardiac output
COHb	Carboxyhemoglobin
COPD	Chronic obstructive pulmonary disease
CPK	Creatine phosphokinase
CrCl	Creatinine clearance
C&S	Culture and sensitivity
CT	Computed tomography
CVS	Cardiovascular system

CXR	Chest x-ray
DDAVP	1-Desamino-(8-D-arginine)-vasopressin
D5NS	5% dextrose in normal saline
D5W	5% dextrose in water
DIC	Disseminated intravascular coagulation
DVT	Deep venous thrombosis
ECF	Extracellular fluid
ECG	Electrocardiogram
EDTA	Disodium edetate
ENDO	Endocrine
ENT	Ears, nose, and throat
ESR	Erythrocyte sedimentation rate
EXT	Extremities
FDP	Fibrin degradation products
F$_{IO_2}$	Fraction of inspired oxygen
FUO	Fever of unknown origin
GI	Gastrointestinal
G-6-PD	Glucose-6-phosphate dehydrogenase
GTT	Glucose tolerance test
GU	Genitourinary
Hb	Hemoglobin
HEENT	Head, eyes, ears, nose, and throat
HIV	Human immunodeficiency virus
HJR	Hepatojugular reflux
HPI	History of present illness
HR	Heart rate
HS	Hora somni (at bedtime)
IBW	Ideal body weight
ICF	Intracellular fluid
ICU	Intensive care unit
ICU/CCU	Intensive care unit/coronary care unit
IDDM	Insulin-dependent diabetes mellitus
IM	Intramuscular
ITP	Idiopathic thrombocytopenic purpura

IV	Intravenous
IVAC	Infusion pump
IVP	Intravenous pyelogram
J	Joule equivalent
JVP	Jugular venous pressure
L	Liter
LDH	Lactate dehydrogenase
LLQ	Lower left quadrant
LOC	Level of consciousness
LP	Lumbar puncture
LUQ	Left upper quadrant
MAO	Monoamine oxidase
MCV	Mean corpuscular volume
MD	Doctor of medicine
MI	Myocardial infarction
MISC	Miscellaneous
MRI	Magnetic Resonance Imaging (formerly NMR)
MSS	Musculoskeletal system
MVP	Mitral valve prolapse
NEURO	Neurological system
NG	Nasogastric
NIDDM	Non-insulin-dependent diabetes mellitus
NMR	Nuclear magnetic resonance (scan)
NPH	Neutral protamine Hagedorn (insulin)
NPO	Nil per os (nothing by mouth)
NS	Normal saline (0.9% saline in water)
NSAID	Nonsteroidal anti-inflammatory drug
NYD	Not yet diagnosed
P/A	Posteroanterior
PAC	Premature atrial contraction
PAT	Paroxysmal atrial tachycardia
PC	After meals
Pco$_2$	Partial pressure of carbon dioxide
PEEP	Positive end-expiratory pressure

PMNs	Polymorphonuclear cells
PND	Paroxysmal nocturnal dyspnea
PO	Per os (by mouth)
Po$_2$	Partial pressure of oxygen
PR	Per rectum
PRN	As necessary
PT	Prothrombin time
PTH	Parathyroid hormone
PTT	Partial thromboplastin time
PUD	Peptic ulcer disease
PVC	Premature ventricular contraction
QHS	At bedtime
QID	Four times a day
RA	Rheumatoid arthritis
RAD	Right axis deviation
RBBB	Right bundle branch block
RBC	Red blood cell
RESP	Respiratory system
RLQ	Right lower quadrant
RN	Registered nurse
ROM	Range of motion
RR	Respiratory rate
RTA	Renal tubular acidosis
RUQ	Right upper quadrant
RV	Right ventricle
S3	Third heart sound
SAH	Subarachnoid hemorrhage
SBE	Subacute bacterial endocarditis (infective endocarditis)
SC	Subcutaneous
SI	International System of Units
SIADH	Syndrome of inappropraite antidiuretic hormone
SL	Sublingual
SLE	Systemic lupus erythematosus
SOB	Shortness of breath

SSS	Sick sinus syndrome
stat	Immediately
STS	Serological test for syphilis
SVT	Supraventricular tachycardia
T₃	Triiodothyronine
T₄	Thyroxine
TB	Tuberculosis
TBW	Total body water
TCA	Tricyclic antidepressants
TIA	Transient ischemic attack
TKVO	To keep vein open
tPA	Tissue plasminogen activator
TPN	Total parenteral nutrition
TSH	Thyroid stimulating hormone
TTP	Thrombotic thrombocytopenic purpura
URTI	Upper respiratory tract infection
UTI	Urinary tract infection
VP	Ventriculoperitoneal
VSD	Ventricular septal defect
WBC	White blood count
ZN	Ziehl-Neelsen

CONTENTS

■ LABORATORY-RELATED PROBLEMS: THE COMMON CALLS

■ APPENDIX

INTRODUCTION

APPROACH TO THE DIAGNOSIS AND MANAGEMENT OF ON-CALL PROBLEMS

Clinical problem solving is an important function required by the physician on call. Historically, a physician approaches the diagnosis and management of a patient's problems with an ordered, structured system (e.g., history taking, physical examination, review of available tests, and x-rays) before formulation of the provisional and differential diagnoses and the management plan. The history and physical examination may take 30 to 40 minutes for an otherwise well patient with a single problem coming to the family physician for the first time, or they may take 60 to 90 minutes for a geriatric patient with multiple complaints. Clearly, if the patient arrives at the emergency department unconscious, having been found on the street, the chief complaint is coma, and the HPI is limited to the minimal information provided by the ambulance attendants or by the contents of the patient's wallet. In this situation, physicians are trained to proceed with examination, investigation, and treatment concurrently. How this is to be achieved is not always clear, although there is agreement on the steps that should be completed within the initial 5 to 10 minutes.

The physician is first confronted with on-call problem solving in the final years of medical school. It is at this stage that the structured history taking and physical examination system directs the student's approach in evaluating a patient. The medical student is faced with well-defined problems when on call (e.g., fall-out-of-bed, fever, chest pain) yet feels ill equipped to begin clinical problem solving unless it involves "the complete history and physical." Anything less than the 60-minute (usually more) "admission history and physical" engenders guilt over a task only partially completed, yet not every on-call problem can involve 60 minutes or more of the physician's time, since inadequate treatment time will be given to sick patients because of the unnecessary time spent on relatively minor problems.

The approach recommended in this book offers a structured system but one that can be logically adapted to most situations. It is intended as a practical guide to assist in efficient clinical problem solving when on call. Chapters so related are divided into four parts as follows.

1. Phone call
2. Elevator thoughts

3. Major threat to life
4. Bedside

PHONE CALL

Most problems confronting the physician on call are first communicated by telephone. The physician must be able to determine the severity of the problem over the telephone, since it is not always possible to immediately assess the patient at the bedside. Patients must be evaluated in order of priority. The phone call section of each chapter is divided into three parts as follows.

1. Questions
2. Orders
3. Inform RN

The questions are selected to assist in determining the urgency of the problem. Orders are suggested that will help expedite the investigation and management of urgent situations. Finally, the RN is informed of the physician's anticipated time of arrival at the bedside and the responsibilities of the RN in the interim.

ELEVATOR THOUGHTS

Since the physician on call is not usually on the floor when he or she is informed of a problem that requires assessment, the time spent travelling to the ward, which may be up to 10 minutes in some large hospitals, may be used efficiently to consider the differential diagnosis of the problem at hand. Since time is spent standing still in the elevator, the term "elevator thoughts" has been coined to summarize the directed differential diagnosis. It should be emphasized that the differential diagnosis lists that are offered are not exhaustive but rather focus on the most common or the most serious (life-threatening) causes that should be considered in hospitalized patients.

MAJOR THREAT TO LIFE

Identification of the major threat to life that each problem presents provides a focus for the subsequent effective investigation and management of the patient. The major threat to life posed by each problem follows logically from a consideration of the differential diagnosis. Rather than arriving at the bedside with a memorized list of possible diagnoses, an appreciation of the one or two most likely threats to life is more useful and relevant in directing one's questions and physical examination. This mental process serves to ensure that the most serious life-threatening possibility in each clinical scenario is both considered and sought after in the initial evaluation of the patient.

BEDSIDE

The protocols for what to do on arrival at the bedside are divided into the following parts.

- Quick look test
- Airway and vital signs
- Selective history
- Selective physical examination
- Selective chart review
- Management

The bedside assessment should begin with the quick look test and airway and vital signs. The quick look test is a rapid visual assessment that may enable the physician to categorize the patient's condition into one of three degrees of severity: well (comfortable), sick (uncomfortable or distressed), or critical (about to die). Next is assessment of the airway and vital signs, important in the evaluation of any potentially sick patient. Because of the nature of the various problems that require assessment when on call, the order of the remaining parts is not uniform. For example, Chapter 5 *Abdominal Pain* follows the expected sequence of Selective History and Chart Review, Selective Physical Examination, and Management, whereas Chapter 23 *Seizures* follows the sequence of Management I, Selective Physicial Examination I, Selective History and Chart Review, Selective Physical Examination II, and Management II. Occasionally, the Selective Physical Examination and Management sections are subdivided. This division allows for the first focus on the urgent, life-threatening problem, leaving the less urgent problems to be reviewed in the second subdivision.

It is hoped that the principles and protocols offered for clinical problem solving of common on-call problems will provide a logical, efficient system for the assessment and management of patients in the hospital.

2

DOCUMENTATION OF ON-CALL PROBLEMS

Accurate, concise documentation of on-call problems at night is essential for the continued efficient care of hospitalized patients. In many instances, the patient you are asked to see at night will not be known to you, and you may not be involved in their continuing care after your night on call. Some problems can be handled safely over the telephone, but in the majority of situations, a selective history and physical examination will be required to correctly diagnose and treat the problem. Documentation is recommended on every patient you examine. If the problem is straightforward your note can be brief, and if the problem is complicated, your note should be concise yet complete.

Begin by recording the date, time, and who you are, e.g., Aug. 10, 1993, 0200H. "Medical student on-call note" or "Resident on-call note."

State who called you and at what time you were called, e.g., Called to see patient by RN at 0130H because the patient "fell out of bed."

If your assessment is delayed by more urgent problems, say so. A brief one or two sentence summary of the patient's admission diagnosis and major medical problems should follow.

This 74-year-old woman with a history of chronic renal failure, NIDDM, and rheumatoid arthritis was admitted 10 days ago with increasing joint pain.

Next, describe the HPI of the "fall out of bed" both from the patient's viewpoint and from that of any witnesses. The HPI is no different from the HPI you would document in your admission history, e.g.

HPI. The patient was on the way to the bathroom to void, tripped on her bathrobe, and fell to the floor, landing on her left side. She denied palpitations, chest pain, lightheadedness, nausea, and hip pain. There was no difficulty walking unaided and no pain afterward. The fall was not witnessed. The RN found the patient lying on the floor. Vital signs were normal.

If your chart review has relevant findings, include these in your HPI, e.g.

Three previous "falls out of bed" on this admission. Patient has no recall of these events.

Documentation of your examination should be selective. A call regarding a fall out of bed requires you to examine relevant components of the vital signs, head and neck, cardiovascular, musculoskeletal, and neurological systems.

It is not necessary to examine the respiratory system or the abdomen unless there is a second separate problem (e.g., you arrive at the bedside and find the patient febrile). On-call problems should not require you to take a complete history and conduct a complete physical examination. These were done when the patient was admitted. Your history, physical examination, and chart documentation should be directed (i.e., problem oriented). It may be useful to underline the positive physical findings both for yourself (it aids your summary) and for the housestaff who will be following the patient in the morning.

Physical Examination

VITALS	BP 140/85
	HR <u>104</u>/min
	RR <u>36</u>/min
	Temp <u>38.9</u> PO

HEENT	No tongue or cheek lacerations
	No hemotympanum
CVS	Pulse rate and rhythm normal; JVP 2 cm > SA
MSS	No skull or face lacerations or hematomas
	Spine and ribs normal
	Full, painless ROM of all 4 limbs
	Reflexes ⎫
	Motor ⎬ Normal
	Sensory ⎭
NEURO	Alert. Oriented to time, place, and person

Relevant laboratory, ECG, or x-ray findings should be documented. Again it is useful to underline abnormal findings, e.g.

- Glucose   7.2 mmol/L
- Sodium   141 mmol/L
- Potassium   3.9 mmol/L
- Calcium   Not available
- Urea   <u>12 mmol/L</u>
- Creatinine <u>180 mmol/L</u>

Your diagnostic conclusion, regarding the problem for which you were called, must be clearly stated. It is not enough to write "patient fell out of bed." The RN could have written that without your even having seen the patient. The information gathered must be synthesized to achieve the highest level of diagnostic integration plausible. This provisional diagnosis should be followed by a differential diagnosis in order of the most likely alternative explanations. In the patient who fell out of bed, your diagnostic conclusion might be as follows.

1. "Fall out of bed" due to difficulty reaching the bathroom to void (?diuretic-induced nocturia, ?contribution of hs sedation)
2. Large hematoma (7 × 9 cm) left thigh

Your plan must be clearly stated, both the measures taken during the night and the investigations or treatment you have organized for the morning. Avoid writing "Plan—see orders." It is not always obvious to the staff taking over the next day why certain measures were taken. If you informed the intern, resident, or attending physician of the problem, document with whom you spoke and the recommendations given. Record whether any of the patient's family members were informed of the problem and what they were told. Finally, sign or print your name clearly so the staff know who to contact should they have any questions about the management of this patient the following day.

3

ASSESSMENT AND MANAGEMENT OF VOLUME STATUS

The assessment of volume status is an integral part of the physical examination. You will find in your years as a medical student and intern and later as a practicing physician that this skill plays a key role in helping to choose the appropriate investigation and management in many clinical situations.

Ideally, this skill is best learned at the bedside. However, some background knowledge will help you in the accurate assessment and interpretation of a patient's volume status.

First, terminology must be clarified. The human body is composed mostly of water (Fig. 3–1). In fact, *total body water* (TBW) makes up 60% of the weight of the adult male. Of this, two thirds is *intracellular fluid* (ICF), and one third is *extracellular fluid* (ECF), i.e., water that is outside of cells. Of the extracellular fluid, 66% is *interstitial fluid*, such as fluid bathing the cells, cerebrospinal fluid, and intraocular fluid. Only 7% of total body weight is *intravascular fluid* (plasma). Clinically, it is the extracellular fluid, consisting of intravascular and interstitial fluids, that one is trying to assess when determining the volume status of a patient.

■ ASSESSMENT OF VOLUME STATUS

There are only three basic states of volume status that a patient can have: volume depleted, normovolemic (euvolemic), and volume overloaded. On approaching the bedside, ask yourself whether the patient is volume depleted, normovolemic, or volume overloaded.

Quick Look Test

Does the patient look well (comfortable), sick (uncomfortable or distressed), or critical (about to die)?

In most instances as you enter the patient's room and first see the patient, it will become apparent whether there is a serious fluid balance abnormality. Patients who are seriously volume depleted look wan, drawn, and tired, whereas patients who are volume overloaded look uncomfortable, anxious, and restless. Of course, these are general guidelines only, and a more detailed physical examination is required.

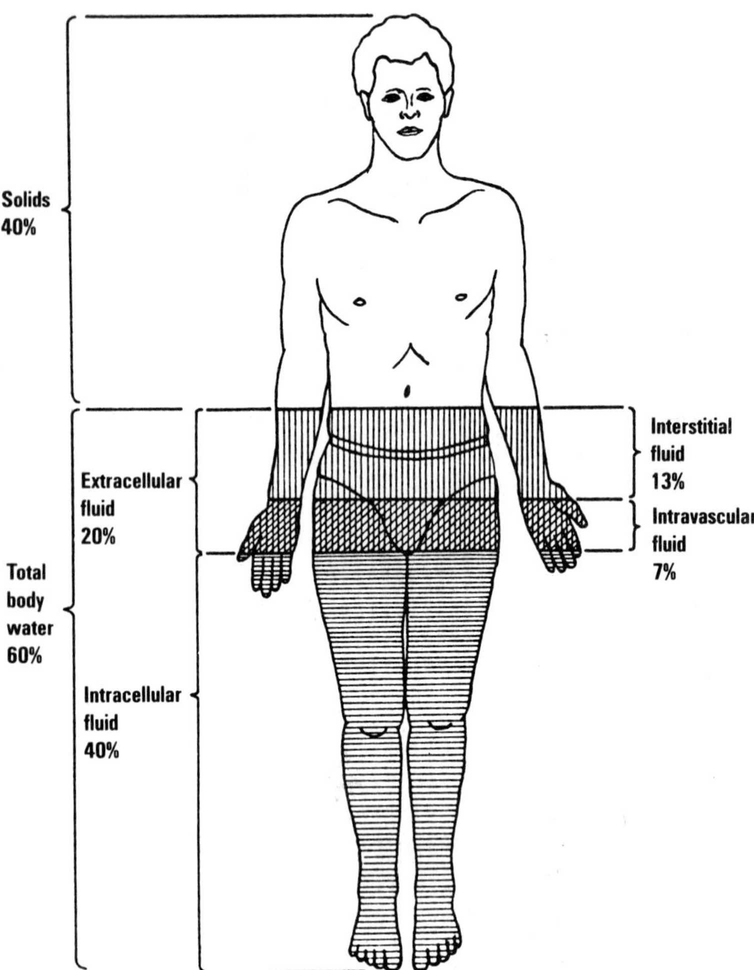

Figure 3–1 □ Body fluid compartments.

Vital Signs

In most cases, simply taking the patient's vital signs will help you determine whether or not there is significant volume depletion.

Measure the heart rate and blood pressure first with the patient supine and then after the patient stands for 1 minute. If the patient is unable to stand alone, ask for assistance or have the patient sit up and dangle his legs over the side of the bed. If the patient is hypotensive in the supine position, this maneuver is not necessary.

An increase in heart rate > 15 beats/min, a fall in systolic blood pressure > 15 mm Hg, or any fall in diastolic blood pressure signifies the presence of postural hypotension, which may indicate *intravascular volume depletion.*

A patient with autonomic dysfunction (e.g., beta blockers, diabetic neuropathy, Shy-Drager syndrome) may also have a pronounced postural fall in BP but without the expected degree of compensatory tachycardia. Unlike the volume depleted patient, however, there should be no other features of extracellular fluid deficit in the patient with uncomplicated autonomic dysfunction.

A resting tachycardia may be seen with either volume depletion or volume overload. *Volume depletion* results in a low stroke volume. As can be seen from the following formula, the patient must, therefore, generate a tachycardia in order to maintain cardiac output.

$$\text{Cardiac output} = \text{Heart rate} \times \text{Stroke volume}$$
$$\text{CO} = \text{HR} \times \text{SV}$$

The volume overloaded patient must also generate a tachycardia in an effort to increase forward flow and thereby relieve the lungs of pulmonary congestion. A *normovolemic* patient without other complicating features will have a normal heart rate.

Measure the respiratory rate. The most important feature to look for when measuring the respiratory rate is tachypnea, which may be seen in the volume overloaded patient in whom pulmonary edema has developed.

Selective Physical Examination

HEENT *Look at the oral mucous membranes.* The adequately hydrated patient has moist mucous membranes. It is normal for a small pool of saliva to collect at the undersurface of the tongue in the area of the frenulum, and this should be looked for.

RESP *Listen for crackles.* Pulmonary edema with bilateral basilar crackles and, occasionally, wheezes or pleural effusions may be a manifestation of the volume overloaded patient.

CVS *Look at the neck veins.* Examination of the internal jugular veins is one of the most helpful components of the volume status examination. The JVP may be assessed with the patient at any inclination from 0 degrees to 90 degrees. However, it is easiest to begin looking for the JVP pulsation with the patient at a 45 degree inclination. If, at 45 degrees, you are unable to visualize the neck veins, this usually signifies that the JVP is either very low (in which case you will need to lower the head of the bed) or very high (in which case you may need to sit the patient upright in order to see the top of the column of blood in the internal jugular vein). Once the internal jugular vein pulsation is identified, measure the perpendicular distance from the sternal angle to the top of the column of blood (Fig. 3–2). This distance represents the patient's JVP in centimeters of H_2O above the sternal angle. Its value represents a composite of the volume of venous return to the heart, the central venous pressure, and the efficiency of right atrial and right ventricular emptying.

A JVP of 2 to 3 cm above the sternal angle is normal in the adult patient. A significantly *volume depleted* patient will have flat neck veins, which may fill only when the patient is placed in the Trendelenburg position. A *volume overloaded* patient will usually have an elevated JVP greater than 3 cm above the sternal angle.

Listen for an S_3. An S_3 is most often associated with the volume overloaded state and, sometimes, may be heard only in the left lateral position.

ABD *Examine the liver.* An enlarged, tender liver and a positive hepatojugular reflux may be manifestations of the volume overloaded state.

SKIN *Check the skin turgor.* Evaluating the skin turgor in an adult is best performed by raising a fold of skin from the anterior chest area over the sternal angle. In a normovolemic patient, the skin should return promptly to its usual position. A sluggish return suggests an *interstitial fluid def-*

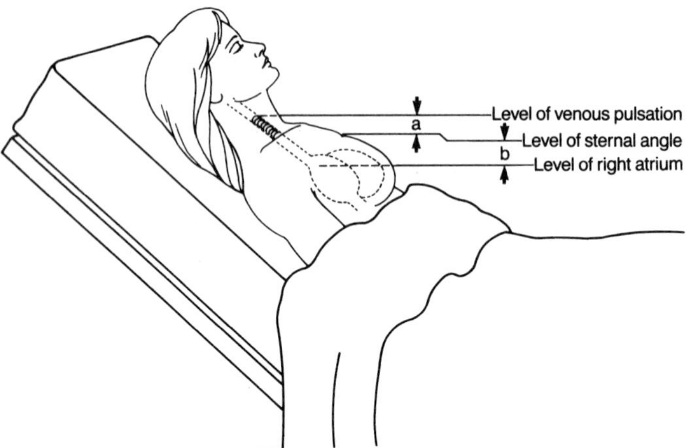

Figure 3–2 □ Measurement of jugular venous pressure. a, The perpendicular distance from the sternal angle to the top of the column of blood and b, the distance from the center of the right atrium to the sternal angle, commonly accepted as measuring 5 cm, regardless of inclination.

icit. Taut, nonpliable skin, which cannot be raised in a fold, suggests *interstitial fluid excess.*
Look at the skin creases and check for edema. Accentuated skin creases from bedsheets' pressing against the posterior thorax and sacral or pedal edema indicate *interstitial fluid excess.*

Selective Chart Review

Sometimes, it is difficult to decide at the bedside whether or not a patient's volume status is normal. There are then a few things in the chart that may help guide you in a difficult case.

Look at the Creatinine/Urea Ratio.   A ratio of less than 12 (calculated in SI units) is suggestive of volume depletion.

Examine the Fluid Balance Records.   Unfortunately, fluid balance records often are notoriously inaccurate. However, if well-kept records are present, a number of clues may be found. A patient who is taking in very little fluid (whether orally or intravenously) may well be volume depleted. A patient whose urine output is greater than 20 ml/h is probably not volume depleted. A net positive intake of several liters over a few days may be indicative of fluid retention with concomitant volume overload.

In the Volume Depleted Patient, Look at the Chart for Contributing Causes.

GI losses	Vomiting
	Nasogastric suction
	Diarrhea
Urinary	Diuretics
losses	Osmotic diuresis (hyperglycemia, mannitol administration, hypertonic IV contrast material)
	Postobstructive diuresis
	Diabetes insipidus
	Recovery phase of acute tubular necrosis
	Adrenal insufficiency
Surface	Skin (increased sweating due to fever, evaporation
losses	in burn patients)
	Respiratory tract (hyperventilation, nonhumidified inhalation therapy)
Fluid	Pancreatitis
sequestration	Ileus
	Burns
Blood losses	GI tract
	Surgical
	Trauma
	Iatrogenic (laboratory sampling)
Other	Inadequate oral or parenteral intake

■ CLASSIC STATES OF VOLUME STATUS

It is a rare occasion when a patient has every feature of volume depletion or volume overload. Still, it is useful when examining a patient to carry a mental picture of the three "classic" states of volume status.

■ *The Classic Volume Depleted Patient*
Quick Look Test

The patient looks wan, tired, and drawn.

Vital Signs

HR	Resting tachycardia
	Postural rise in HR >15 beats/min
BP	Normal or low resting BP
	A postural drop in systolic BP >15 mm Hg or any drop in diastolic BP
RR	Normal
HEENT	Dry oral mucous membranes
RESP	Clear
CVS	JVP flat
	No S_3
ABD	Normal
SKIN	Poor turgor
	No edema

■ *The Classic Volume Overloaded Patient*
Quick Look Test

The patient looks sick and short of breath. Often he or she will be sitting upright and appear uncomfortable, anxious, and restless.

Vital Signs

HR	Resting tachycardia
	Postural rise in HR <15 beats/min
BP	May be low, normal, or high
	No postural fall in systolic or diastolic BP
RR	Tachypnea
RESP	Crackles bilaterally at bases
	±Wheezing
	±Pleural effusions
CVS	JVP >3 cm above the sternal angle
	S_3 present
ABD	Positive hepatojugular reflux
	±Enlarged tender liver
EXT	Accentuated skin folds on posterior thorax
	Sacral or pedal edema

■ *The Classic Patient with Normal Volume Status*

Quick Look Test

The patient looks well.

Vital Signs

HR	Normal
	Postural rise in HR <15 beats/min
BP	Normal
	Postural fall of systolic BP <15 mm Hg and no fall in diastolic BP
RR	Normal
HEENT	Moist oral mucous membranes
RESP	Clear
CVS	JVP 2 to 3 cm above the sternal angle
	No S_3
ABD	Normal
EXT	No edema

■ CHOOSING THE CORRECT INTRAVENOUS FLUID

Selection of an appropriate intravenous fluid for a particular clinical situation need not be a guessing game. A basic understanding of physiology will help to make your fluid management decisions rational and effective.

Water is important in the body because it serves as a *solvent* for a variety of solutes. *Solutes* can be either electrolytes or nonelectrolytes.

Electrolytes are substances in which the molecules disassociate into charged components (ions) when placed in water, and they include the following commonly measured substances.

Sodium Potassium Calcium Magnesium	Cations
Chloride Bicarbonate	Anions

In physiological solutions, the total number of cations always equals the total number of anions.

Nonelectrolytes are solutes that have no electrical charges, and they include such substances as glucose and urea.

As mentioned previously, intravascular volume is mostly made up of *water*, which acts as a solvent to dissolve and transport electrolytes and nonelectrolytes. Water is able to move from one body compartment to the next by the process of *osmosis*. When two solutes are separated by a semipermeable membrane, such as a cell membrane, water will tend to flow across the membrane from the solution of lower concentraton to that of higher con-

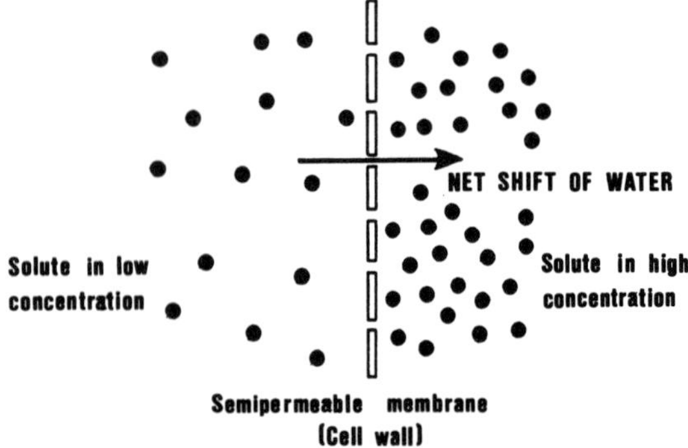

Figure 3–3 □ Osmosis. Water flows across a semipermeable membrane to equalize solute concentrations on either side of the membrane.

centration, the net effect being to equalize the solute concentration on each side of the membrane (Fig. 3–3).

Suppose you were seeing a patient in whom you had decided to infuse a liter of pure water without any solutes. What would happen to the patient's red blood cells? Understanding the process of osmosis allows you to reason that since the solute concentration inside the red blood cells is vastly higher than that in the water infused, water would move across the cell membrane into the red blood cells (Fig. 3–4). There is a limit to how much the red blood cell membrane can stretch, and eventually the red blood cells would burst. Similarly, you can see that if a hypertonic solution was infused directly into the patient's vein, the red blood cells would shrink (crenate) as water moved out of the red blood cells and into the surrounding solution.

For these reasons, most intravenous fluids that are prepared for hospital use are usually close to isotonic; i.e., they have the same solute concentration as the blood to minimize such fluid shifts. Although cell membranes allow water to pass freely by the process of osmosis, such membranes fortunately limit the passage of solutes to a varying degree. Some solute molecules cross membranes more readily than others, depending on their size and physical properties.

In hospitalized patients, there are only three solutes that you

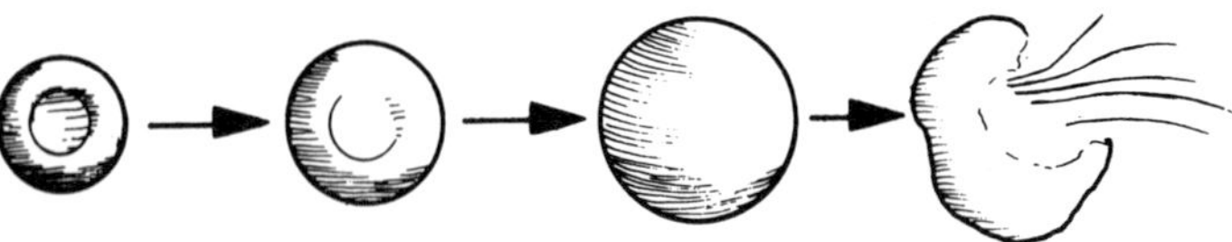

Figure 3–4 □ Osmosis. Effect of infusion of pure water on RBC volume.

need to know about to effectively diagnosis and treat disorders of fluid balance. Glucose distributes widely throughout both intracellular and extracellular spaces, whereas sodium is limited primarily to the extracellular space. Albumin remains largely within the intravascular space. The distribution that these three solutes have is a fundamental principle you will find useful in guiding your decisions about choice of fluid therapy.

D5W consists of 50 g of dextrose dissolved in 1 L of water. It has an osmolality of 252 mOsm/L, which will prevent the patient's red blood cells from shrinking or swelling. Dextrose can be expected to equilibrate rapidly among the intravascular, interstitial, and intracellular spaces, and water will follow along quickly by osmosis.

NS is another commonly employed intravenous solution. It has an osmolality of 308 mOsm/L and, although slightly hypertonic, is not different enough from blood tonicity to cause cell shrinkage. NS will stay predominantly in the extracellular space somewhat longer than a glucose infusion because sodium does not readily move intracellularly.

Albumin and *plasma* will stay in the intravascular space for many hours, since albumin is a large molecule that does not easily traverse the endothelial pores of the blood vessels. The half-life of albumin within the intravascular space is 17 to 20 hours.

From this knowledge of solutes and their membrane permeability, it will be easy to make logical choices regarding fluid management.

In patients with *intravascular volume depletion*, the goal of treatment is to correct and maintain adequate intravascular volume and tissue perfusion. Hence, the volume depleted patient could be treated with intravenous NS, albumin, or plasma. Because NS is more readily available and much less expensive, it is the treatment of choice for the initial resuscitation of the volume depleted patient. Infusing D5W would be of little benefit, since the glucose and water would rapidly distribute throughout the intravascular, interstitial, and extravascular spaces.

In patients with *extravascular volume excess*, the goal of treatment is to improve and maintain adequate cardiac function and tissue perfusion. These usually require the use of preload reducing measures, as outlined in Chapter 24, page 238. However, because these patients are often critically ill, they require intravenous access for medication administration. The best choice of fluid to give, usually at a TKVO rate, is D5W, which will very quickly leave the intravascular space. Infusing NS or albumin could worsen the patient's condition by further increasing intravascular volume. This is why cardiac patients, who are at risk for volume overload, usually are given an IV of D5W when IV access is required for administration of medication.

Another IV solution, "⅔rds ⅓rd," contains 33 g/L of glucose

and 51 mmol/L each of sodium and chloride and is approximately isotonic at 269 mosmol/L. Although there is no particular physiologic basis for its use, it has been popularized as a maintenance IV solution for patients in whom adequate oral intake cannot be met.

REMEMBER

Volume status abnormalities should be corrected at a rate similar to the rate at which they developed. Biological systems are more responsive to rates of change than to absolute amounts of change. It is safest to correct half the deficit and then reevaluate. There is no substitute for frequent repeated examination of the patient when trying to effect changes in volume status.

Occasionally, you will be faced with a patient in whom there is a discrepancy between the two compartments of the extracellular fluid, e.g., the patient with a decreased intravascular volume but an excess of interstitial fluid (i.e., edema). This discrepancy is most commonly seen in states of marked hypoalbuminemia.

Fluid transfer from the intravascular space to the interstitial space depends on the permeability of the capillary bed, how much hydrostatic pressure is being exerted to force fluid out of the intravascular space, and the difference in *oncotic pressure* between the intravascular and interstitial spaces (Fig. 3–5).

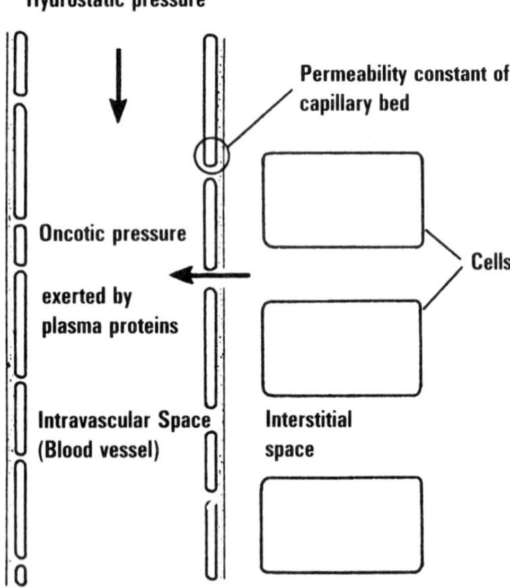

Figure 3–5 □ Factors influencing fluid transfer between the intravascular and extravascular spaces.

Oncotic pressure is exerted by *plasma protein* (i.e., albumin). There is little, if any, protein in the interstitium, and hence the intravascular oncotic pressure exerted by albumin tends to draw water out of the interstitium and into the intravascular space. This knowledge becomes important in the occasional patient who has intravascular volume depletion as assessed by your clinical examination, together with interstitial fluid excess (i.e., edema). To help shift fluid from the interstitium to the intravascular space in such a patient, a logical choice is to administer IV albumin. Artificial plasma expanders (e.g., dextran, hetastarch) also may be used. They are high molecular weight glucose polymers that remain in the intravascular space because of their large size.

Remember that oncotic pull comes from albumin. It does not come from sodium, so NS is not an appropriate fluid to give in this situation. It does not come from red blood cells, so a blood transfusion is not an appropriate fluid to give. Note that albumin is available in two concentrations—5% and 25%. The 25% albumin is the preferred concentration when trying to effect a shift in fluid from the interstitial space to the intravascular space.

Unfortunately, albumin, plasma, and artificial plasma expanders are expensive, and their effect in removing edema fluid is transient. Hence, their continued use for this indication is controversial. Certainly, the best way to correct edema in a patient with a decreased intravascular volume but an excess of interstitial fluid is to correct the underlying cause of interstitial volume excess. In most cases, the cause is hypoproteinemia (e.g., malabsorption, liver disease, nephrotic syndrome, protein losing enteropathy).

In summary, most disorders of fluid balance can be treated logically and successfully by employing the simple principles of water and solute transfer across cell membranes (See Table 3–1 for a listing of the commonly used IV fluids.)

Table 3–1 □ COMMONLY USED INTRAVENOUS FLUIDS

	Glucose (g/L)	Na (mmol/L)	Cl (mmol/L)	K (mmol/L)	Ca (mmol/L)	Lactate (mmol/L)	Approximate Osmolality (mosmol/L)
D5W	50	—	—	—	—	—	252
D10W	100	—	—	—	—	—	505
D20W	200	—	—	—	—	—	1010
D50W	500	—	—	—	—	—	2525
"⅔rds ⅓rd"	33	51	51	—	—	—	269
0.45% NaCl (½ NS)	—	77	77	—	—	—	154
0.9% NaCl (NS)	—	154	154	—	—	—	308
D5NS	50	154	154	—	—	—	560
Ringer's lactate	—	130	109	4	3	28	272
Albumin	—	145	145	Available in 5% concentrations (50, 250, or 500 ml) or 25% concentrations (20, 50, or 100 ml)			
Fresh frozen plasma (FFP)	200 ml plasma that has been separated from whole blood and frozen within 6 hours of collection. FFP contains all coagulation factors.						
Stored plasma	200 ml of plasma that has been separated from whole blood within 72 hours of collection. Contains all coagulation factors except V and VIII.						

4

AIDS AND THE HOUSE OFFICER

The risk of transmission of HIV from patient to health care worker is extremely low. The rate of transmission is less than 0.5% after direct inoculation of infected blood through a needlestick injury and even lower after other types of exposure.

Hepatitis represents a risk of transmission that is 25 times that of HIV. In the USA, 200 to 300 health care workers die of hepatitis annually. Hepatitis B prophylaxis is, therefore, recommended for all potentially exposed staff.

Risk of exposure to HIV and hepatitis virus can be minimized by adhering to straightforward practices referred to as "blood and body fluid precautions." Table 4–1 will familiarize you with these precautions.

Despite attention to safe practices, you may, in the course of your training, suffer accidental exposure to potentially infectious blood or body fluids. Your hospital should have an established policy for helping you, and you should contact the appropriate individual if you have been accidentally exposed.

The following general guidelines are recommended if you have been exposed to blood or body fluids.

■ FIRST AID

1. Seek assistance from a more senior member of staff.
2. Immediately cleanse the contaminated site.
   a. *Needlestick:* Wash well with detergent and water; promote passive bleeding; soak in 1:10 bleach solution for 5 minutes.
   b. *Skin contamination:* Wash well with detergent and water.
   c. *Mucous membrane or eye contact:* Rinse well with water or saline.
3. Save instrument, without washing, in a Sharps container.
4. Report immediately to the designated officer responsible for helping you.

■ IMMEDIATE MANAGEMENT

Treatment of parenteral exposure (i.e., nonintact skin, mucous membrane, or skin puncture) may include

1. Tetanus prophylaxis, as required.
2. Serologic testing of the patient and you, with follow-up vaccination if you are negative and have not been vaccinated for hepatitis B. *Continued on p. 24.*

Table 4–1 □ **UNIVERSAL PRECAUTIONS TO PREVENT TRANSMISSION OF HIV**

Universal Precautions

Because a medical history and physical examination cannot reliably identify all patients infected with HIV or other blood-borne pathogens, blood and body fluid precautions should be consistently used for all patients, especially those in emergency care settings in which the risk of blood exposure is increased and the infection status of the patient is usually not known.

1 Use appropriate barrier precautions to prevent skin and mucous membrane exposure when exposure to blood, body fluids containing blood, or other body fluids to which universal precautions apply (see below) is anticipated. Wear gloves when touching blood or body fluids, mucous membranes, or nonintact skin of all patients, when handling items or surfaces soiled with blood or body fluids, and when performing venipuncture and other vascular access procedures. Change gloves after contact with each patient; do not wash or disinfect gloves for reuse. Wear masks and protective eyewear or face shields during procedures that are likely to generate droplets of blood or other body fluids to prevent exposure of mucous membranes of the mouth, nose, and eyes. Wear gowns or aprons during procedures that are likely to generate splashes of blood or other body fluids.

2 Wash hands and other skin surfaces immediately and thoroughly following contaminations with blood, body fluids containing blood, or other body fluids to which universal precautions apply. Wash hands immediately after gloves are removed.

3 Take care to prevent injuries when using needles, scalpels, and other sharp instruments or devices, when handling sharp instruments after procedures, when cleaning used instruments, and when disposing of used needles. Do not recap used needles by hand; do not remove used needles from disposable syringes by hand; and do not bend, break, or otherwise manipulate used needles by hand. Place used disposable syringes and needles, scalpel blades, and other sharp items in puncture-resistant disposal containers, which should be located as close to the use area as is practical.

4 Although saliva has not been implicated in HIV transmission, the need for emergency mouth-to-mouth resuscitation should be minimized by making mouthpieces, resuscitation bags, or other ventilation devices available for use in areas in which the need for resuscitation is predictable.

5 Health care workers with exudative lesions or weeping dermatitis should refrain from all direct patient care and from handling patient care equipment until the condition resolves.

Universal precautions are intended to supplement rather than replace recommendations for routine infection control, such as hand washing and use of gloves to prevent gross microbial contamination of hands. In addition, implementation of universal precautions does not eliminate the need for other category- or disease-specific isolation precautions, such as enteric precautions for infectious diarrhea or isolation for pulmonary tuberculosis. Universal precautions are not intended to change waste management programs undertaken in accordance with state and local regulations.

Body Fluids to Which Universal Precautions Apply

Universal precautions apply to blood and other body fluids containing visible blood. Blood is the single most important source of HIV, hepatitis B virus, and other blood-borne pathogens in the occupational setting. Universal precautions also apply to tissues, semen, vaginal secretions, and the following fluids: cerebrospinal, synovial, pleural, peritoneal, pericardial, and amniotic.

Universal precautions do not apply to feces, nasal secretions, sputum, sweat, tears, urine, and vomitus unless they contain visible blood. Universal precautions also do not apply to human breast milk, although gloves may be worn by health care workers in situations in which exposure to breast milk might be frequent. In addition, universal precautions do not apply to saliva. Gloves need not be worn when feeding patients or wiping saliva from skin, although special precautions are recommended for dentistry, in which contamination of saliva with blood is predictable. The risk of transmission of HIV, as well as hepatitis B virus, from these fluids and materials is extremely low or nonexistent.

Use of Gloves for Phlebotomy

Gloves should be effective in reducing the incidence of blood contamination of hands during phlebotomy (drawing of blood samples), but they cannot prevent penetrating injuries caused by needles or other sharp instruments. In universal precautions, all blood is assumed to be potentially infectious for blood-borne pathogens. Some institutions have relaxed recommendations for the use of gloves for phlebotomy by skilled health care workers in settings in which the prevalence of blood-borne pathogens is known to be very low (e.g., volunteer blood donation centers). Institutions that judge that routine use of gloves for all phlebotomies is not necessary should periodically reevaluate their policy. Gloves should always be available for those who wish to use them for phlebotomy. In addition, the following general guidelines apply:

1 Use gloves for performing phlebotomy if cuts, scratches, or other breaks in the skin are present.
2 Use gloves in situations in which contamination with blood may occur—for example, when performing phlebotomy on an uncooperative patient.
3 Use gloves for performing finger or heel sticks on infants and children.
4 Use gloves when training persons to do phlebotomies.

3. HIV assessment and prevention. Procedures regarding the assessment of the source patient vary from institution to institution. At the time of this writing, there has been no proven prophylactic drug regimen to prevent transmission once inoculation has occurred. Your institution may have a formal protocol to follow in the event of exposure, and you should familiarize yourself with such policies. Although as yet unproven, *zidovudine* (AZT) is offered by many institutions. Since AZT therapy may be more effective if given immediately, *the reporting of needlesticks or other exposure to HIV-contaminated fluids should not be delayed.*

PATIENT-RELATED PROBLEMS: THE COMMON CALLS

□ **5** □

ABDOMINAL PAIN

Many patients complain of abdominal pain during their hospital stays. It is essential to distinguish the acute abdominal emergency from the recurrent nonemergency. The former requires urgent medical or surgical intervention, whereas the latter requires thorough, but less urgent, investigation. Avoid ordering analgesics until a preliminary diagnosis is made. Narcotic analgesics may mask the physical findings of an acute abdomen, thereby delaying recognition and treatment of a serious intraabdominal disorder.

PHONE CALL
Questions

1 **How severe is the pain?**
2 **Is the pain localized or generalized?**
3 **What are the vital signs?**
Fever and abdominal pain are suggestive of intraabdominal infection or inflammation.
4 **Is this a new problem?**
5 **What was the reason for admission?**
6 **Is the patient on steroids?**
Steroids may mask the pain and fever attendant with inflammatory processes, tricking you into underestimating the nature or severity of a patient's abdominal pain. If the patient is on steroids even mild abdominal pain should be assessed soon.

Orders

If the abdominal pain is mild and the vital signs are normal, ask the RN to phone immediately if the pain becomes worse before you are able to assess the patient.

Inform RN

"Will arrive at bedside in . . . minutes."

Abdominal pain of acute onset, severe abdominal pain, or pain associated with fever or hypotension requires you to see the patient immediately. Mild recurrent abdominal pain is a less urgent problem and may be attended to in an hour or two if other patient problems of higher priority exist.

ELEVATOR THOUGHTS (What causes abdominal pain?)

The causes of *localized abdominal pain* are numerous. A useful system for approaching the problem is "diagnosis by location." Figure 5–1 illustrates a differential diagnosis by location.

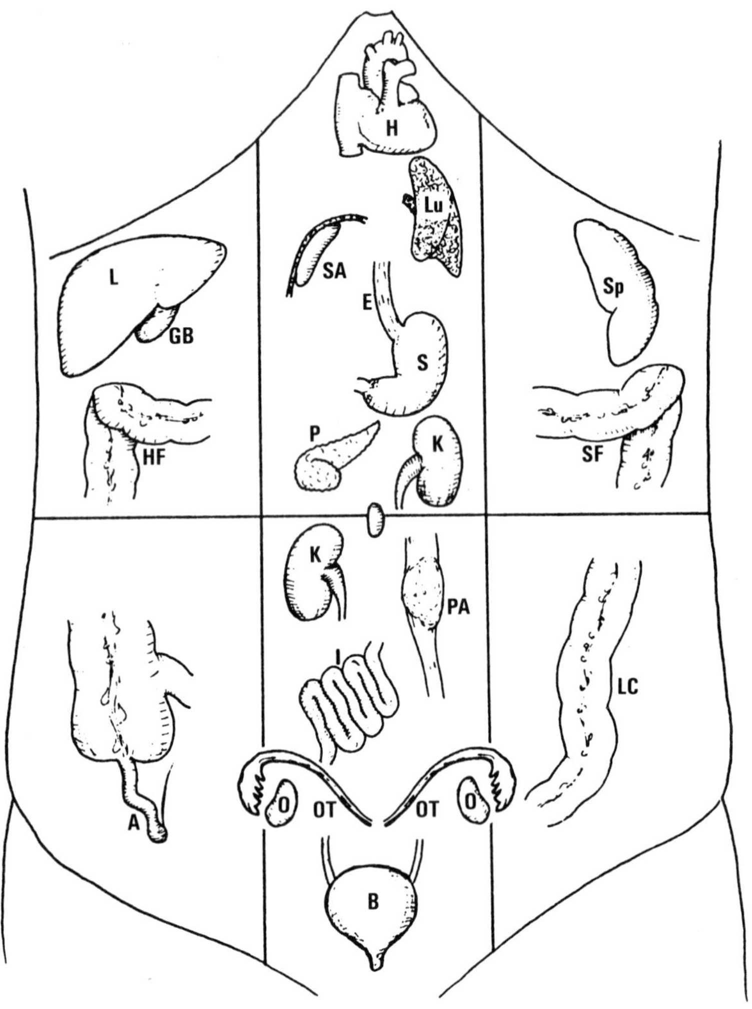

Figure 5–1 □ Differential diagnosis by abdominal quadrant. (See key on opposite page.)

The causes of *generalized abdominal pain* are fewer. Disorders producing either localized or generalized pain are indicated by an asterisk, and additional causes of generalized abdominal pain alone are listed in the legend to Figure 5–1.

Key to Figure 5–1.
Right upper quadrant
  L, Liver (hepatitis, abscess, perihepatitis)
  GB, Gallbladder (cholelithiasis, choledocholithiasis)
  HF, Hepatic flexure (obstruction)
Right lower quadrant
  A, Appendix (appendicitis,* abscess)
  O, Ovary (torsion, ruptured cyst, carcinoma)
Left upper quadrant
  Sp, Spleen (rupture, infarct, abscess)
  SF, Splenic flexure (obstruction)
Left lower quadrant
  LC, Left colon (diverticulitis, ischemic colitis)
  O, Ovary (torsion, ruptured cyst, carcinoma)
Epigastrium
  H, Heart (myocardial infarction, pericarditis, aortic dissection)
  Lu, Lung (pneumonia, pleurisy)
  SA, Subphrenic abscess
  E, Esophagus (esophagitis)
  S, Stomach and duodenum (peptic ulcer)
  P, Pancreas (pancreatitis)
  K, Kidney (pyelonephritis, renal colic)
Hypogastrium
  K, Kidney (renal colic)
  PA, Psoas abscess
  I, Intestine (infection,* obstruction,* inflammatory bowel disease*)
  O, Ovary (torsion, ruptured cyst, carcinoma)
  OT, Ovarian tube (ectopic pregnancy, salpingitis, endometriosis)
  B, Bladder (cystitis, distended bladder)
Generalized abdominal pain
  1. See conditions marked with an asterisk.
  2. Peritonitis (any cause)
  3. Diabetic ketoacidosis
  4. Sickle cell crisis
  5. Acute intermittent porphyria
  6. Acute adrenocortical insufficiency due to steroid withdrawal

---

MAJOR THREAT TO LIFE

- Perforated or ruptured viscus
- Ascending cholangitis
- Necrosis of viscus
- Exsanguinating hemorrhage

A *perforated or ruptured viscus* may result in hypovolemic shock (from third space losses), septic shock (from bacterial peritonitis), or both. Exacerbation of infection from an initial localized site (e.g., *ascending cholangitis*) to septic shock may occur rapidly, i.e., within hours of the patient's first presenting symptom. *Necrosis of a viscus*, as in intussusception, volvulus, strangulated hernia, or ischemic colitis, may cause hypovolemic or septic shock and electrolyte and acid-base disturbances. *Exsanguinating hemorrhage* with hypovolemic shock may result from a ruptured ectopic pregnancy, from a splenic rupture, occasionally from a liver or renal biopsy, or from a misdirected thoracentesis.

Patients with myocardial infarction and aortic dissection occasionally present with abdominal pain. These diagnoses should be considered, especially if no local abdominal signs can be identified.

BEDSIDE
Quick Look Test

Does the patient look well (comfortable), sick (uncomfortable or distressed), or critical (about to die)?

Appearances are often deceptive in acute abdominal disease. *If the patient has recently received narcotic analgesics or high-dose steroids, he or she may appear well despite a serious underlying problem.*

Patients suffering from severe colic or intraperitoneal hemorrhage are often restless, in contrast to those suffering peritonitis, who lie immobile, avoiding movement that exacerbates the pain. With peritonitis, patients may have their knees drawn up to reduce abdominal tension.

Airways and Vital Signs

What is the BP?

Hypotension associated with abdominal pain is an ominous sign suggestive of impending hypovolemic, hemorrhagic, or septic shock.

Are there postural changes (lying and standing) in the BP and HR?

If there are postural changes, recheck the BP and HR with the patient standing. A drop in BP that is associated with an increased heart rate (>15 beats/min) suggests volume depletion.

What is the temperature?

Fever associated with abdominal pain is suggestive of intraabdominal infection or inflammation. However, the lack of fever in the elderly patient or in the patient receiving an antipyretic or immunosuppressive drug does not rule out infection.

Selective History and Chart Review

Diagnosis is often dependent on a careful history addressing (1) the pain at onset and its subsequent progression, (2) any associated symptoms, and (3) the past history.

Pain

Is the pain localized?

The location of maximum intensity of the pain can provide a clue to the site of origin (Fig. 5–1). Remember that a patient may complain of diffuse abdominal pain, but on careful examination, the pain will be found to be localized.

How is the pain characterized (e.g., severe or mild, burning or knifelike, constant or waxing-and-waning, as in colic)?

There are characteristic descriptions of pain associated with certain diseases as follows: the pain of peptic ulcer tends to be burning, that of a perforated ulcer is sudden, constant, and severe, that of biliary colic is sharp, constricting ("taking one's breath away"), that of acute pancreatitis is deep and agonizing, and that of obstructed bowel is gripping, with intermittent worsening.

Did the pain develop gradually or suddenly?

The severe pain of colic (renal, biliary, or intestinal) develops in hours. An acute onset with fainting suggests perforation of a viscus, strangulation of the gut, ruptured ectopic pregnancy, torsion of an ovarian cyst, or biliary or renal colic.

Has the pain changed since its onset?

A ruptured viscus initially may be associated with localized pain, which subsequently shifts or becomes generalized, with the development of chemical or bacterial peritonitis.

Does the pain radiate?

Radiation of the pain (i.e., referred pain) occurs to the dermatome or cutaneous areas supplied by the same sensory cortical cells as the deep-seated structure (Fig. 5–2). For example, the diaphragm is supplied by the cervical roots C3, C4, and C5. Many upper abdominal or lower thoracic conditions that cause irritation of the diaphragm refer pain to the cutaneous supply of C3, C4, and C5, i.e., the shoulder and the neck. The liver and gallbladder are derived from the right 7th and 8th thoracic segments. Thus, biliary colic frequently refers pain to the inferior angle of the right scapula.

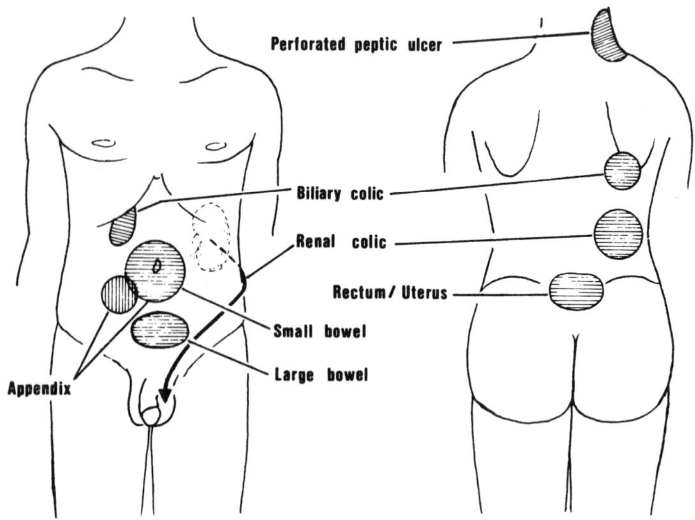

Figure 5–2 □ Common sites of referred pain.

Are there any aggravating factors?

Pain that increases with meals, decreases with passage of bowel movements, or both suggests a hollow gut origin. An exception is pain from duodenal ulcer, which is often relieved by the ingestion of food. Pain that increases with inspiration suggests pleuritis or peritonitis, and pain that is aggravated by micturition suggests a urogenital cause.

Associated Symptoms

Is there any associated nausea or vomiting?

Vomiting occurring with the onset of pain frequently accompanies acute peritoneal irritation or perforation of a viscus. It is also commonly associated with acute pancreatitis or obstruction of any muscular hollow viscus. Pain relieved by vomiting suggests hollow gut origin, e.g., bowel obstruction. Vomiting many hours after the onset of abdominal pain may be a clue to intestinal obstruction or ileus.

What is the nature of emesis?

Brown, feculent emesis is pathognomonic of bowel obstruction, either paralytic or mechanical. Frank blood is suggestive of an upper GI bleed. Vomiting food after fasting is consistent with gastric stasis or gastric outlet obstruction.

Is there any associated diarrhea?
Diarrhea and abdominal pain are seen in infectious gastroenteritis, ischemic colitis, appendicitis, and partial small bowel obstruction. Diarrhea alternating with constipation is a common symptom of diverticular disease.

Is there associated fever or chills?
Check the temperature record since admission. Check the medication sheet for antipyretic, steroid, or antibiotic drugs, since fever may be masked by the administration of these medications.

Past History and Chart Review

Is there a history of peptic ulcer disease or antacid ingestion?
Peptic ulcer disease is a chronic, recurring disease. History repeats itself!

Is there a history of blunt or penetrating trauma to the abdomen? Has there been a liver or kidney biopsy or a thoracentesis since admission?
A subcapsular hemorrhage of the spleen, liver, or kidney may result in hemorrhagic shock 1 to 3 days later.

Is there a history of alcohol abuse and ascites?
Spontaneous bacterial peritonitis must always be considered in the alcoholic patient with ascites and fever.

Is there a history of coronary or peripheral vascular disease?
Atherosclerosis is a diffuse process and may affect the vascular supply to several body systems. In addition to the possibility of a myocardial infarction occurring with abdominal pain, ischemic colitis due to atherosclerosis of the mesenteric arteries should be considered.

If the patient is a premenopausal female, ask the date of the last normal menstrual period.
Abdominal pain associated with a missed period raises the possibility of an ectopic pregnancy. Hypotension in this situation suggests a ruptured ectopic pregnancy, a life-threatening situation.

Is there a history of previous abdominal surgery?
Adhesions are responsible for 70% of bowel obstructions.

Is the patient anticoagulated?
Intraabdominal hemorrhage may occur in the anticoagulated patient, especially if there is a history of peptic ulcer disease.

Is there a history of aspirin, or NSAID, alcohol, or other ulcerogenic drug use?

Selective Physical Examination

VITALS	Repeat now
HEENT	Icterus (cholangitis, choledocholithiasis)
	Spider nevi (risk of spontaneous bacterial peritonitis if ascites is present)
RESP	Generalized or localized restriction of abdominal wall movement in respiration (localized or generalized peritoneal effusion)
	Stony dullness to percussion, decreased breath sounds, decreased tactile fremitus (pleural effusion)
	Dullness to percussion, diminished or bronchial breath sounds, crackles (consolidation and pneumonia)
CVS	Decreased JVP (volume depletion)
	New onset of dysrhythmia, mitral insufficiency murmur or S_4 (myocardial infarction)
ABD	Before examining the abdomen, make sure your hands are warm and make sure the head of the bed is flat. It

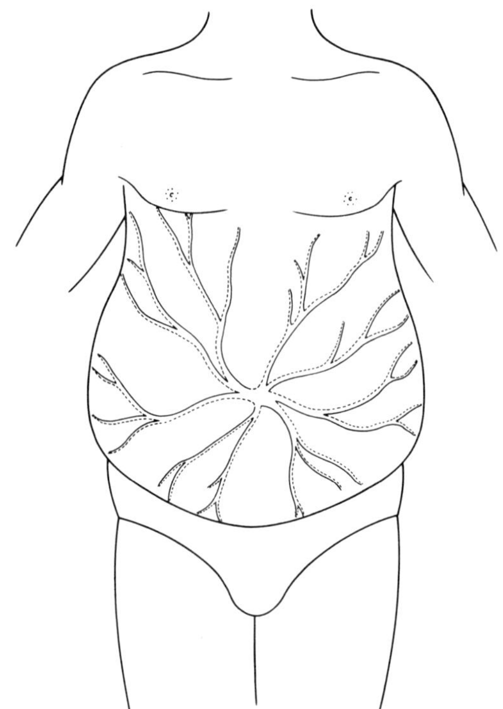

Figure 5–3 □ Caput medusae is a manifestation of portal hypertension.

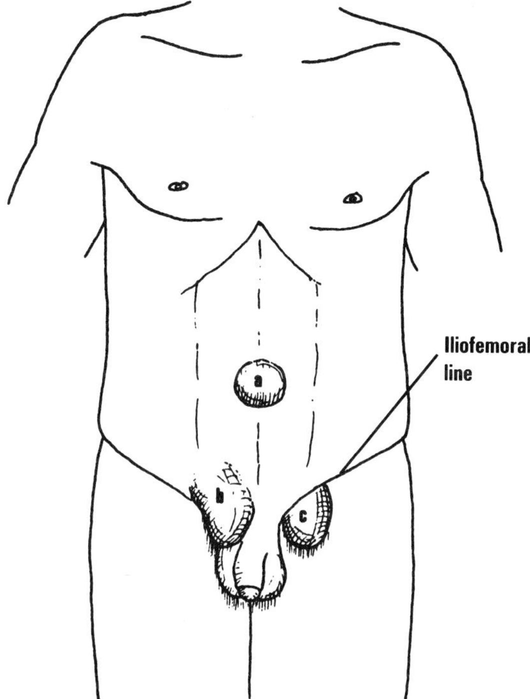

Figure 5–4 □ Hernial orifices. a, Umbilical hernia; b, inguinal hernia; c, femoral hernia. Note that the "bulge" of the inguinal hernia begins superiorly to the inguinal ligament, whereas the "bulge" of the femoral hernia originates inferiorly to the inguinal ligament.

may be helpful to flex the patient's hips to relax the abdominal wall. When examining for tenderness, begin in a nonpainful region.

Visible peristalsis (bowel obstruction)

Bulging flanks (ascites)

Caput medusa (Fig. 5–3) (portal hypertension and increased risk of spontaneous bacterial peritonitis)

Loss of liver dullness (perforated viscus)

Localized tenderness, masses (Fig. 5–1)

Rigid abdomen, guarding, rebound tenderness (peritonitis)

Shifting dullness, fluid wave (ascites)

Absent bowel sounds (paralytic ileus or late bowel obstruction)

Check all hernia orifices (strangulated hernia) (Fig. 5–4)

Murphy's sign (cholecystitis) (Fig. 5–5)

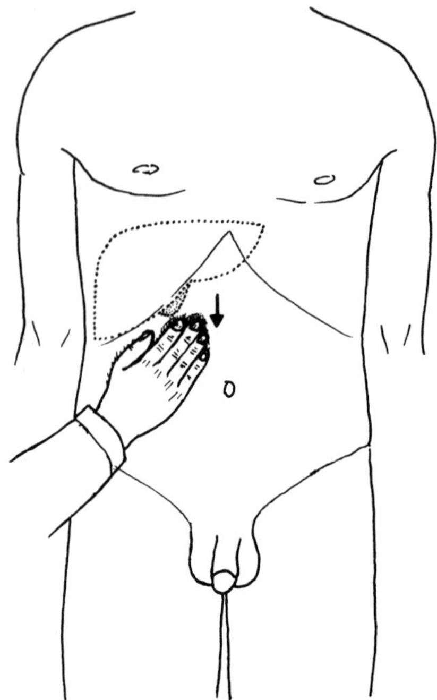

Figure 5–5 □ Murphy's sign. A positive Murphy's sign is manifested by pain and inspiratory arrest when the patient takes a deep breath while the examiner applies pressure against the abdominal wall in the region of the gallbladder. A positive Murphy's sign is often seen in the presence of cholecystitis.

	Psoas sign (retrocecal appendicitis) (Fig. 5–6)
	Obturator sign (retrocecal appendicitis) (Fig. 5–7)
RECTAL	Tenderness (rectrocecal appendicitis, prostatitis)
	Mass (rectal carcinoma)
	Rectal fissure (Crohn's disease)
	Stool positive for occult blood (ischemic colitis, peptic ulcer)
PELVIC	Tenderness (ectopic pregnancy, ovarian cyst, or pelvic inflammatory disease)
	Mass (ovarian cyst or tumor)

Management

Your assessment and investigation thus far may not have led you to a specific diagnosis of the etiology of the patient's abdominal pain. You will, however, have been able from your physical examination to determine whether the patient has developed shock, the most serious of potential complications from disorders that cause abdominal pain.

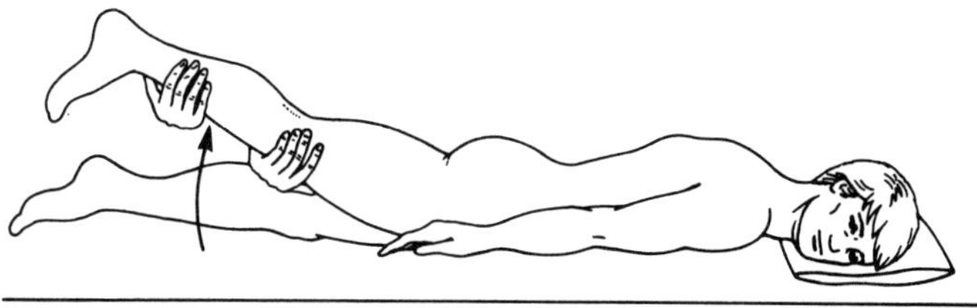

Figure 5–6 □ Psoas sign. A positive psoas sign is manifested by abdominal pain in response to passive hip flexion. (This test also may be performed with the patient lying on his or her side.) This sign is often present in patients with retrocecal appendicitis or a psoas abscess.

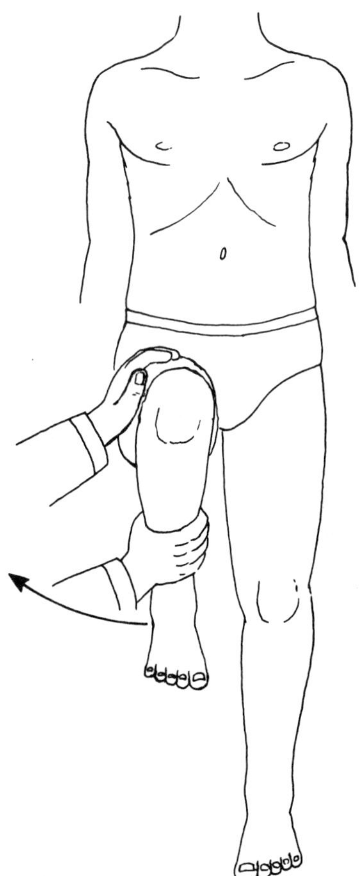

Figure 5–7 □ A positive obturator sign is manifested by abdominal pain in response to passive internal rotation of the right hip from the 90 degree hip/knee flexion position, when the patient is supine. This sign is often present in patients with retrocecal appendicitis.

Shock.   The initial treatment of either *hypovolemic or septic shock* is the same and is aimed at immediate expansion of the intravascular volume.

1. Rapid volume repletion can be achieved using normal saline or Ringer's lactate (500 ml IV as rapidly as possible, followed by an IV rate titrated to the JVP and vital signs).
2. Blood should be drawn for a stat crossmatch for 4 to 6 units of packed RBCs, Hb, PT, aPTT, and platelet count. Baseline values of electrolytes, urea, creatinine, blood glucose, amylase, and WBC and manual differential also are useful. Two sets of blood cultures should be drawn if septic shock is suspected.
3. If hemorrhagic shock is suspected, packed RBCs should be given in place of, or in addition to, the crystalloid, NS, or Ringer's lactate as soon as the crossmatch has been completed.
4. When shock occurs in the setting of a disorder causing abdominal pain, urgent surgical consultation is almost always required. Ensure that the patient is NPO. Consider inserting an NG tube if the patient is vomiting.
5. As resuscitation measures are being initiated, additional investigations can be arranged, as follows:

    a. Order three radiographic views of the abdomen (A/P abdomen supine and erect or lateral decubitus and P/A chest erect). If the patient looks unwell or critical, these x-rays will need to be done on a stat portable basis.
    Toxic megacolon is manifested by an increase in diameter of the midtransverse colon (>7 cm) and a mucosal pattern of thumbprinting or thickening. This condition is a medical or surgical emergency. Look for air under the diaphragm in the chest film or between the viscera and subcutaneous tissue in the lateral decubitus film. This sign is indicative of a *perforated viscus*.
    b. If septic shock is suspected, specimens for Gram's stain, culture, and sensitivity testing should be obtained immediately from sputum if available, urine, which may require in/out catheterization, and wounds. If there is ascites, an immediate diagnostic paracentesis should be performed.

6. Once culture specimens have been obtained in a case of suspected septic shock, empiric, broad-spectrum antibiotics (ampicillin and aminoglycoside, plus metronidazole or cefoxitin) should be started immediately, to treat infection due to coliforms and gut anaerobes.

Acute "Surgical" Abdomen.   If the patient is not in shock or has now been successfully resuscitated from shock, you must consider the possible underlying conditions responsible for the complaint of abdominal pain. Of utmost importance at this point is to determine whether the patient has an acute "surgical" (i.e., requiring surgery) abdomen.

PERFORATED OR RUPTURED VISCUS. Finding air under the diaphragm on the upright CXR or between the viscera and subcutaneous tissue on the lateral decubitus film indicates a perforated or ruptured viscus. Immediate surgical consultation is required. Ensure that the patient is NPO.

INTRAABDOMINAL HEMORRHAGE. Abdominal pain due to an intraabdominal hemorrhage almost always requires immediate surgical consultation. Ensure that the patient is kept NPO and that blood has been sent for a stat crossmatch for 4 to 6 units of packed RBCs.

RUPTURED INTRAABDOMINAL ABSCESS. An intraabdominal abscess that has ruptured often results in acute peritonitis and, if left untreated, may progress to septic shock. Urgent surgical consultation for proper drainage is required. Make sure the patient is kept NPO.

NECROSIS OF A VISCUS. Necrosis of an intraabdominal viscus due to intussusception, volvulus, strangulated hernia, or ischemic colitis requires urgent surgical consultation. Ensure that the patient is kept NPO.

Other Conditions. Other specific conditions that may not cause an acute "surgical" abdomen are common and should be considered if none of the above-mentioned conditions is present. Each has features requiring specific attention when on-call.

PANCREATITIS. Pancreatitis should be suspected in the alcoholic patient with abdominal pain but with no evidence of an upper GI bleed or ascites. The abdominal x-ray films may reveal a sentinel loop, colonic distention, a left pleural effusion, or calcification within the pancreas (Fig. 5–8). An elevated amylase level supports the diagnosis, but a normal amylase level does not exclude the possibility of pancreatitis. The patient should be NPO. IV fluids with NS should be ordered to replace any losses. Narcotic analgesia usually will be required. *Meperidine* (Demerol) 50 to 150 mg IM or SC q3–4h PRN is the drug of choice, since morphine can cause spasm of the sphincter of Oddi. If the patient develops a fever, an abdominal ultrasound scan should be ordered to search for a possible pancreatic abscess.

INTRAABDOMINAL ABSCESS. A contained intraabdominal abscess will require delineation by either ultrasound or CT scan. This can be arranged in the morning provided the patient is otherwise stable. Subphrenic and psoas abscesses will require decompression. Hepatic abscesses may be drained percutaneously under ultrasound guidance or surgically. Splenic abscesses usually require splenectomy.

PEPTIC ULCER DISEASE OR GASTRITIS. Cases of suspected peptic ulcer disease or gastritis should be considered for endoscopy. H_2

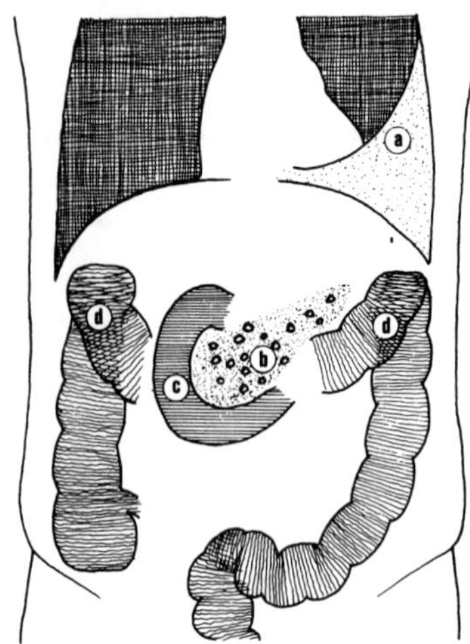

Figure 5–8 □ Radiographic features of pancreatitis. a, Left pleural effusion; b, calcification within the pancreas; c, sentinel loop; d, colonic distention.

blockers should be started as follows: *cimetidine* (Tagamet) 300 mg IV or PO q6–8h (300 mg IV BID in renal failure) or *ranitidine* (Zantac) 50 mg IV q8h or 150 mg PO BID (50 mg PO or IV BID in renal failure). Antacids are contraindicated if endoscopy is to be performed, since antacids coat the lining of the stomach, obscuring the endoscopist's view of mucosal lesions.

PYELONEPHRITIS. Pyelonephritis requires empiric IV antibiotics (ampicillin and an aminoglycoside) until the specific organism has been identified.

RENAL STONES. Patients with renal stones may be managed medically with narcotic analgesics after the diagnosis has been confirmed with an IVP. Surgical removal, basket extraction, or lithotripsy may be required if the stone has not passed within a few days or if an associated persistent infection is present.

INFECTIOUS GASTROENTERITIS. Infectious gastroenteritis may require specific antibiotics if the stool culture results reveal a bacterial cause. Viral gastroenteritis is treated supportively with IV fluids. *Clostridium difficile* infection should be suspected in any patient developing diarrhea during or after a course of antibiotics. Sigmoidoscopy may reveal a characteristic pseudomembrane, in which case *metronidazole* 500 mg PO q6h or *vancomycin* 125 to 500 mg q6h may be instituted before confirmation by *C. difficile* culture or toxin assay.

OVARIAN CYST, TUMOR, OR SALPINGITIS. These are best managed by referral to a gynecologist.

■ ABDOMINAL PAIN IN THE AIDS OR IMMUNOSUPPRESSED PATIENT

Symptoms, such as chronic abdominal pain, nausea, and vomiting, are common in the critically ill AIDS or immunosuppressed patient. Many AIDS patients already appear chronically ill, and this must be factored into one's assessment of the cause of abdominal pain. Many also will already have abnormalities in baseline laboratory values, making *changes* in laboratory parameters more important than absolute values.

The following features are pertinent in the evaluation of abdominal pain in the AIDS or immunosuppressed patient:

1. Fever is a sensitive sign of infection in the AIDS patient with abdominal pain. Unfortunately, it is a nonspecific finding in the AIDS patient and may be due to nonabdominal occult infections or due to HIV itself. AIDS patients with temperatures $\geq 38.5°C$ should have blood cultures drawn twice, although frequently no etiologic agent is isolated.
2. AIDS and immunocompromised patients commonly suffer from leukopenia due to the effect of HIV suppression of the bone marrow and to drugs. Thus, even a normal WBC, especially if accompanied by a left shift, should be interpreted as a sign of possible infection in the AIDS patient with fever and abdominal pain.
3. Bowel wall ulceration or perforation due to *cytomegalovirus (CMV)* infection is a common cause of an acute surgical abdomen in the AIDS patient. CMV can also cause hepatitis, pancreatitis, and gastritis in this patient population.
4. Causes of small bowel obstruction that should be considered include bulky lymphadenopathy due to TB or to *Mycobacterium avium-intracellulare* and tumors such as bowel lymphoma.
5. Pancreatitis is an unusual cause of abdominal pain in AIDS patients and, when seen, may be a side effect of *pentamidine* or *trimethoprim-sulfamethoxasole,* two drugs commonly used to treat *Pneumocystis carinii* pneumonia.

■ ABDOMINAL PAIN IN THE ELDERLY

The investigation and management of abdominal pain in the elderly patient should proceed along the same lines as for other patient groups. Of note in the elderly is that abdominal pain may be very mild despite the presence of an acute abdomen. One should not underestimate the seriousness of mild abdominal pain in the elderly, especially if associated with acute confusion, fever, an elevated WBC, or a metabolic acidosis.

Two conditions causing abdominal pain that are usually unique to the elderly are *colonic perforation due to diverticular disease* and *mesenteric ischemia* due to atherosclerosis.

6

CHEST PAIN

In developed countries, where coronary artery disease is the leading cause of death, it is not surprising that when a patient complains of "chest pain," you will wonder whether the patient is having angina or, worse yet, a heart attack. There are, however, several other equally serious causes of chest pain that may go undiagnosed if not specifically looked for. In the assessment of chest pain, history taking is your most powerful tool.

PHONE CALL

Questions

1 **How severe is the pain?**
2 **What are the vital signs?**
3 **What was the reason for admission?**
4 **Does the patient have a past history of angina or myocardial infarction? If yes, is the pain similar to their usual angina or previous infarction?**

Orders

If myocardial ischemia is suspected

1. ECG stat.
2. Oxygen by face mask or nasal prongs at 4 L/min. If the patient is a CO_2 retainer, you will have to be cautious when giving oxygen (maximum FIO_2 0.28 by mask or 2 L/min by nasal prongs).
3. Nitroglycerin 0.3 mg SL q5min, provided the systolic BP is > 90 mm Hg.
4. Ask the RN to take the patient's chart to the bedside.

Inform RN

"Will arrive at bedside in . . . minutes."

Most causes of chest pain are diagnosed by history. It is impossible to obtain an accurate and relevant history by speaking to the RN over the phone. The history must be taken first hand from the patient. Because some causes of chest pain represent medical emergencies, the patient should be assessed immediately.

ELEVATOR THOUGHTS (What causes chest pain?)

CARDIAC   Angina
Myocardial infarction
Aortic dissection
Pericarditis

RESP	Pulmonary embolism or infarction
	Pneumothorax
	Pleuritis (± pneumonia)
GI	Esophageal spasm, reflux, esophagitis
	Peptic ulcer disease
MSS	Costochondritis
	Rib fracture
SKIN	Herpes zoster

MAJOR THREAT TO LIFE

- Myocardial ischemia or infarction
- Aortic dissection
- Pneumothorax
- Pulmonary embolus

Cardiogenic shock or fatal dysrhythmias may occur as a result of myocardial infarction. Aortic dissection may result in death from cardiac tamponade, aortic rupture, or myocardial infarction and may damage other organ systems by compromising the vascular supply. Pneumothorax and pulmonary embolism cause hypoxia.

BEDSIDE
Quick Look Test

Does the patient look well (comfortable), sick (uncomfortable or distressed), or critical (about to die)?

Most patients with chest pain from myocardial infarction or ischemia look pale and anxious. If the patient looks well, suspect esophagitis or a musculoskeletal problem, such as costochondritis.

Airway and Vital Signs

What is the BP?

Most patients with chest pain will have a normal BP. Hypotension may be seen with myocardial infarction, massive pulmonary embolism, or tension pneumothorax. Hypertension, occurring in association with myocardial ischemia or aortic dissection, should be treated urgently (see Chapter 16, p. 141).

What is the HR?

Does the patient have tachycardia? Severe chest pain of any cause may result in sinus tachycardia. Heart rates >100/min should alert you to the possibility of a tachydysrhythmia, such as atrial fibrillation, PAT, or ventricular tachycardia, which may require immediate cardioversion.

Does the patient have bradycardia? Bradycardia in a patient with chest pain may represent sinus or AV nodal ischemia (as may be seen with myocardial infarction) or beta blockade or calcium channel blockade due to drugs. Immediate treatment of bradycardia is not required unless the rate is extremely slow (< 40/min) or the patient is hypotensive (see Chapter 18, p. 153).

What is the breathing pattern?

Tachypnea may accompany any type of chest pain. Shallow, painful breathing suggests a pleural or musculoskeletal cause (pleuritis, pneumothorax, costochondritis).

What does the ECG show?

Coronary artery disease is common. Many patients seen at night with chest pain will have myocardial ischemia or infarction. Remember, a normal ECG does not rule out the possibility of angina or myocardial infarction. Since thrombolysis is most effective when given within the first 4 hours of chest pain, if a myocardial infarction is suspected from the ECG, call your resident *immediately* to assess the patient for possible thrombolytic therapy.

Management I

Is the patient receiving oxygen?

Ensure that the patient is receiving oxygen at an appropriate concentration.

Does the patient have chest pain now? If myocardial ischemia is suspected, proceed as follows.

Chest pain and systolic BP > 90 mm Hg
- If the last dose of sublingual nitroglycerin was given > 5 minutes ago, give another dose immediately.
- If the patient was receiving 0.3 mg and it made no difference in the chest pain, increase the dose to 0.6 mg.
- If the pain continues despite three doses of nitroglycerin, ask the RN to draw up 10 mg (1 ml) of morphine into a syringe diluted with 9 ml of NS. Give the *morphine* in 2 to 4 mg aliquots IV until the pain is relieved, provided the systolic BP is > 90 mm Hg.

  Morphine sulfate may cause hypotension or respiratory depression. Take the BP and RR before each dose is given. If necessary, *naloxone hydrochloride* (Narcan) 0.2 to 2 mg IV or SC may be given q5min to a total of 10 mg to reverse these side effects. Nausea or vomiting may also occur and usually can be controlled with *dimenhydrinate* (Dramamine, Gravol) 25 mg IV or 50 mg PO q4h PRN.

- If the chest pain requires administration of morphine, arrange for assessment by the ICU/CCU team as soon as possible.

Chest pain and systolic BP < 90 mm Hg
- What is the patient's normal BP? If the systolic BP is normally 90 mm Hg, you may proceed cautiously with sublingual ni-

troglycerin 0.3 mg, as described, provided there is no further drop in the BP.

- If the hypotension is an acute change, establish IV access immediately with a large-bore IV (size 16 if possible). Refer to Chapter 18, p. 155, for management of hypotension.

If the patient looks sick or critical
Establish IV access using D5W if not already done.
Draw ABG sample.

Selective History and Chart Review

How does the patient describe the pain? Is the pain the same as the patient's usual angina?
Crushing, squeezing, viselike pain or pressure is characteristic of myocardial infarction. Severe tearing or ripping pain is characteristic of an aortic dissection.

Is the chest pain worse with deep breathing or coughing?
Pleuritic chest pain suggests pleuritis, pneumothorax, rib fracture, pericarditis, pulmonary embolism, pneumonia, or costochondritis.

Does the pain radiate?
Radiation of pain to the back suggests myocardial ischemia, infarction, or aortic dissection distal to the left subclavian artery. Dissection proximal to the left subclavian artery characteristically causes nonradiating anterior chest pain. Review the chest x-ray as soon as possible, looking specifically for a widened mediastinum. Suspected aortic dissection requires you to proceed urgently with the appropriate investigation and management (see pp. 46 and 141).

Is there any associated nausea, vomiting, diaphoresis, or light-headedness?
Cardiogenic nausea and vomiting are associated with larger myocardial infarctions but do not suggest a particular location, as previously thought.

Is the chest pain worse with swallowing?
Chest pain that is made worse by swallowing suggests an esophageal disorder or pericarditis.

Selective Physical Examination

VITALS	Repeat now
HEENT	Blindness (aortic dissection)
	White exudate in oral cavity or pharynx (thrush with possible concomitant esophageal candidiasis)

RESP	Crackles (CHF secondary to acute MI or pulmonary embolism, pneumonia)
	Consolidation and pleural effusion (pulmonary infarction or pneumonia)
CVS	Unequal upper limb BP or diminished femoral pulses (aortic dissection)
	Elevated JVP (right ventricular failure secondary to MI or cor pulmonale, tension pneumothorax)
	Right ventricular heave (cor pulmonale)
	Left ventricular heave (CHF)
	Loud P_2 (cor pulmonale), S_3 (CHF)
	Mitral insufficiency murmur (papillary muscle dysfunction)
	Aortic insufficiency murmur (proximal aortic dissection)
	Pericardial rub (pericarditis)
	Pericardial rubs are biphasic or triphasic scratching sounds that vary with position.
ABD	Guarding, rebound tenderness (perforated ulcer)
	Epigastric tenderness (peptic ulcer disease)
	Generalized abdominal pain (mesenteric infarction from aortic dissection)
CNS	Hemiplegia (aortic dissection)
SKIN	Unilateral maculopapular rash or vesicles in a dermatomal pattern (herpes zoster)

Management II

Angina.   If angina has been relieved with 1 to 3 nitroglycerin tablets, review the precipitating cause. An adjustment in the antianginal medication may be required and should be made in consultation with your resident and attending physician. However, if the angina occurred at rest, or this is the first episode of angina, the patient should be assessed by the ICU/CCU staff regardless of whether the pain was relieved with ≤ 3 nitroglycerin tablets.

If the angina required more than three doses of nitroglycerin or IV morphine, serial cardiac enzymes and ECGs should be ordered. If the clinical impression is of possible myocardial infarction, the patient should be transferred to the ICU/CCU for continuous ECG monitoring.

Myocardial Infarction.   If a myocardial infarction is suspected by history or ECG changes (see p. 331), the patient should be transferred to the ICU/CCU as soon as possible. In addition to morphine, ongoing myocardial ischemia may require treatment with IV nitroglycerin or beta blockers. The patient also should be evaluated immediately for possible thrombolytic therapy.

Aortic Dissection.   Suspicion of aortic dissection requires urgent investigation and management as follows.

1. Arrange for an urgent CT scan of the thorax or a transesoph-

ageal echocardiogram. If neither of these can be performed within the next hour, a transthoracic echocardiogram may detect a dilated aortic root, aortic valvular insufficiency, or a pericardial effusion. Occasionally, an aortic dissection flap also is visualized by this procedure.

2. Draw blood for a stat crossmatch for 6 to 8 units of packed RBCs on hold, electrolytes, urea, creatinine, glucose, CBC and differential, PT, and aPTT.
3. Review the ECG for evidence of an acute MI. This finding suggests aortic dissection involving the coronary ostia.
4. The patient should be transferred to the ICU/CCU as soon as possible for careful control of blood pressure (see Chapter 16, p. 141).
5. Surgical consultation should be obtained early when the diagnosis of dissection is entertained. The diagnosis can be confirmed by aortography.

Pericarditis.   Patients with suspected pericarditis should have nonurgent echocardiograms performed to look for pericardial effusions or signs of hemodynamic compromise. *Indomethacin* (Indocin) 50 mg PO TID or *aspirin* 650 mg PO QID are helpful.

NSAIDs are contraindicated in the patient who has the syndrome of aspirin sensitivity, nasal polyps, and bronchospasm, in the patient who is anticoagulated, and in the patient who has active peptic ulcer disease. Because of their sodium-retaining properties, caution should be used in giving NSAIDs to patients in CHF. NSAIDs also should be used with caution in patients with renal insufficiency, since these drugs may inhibit renal prostaglandins, which are responsible for maintaining renal perfusion in those with prerenal conditions. Sulindac (Clinoril) may not have this effect.

Pulmonary Embolus.   The management of pulmonary embolus is discussed in Chapter 24, p. 242.

Pneumothorax.   A pneumothorax may require chest tube drainage depending on its size. If the patient develops a tension pneumothorax, immediate treatment is necessary to relieve the pressure using a 16-gauge IV catheter as described on p. 177.

Pneumonia.   Suggested antibiotics for pneumonia are discussed in Chapter 24, p. 244 and should be chosen according to the Gram's stain results and patient's characteristics.

Esophagitis.   Esophagitis may be treated with antacids. Choose carefully. Magnesium-containing antacids (Gelusil, Maalox) may cause diarrhea, whereas antacids containing solely aluminum (Amphogel, Basalgel) may cause constipation. Do not substitute one GI complaint for another! *Gelusil* 30 to 60 ml 1 hour and 3 hours after meals and qhs is a standard antacid order. More frequent doses may be required if the pain is severe. Elevation of the head of the bed may also be helpful.

Esophageal candidiasis will not respond to antacids. Immunocompromised patients may experience severe chest pain from this condition. Diagnosis should be confirmed by endoscopy. Treatment with *nystatin* (Mycostatin) 400,000 to 600,000 units PO (swish and swallow) QID is usually effective. However, in the AIDS or immunocompromised patient, *clotrimazole* (Canesten) 10 mg troche PO QID or *ketoconazole* 200 to 400 mg PO daily is more effective.

Peptic Ulcer.   A patient with suspected peptic ulcer disease should be referred for a possible endoscopic evaluation in the morning.

Costochondritis.   Costochondritis may be treated with an NSAID, such as *naproxen* (Naprosyn) 250 mg PO BID.

NSAIDs are contraindicated in the patient who has the syndrome of aspirin sensitivity, nasal polyps, and bronchospasm, in the patient who is anticoagulated, and in the patient who has active peptic ulcer disease. Because of their sodium-retaining properties, caution should be used in giving NSAIDs to patients in CHF. NSAIDs also should be used with caution in patients with renal insufficiency, since these drugs may inhibit renal prostaglandins, which are responsible for maintaining renal perfusion in those with prerenal conditions. Sulindac (Clinoril) may not have this effect.

Herpes Zoster.   Unilateral chest pain in a dermatomal distribution may precede the typical skin lesions of herpes zoster (shingles) by 2 or 3 days. The rash begins as a reddened, maculopapular area, which rapidly evolves into vesicular lesions. Treatment of acute herpes zoster neuritis may be difficult and often requires narcotic *analgesics, amitriptyline hydrochloride,* and in some cases *steroids.* In the immunocompromised or AIDS patient, *vidarabine* 15 mg/kg IV daily, given over 12 hours, may hasten healing of skin lesions and diminish the incidence of complications, such as varicella-zoster pneumonitis, meningoencephalitis, or hepatitis.

7

COMBATIVENESS:
THE OUT-OF-CONTROL PATIENT

Every once in a while, you will be paged by an exasperated nurse who has been trying to reason with an out-of-control patient. We are not referring here to the moody or uncooperative patient—we are referring to the hostile individuals whose temporary behavior poses a real physical threat to themselves, other patients, or hospital staff. Your job here is not to act as the strong-arm of the hospital law. Your role is to deem which medical reasons, if any, are responsible for the patient's behavior and to administer appropriate treatment.

PHONE CALL
Questions

1 **What was the reason for admission?**
2 **What medications is the patient taking now?**
3 **Is there an obvious reason for the patient's combative behavior?**
4 **What measures have been employed thus far to calm or reason with the patient?**
5 **What additional hospital personnel are there to help you now?**
6 **What is the patient's estimated height and weight?**

Orders

1. Ask the RN to phone the hospital's security personnel now, if not already done. Your job is not to hurry to the ward to help hold the patient down. Your role is to determine the cause of the patient's behavior and institute appropriate treatment.
2. *Haloperidol* (Haldol) 1 to 10 mg IM stat. By the time the RN has phoned you, he or she has usually wrestled with the patient for 10 to 20 minutes, employed the aid of orderlies, and tried everything at his or her immediate disposal. The RN by this time is desperate for a medication order, and providing the patient is not allergic, haloperidol is a good choice.

    The initial dose depends on the patient's height and body weight: 1 mg IM may suffice for the elderly patient of slight build, whereas 10 mg IM may be necessary for the young, large, football player.

Inform RN

"Will arrive at the bedside in . . . minutes."

The out-of-control patient requires your immediate attention.

49

ELEVATOR THOUGHTS (What causes dangerously combative behavior?)

Any confusional state due to an acute or chronic medical or psychiatric condition can result in temporary hostile or combative behavior. How an individual reacts in a given situation is often a reflection of his or her premorbid personality. The most common out-of-control patient is a young individual who feels frustrated, confined, and overwhelmed by the illness and the hospital environment. A second common out-of-control patient is the elderly person who becomes disoriented and combative, particularly at night (the sundown phenomenon).

Numerous other medical conditions may set off this behavior in any hospitalized patient and should be carefully looked for. These include intracranial disease, systemic disorders (drugs, organ failure, metabolic and endocrine disorders, infections and inflammation), and psychiatric disorders. Once the patient is safely approachable, these conditions should be carefully searched for (see Chapter 8, pp. 54–55).

MAJOR THREAT TO LIFE

Physical Injury

Patients who are acutely agitated and hostile are not reasoning properly and appear to be "looking for a fight." The typical out-of-control patient will have pulled out the IVs, NG tubes, or Foley's catheter and will be cursing, threatening, and pummeling at any hospital personnel within striking distance. The patient loses regard for his or her own safety and risks both new injury and worsening of the underlying medical condition that necessitated the hospitalization.

BEDSIDE

Quick Look Test

Does the patient look well (comfortable), sick (uncomfortable or distressed), or critical (about to die)?

The combative patient looks very much alive, agitated, and (often) ready for a fight!

Stand back from the situation for a moment and observe the patient. You must judge from a distance how dangerous the patient is and what immediate measures will be required to calm the patient and regain control. Look for any obvious signs of conditions that may require specific treatment.

- Is the patient cyanotic or having difficulty breathing (hypoxia)?
- Does the patient appear to be hallucinating (drug intoxication or withdrawal)?
- Is the patient in pain?

Management

The first priority is to calm the patient and regain control of the situation. In performing this task, the first rule is to remain calm yourself. It is not necessary to jump into the brawl, and you will be far more effective by using your head in this situation.

1. Some patients will become calm simply because "the doctor" has arrived, and they will feel less helpless and more in control of themselves with a physician there to address their immediate concerns. You will be able to judge in the first 30 seconds whether you are lucky enough for this to be the situation.

2. Some patients are so completely out of control that calm reasoning is futile. These patients may require temporary physical restraints while medication is being given. You may try to explain to the patient that you are going to give him or her "a shot" to calm him down and make him feel better. If he or she does not allow you to approach because of aggressive behavior, the patient will need to be held down while medication is administered. Continued restraint may be required until the medication takes effect. Should you need to physically restrain a violent individual, the general rule is to have at least one person per limb plus one.

   If the patient has already been given the haloperidol that you ordered over the phone, and is still out of control, physical restraints may be necessary. Allow adequate time for the medication administered to take effect. If the patient remains agitated, you may give additional doses of *haloperidol* 1 to 3 mg PO or IM until adequate sedation is achieved. Always use the lowest effective dosage.

   The two main acute side effects of haloperidol are hypotension and the occasional acute dystonic reaction (spasm of the face, tongue, back, or neck). The hypotension is usually postural, and once the patient is cooperative, he or she should be assisted when initially going from the supine to the upright position. Acute dystonic reactions usually respond to *diphenhydramine* 25 to 50 mg PO, IM, or IV or *benztropine mesylate* 1 to 2 mg PO, IM, or IV.

   If haloperidol is not available, a good alternative choice is *chlorpromazine* (Thorazine) 25 to 50 mg PO or IM q3–4h.

   Hypotension may be particularly pronounced with IM chlorpromazine and may respond to fluid administration with NS. The treatment for acute dystonic reactions is the same as for haloperidol.

3. Benzodiazepines or barbiturates should be avoided, since although they have valuable sedative properties, they tend to cloud consciousness and may actually compound the behavioral problem.

4. Call the patient's family, explain what has happened, and see if the family can shed any light on the patient's behavior. If physical restraints (wrist and ankle restraints or a posey) have been required, inform the family immediately and reassure them that you anticipate that the restraints will be required only temporarily. Emphasize that these measures are being employed only temporarily to protect the patient from injuring himself or herself. There is no better way to upset an uninformed and unsuspecting family than to have them walk into their loved one's room the next day and find the patient "tied down" to the bed.

5. Once the acute crisis is over, a thorough evaluation for underlying causes of confusion (any of which may lead to combative behavior) should be undertaken (see Chapter 8). Once the patient is safely approachable, a directed physical examination looking for life-threatening (see p. 55) or correctable causes (see p. 58) of confusion should be performed. You will have to use your judgment, since sometimes these patients are best left alone to sleep for a while. Just as often, however, the recently out-of-control patient will be grateful for the additional attention received from a concerned medical student or physician.

8

CONFUSION/DECREASED LEVEL OF CONSCIOUSNESS

Confusion is a common problem in hospitalized patients, especially among the elderly. Unfortunately, the terms delirium, toxic psychosis, acute brain syndrome, and acute confusional state often are used interchangeably to refer to any cause of confusion. When the term metabolic encephalopathy is used, it implies that the confusion is not due to psychiatric disorders or structural intracranial lesions.

The two recommended terms are delirium and dementia. *Delirium* is characterized by restlessness, agitation, clouding of consciousness, and in some patients, bizarre behavior, hallucinations, delusions, and illusions. *Dementia* refers to a state of irreversible loss of memory and a global cognitive deficit. The level of consciousness is an important distinguishing feature between delirium and dementia. Delirium is characterized by a clouding of consciousness (a decreased clarity of awareness of the environment), whereas dementia is associated with a normal level of consciousness. Also, the signs of delirium fluctuate, whereas the confusion seen with dementia is more constant.

Drowsiness, *stupor*, and *coma* refer to various degrees of unresponsiveness or diminished levels of consciousness.

PHONE CALL

Questions

1 **Clarify the situation. In what way is the patient confused?**
2 **What are the vital signs?**
3 **Has there been a change in the level of consciousness?**
4 **Have there been previous episodes of confusion?**
5 **What was the reason for admission?**
6 **Is the patient diabetic?**
   Confusion can be caused by either too much or too little sugar in the blood. Hypoglycemia (due to excess insulin or oral hypoglycemics) and marked hyperglycemia (due to inadequate insulin or oral hypoglycemic dosage) are prime considerations when confusion occurs in the diabetic patient.
7 **How old is the patient?**
   A 30-year-old patient is much more likely to have a serious yet reversible cause of confusion than an 80-year-old patient receiving multiple medications.

Orders

1. Blood glucose, Chemstrip, or Glucometer reading. Hypoglycemia is a rapidly reversible cause of confusion.
2. O_2 saturation, if pneumonia or a respiratory disorder was the reason for admission. This can be measured by attaching a pulse oximeter to the patient.

Inform RN

"Will arrive at the bedside in . . . minutes."

Confusion in association with fever, decrease in the level of consciousness, or acute agitation (see Chapter 7) requires you to see the patient immediately.

ELEVATOR THOUGHTS (What causes confusion or a decreased level of consciousness?)

Many disorders that begin with confusion may lead to a diminished level of consciousness and, ultimately, coma (note items marked with an asterisk in the following lists). To cause a diminished level of consciousness, both cerebral hemispheres must be affected (e.g., drugs or toxins), or there must be suppression of the brainstem reticular activating system.

CNS (Intracranial)

1. Dementia
   a. Alzheimer's disease (80% to 90% of all dementias)
   b. Multiinfarct dementia
   c. Parkinson's disease
   d. Normal pressure hydrocephalus*
2. Malignancy (primary CNS tumor, CNS metastasis, paraneoplastic syndrome)
3. Head trauma (subdural and epidural hematoma, concussion, cerebral contusion)*
4. Postictal state*
5. TIA/stroke*
6. Hypertensive encephalopathy*
7. Wernicke's encephalopathy (thiamine deficiency)
8. Vitamin B_{12} deficiency

Systemic

Drugs

1. Alcohol withdrawal. Confusion in the alcoholic patient may occur when the patient is intoxicated during early withdrawal, or later as part of delirium tremens.
2. Narcotic and sedative drug excess* or withdrawal. Even "normal" doses of these drugs frequently cause confusion in the elderly.

   3. NSAIDs, including aspirin
   4. Antihypertensives (methyldopa, beta blockers)
   5. Psychotropic medications (tricyclic antidepressants, lithium, phenothiazines, MAO inhibitors, benzodiazepines)*
   6. Miscellaneous (steroids, cimetidine, antihistamines, anticholinergics)

Organ Failure*
   1. Respiratory failure (hypoxia, hypercapnea)
   2. Renal failure (uremic encephalopathy)
   3. Liver failure (hepatic encephalopathy)
   4. CHF (hypoxia), hypertensive encephalopathy

Metabolic*
   1. Hyperglycemia, hypoglycemia
   2. Hypernatremia, hyponatremia
   3. Hypercalcemia

Endocrine
   1. Hyperthyroidism or hypothyroidism*
   2. Hyperadrenocorticism or hypoadrenocorticism

Infection or inflammation
   1. Meningitis,* encephalitis,* brain abscess*
   2. Lyme disease
   3. Cerebral vasculitis (SLE, polyarteritis nodosa)*

Psychiatric Disorders
   1. Mania, depression
   2. Schizophrenia

MAJOR THREAT TO LIFE

- Intracranial mass
- Delirium tremens
- Meningitis

Patients with an *intracranial mass* (e.g., subdural or epidural hematoma, brain abscess, tumor) may initially present with confusion. Patients with untreated *delirium tremens* can suffer a mortality rate of up to 15%. *Meningitis* needs to be recognized early if antibiotic medication is to be effective.

BEDSIDE
Quick Look Test

Does the patient look well (comfortable), sick (uncomfortable or distressed), or critical (about to die)?

Most patients with delirium look sick, whereas most patients with dementia look well.

Airway, Vital Signs, and Chemstrip Results

Is the patient receiving oxygen?
An FiO_2 of > 0.28 given to a patient with COPD may depress the respiratory center, resulting in confusion from hypercapnea.

What is the BP?
Hypertensive encephalopathy is rare; diastolic BP is usually $>$ 120 mm Hg. Confusion in association with a systolic BP < 90 mm Hg may be due to impaired cerebral perfusion secondary to shock. Drug overdose, adrenal insufficiency, and hyponatremia are metabolic causes that should be considered in the hypotensive, confused patient.

What is the HR?
A tachycardia suggests sepsis, delirium tremens, hyperthyroidism, or hypoglycemia, but it may also be seen in any agitated, anxious patient.

What is the temperature?
Fever suggests infection, delirium tremens, or cerebral vasculitis.

What is the respiratory rate?
Confusion in association with tachypnea should alert you to the possibility of hypoxia. Tachypnea with confusion and petechiae in a young patient with a femoral fracture is a classic presentation of fat embolism syndrome.

What is the blood glucose result?
Hypoglycemia is most commonly seen in the patient with diabetes mellitus who has received the usual insulin dose but has not eaten. Rarely, an incorrect dose of insulin, surreptitious insulin use, or an insulinoma is the cause (see Chapter 32, p. 307 for the management of hypoglycemia and p. 303 for the management of hyperglycemia).

Selective Physical Examination I

Is there evidence on physical examination of one of the major threats to life?

HEENT	Nuchal rigidity (meningitis)
	Papilledema (hypertensive encephalopathy, intracranial mass)
	Pupil size and symmetry
	Dilated pupils suggest increased sympathetic outflow, such as may be seen in delirium tremens, whereas pinpoint pupils suggest narcotic excess or recent application of constricting eyedrops.
	Palpate the skull for fractures, hematomas, and lacera-

tions (subdural or epidural hematoma, concussion)
Hemotympanum or blood in the ear canal (basal skull fracture)

NEURO   General appearance—behavior and attitude
Level of consciousness—alert, drowsy
Mood, affect—depressed, agitated, restless
Form of thought—flight of ideas, circumstantiality, loosening of associations, perseveration
Thought content—delusions, concrete thinking
Perceptions—illusions, hallucinations (auditory, visual)
Mental status: A detailed mental status examination is required in the assessment of the confused patient. However, if the patient has a decreased level of consciousness, is agitated or uncooperative, not all the categories discussed subsequently will be appropriate.

Orientation—time, place, and person
Registration—name 3 objects (e.g., apple, pencil, car) and have the patient repeat them
Attention and calculation—serial 7s
Recall—ask for the 3 aforementioned objects (apple, pencil, car)
Language—point to and identify objects; follow a 3-stage command; write a sentence
Long-term memory—birthdate, name of home town, when was WWII?
Judgment—test hypothetical situations

A full neurological examination is required (within the limits posed by the mental status examination).

Is there any tremor (delirium tremens, Parkinson's disease, hyperthyroidism)?
Is there any asymmetry of pupils, visual fields, eye movement, limbs, tone, reflexes, or plantars? Asymmetry suggests structural brain disease.

Management I

Bacterial Meningitis.   If there is a suspicion of bacterial meningitis, refer immediately to Chapter 12, p. 85, for further investigation and management.

Intracranial Lesion.   A structural intracranial lesion (e.g., stroke, tumor, subdural hematoma, or epidural hematoma) should be suspected in the patient with new findings of asymmetry on neurological examination. An urgent CT head scan will help define the intracranial lesion. Prompt referral to a neurosurgeon will be required for a subdural or epidural hematoma and for a cerebellar hemorrhage.

Delirium Tremens.   Delirium tremens (confusion, fever, tachycardia, dilated pupils, diaphoresis) and alcohol withdrawal need to be treated urgently with sedation. Benzodiazepines are of proven benefit. The loading dose of *diazepam* (Valium) is 5 to

10 mg IV at a rate of 2 to 5 mg/min q30–60 min, until the patient is sedated (i.e., drowsy, but rouses when stimulated). The maintenance dose is 10 to 20 mg PO QID, with subsequent tapering. Alternatively, *chlordiazepoxide* 100 mg PO QID for several days, with subsequent gradual tapering of the dose, may be used. *Thiamine* 100 mg PO, IM, or IV daily for up to 3 days, if not already administered during this hospitalization, should be given to prevent the development of Wernicke's encephalopathy in the alcoholic or malnourished patient. If necessary, IV D5NS may then be given to correct volume depletion, following the initial dose of thiamine.

Selective Physical Examination II

Are there other correctable causes of confusion?

VITALS	Hypertension and bradycardia may signify rising intracranial pressure.
	Hypotension may indicate an Addisonian crisis.
	Hypothermia suggests myxedema or alcohol, barbiturate, or phenothiazine intoxication
HEENT	Subhyaloid hemorrhage (SAH)
	Conjunctival and fundal petechiae (fat embolism syndrome) (Fig. 8–1)
	Lacerated tongue or cheek (postictal)
	Goiter (hyperthyroidism or hypothyroidism)
RESP	Cyanosis (hypoxia)
	Barrel chest (COPD with hypoxia or hypercapnea)
	Bibasilar crackles (CHF with hypoxia)
CVS	Elevated JVP
	S_3 (CHF)
	Pitting edema

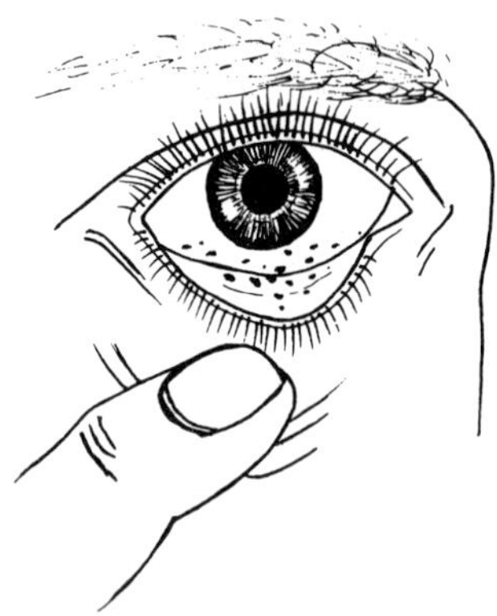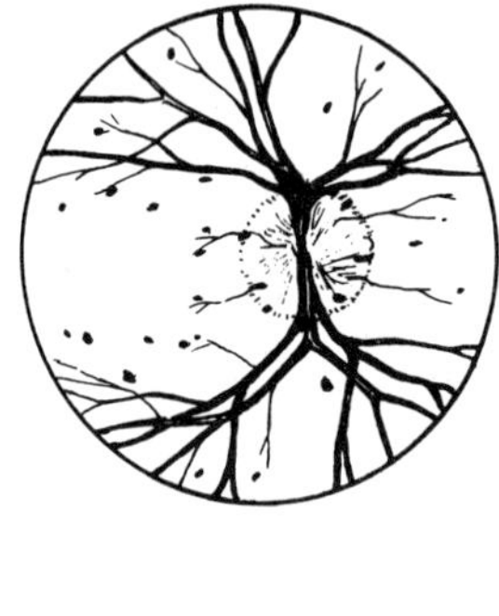

Figure 8–1 □ Conjunctival and fundal petechiae seen in fat embolism syndrome.

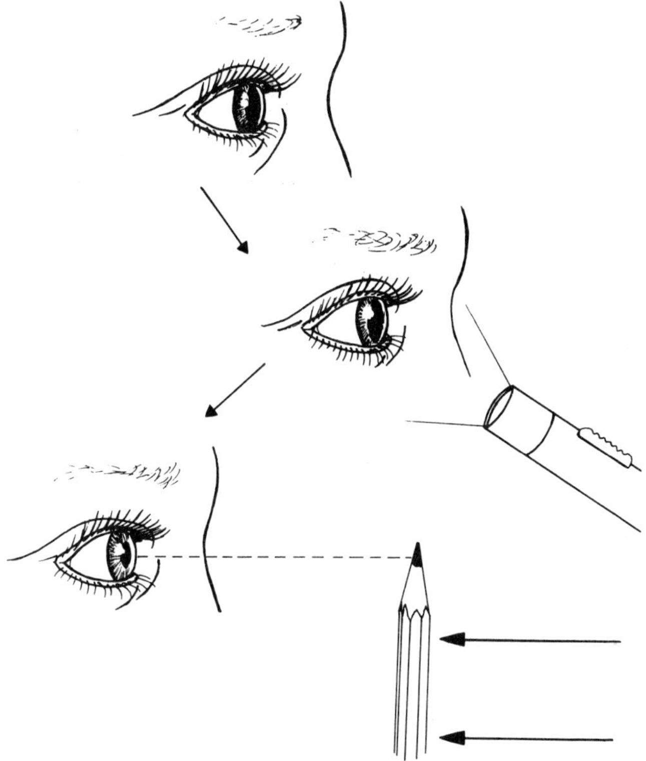

Figure 8–2 □ Argyll Robertson pupils. Pupils do not react to light, but they accommodate.

ABD	Costovertebral angle tenderness (pyelonephritis) Liver, spleen, or kidney tenderness (infection) Guarding, rebound tenderness (intraabdominal infection) Shifting dullness, dilated superficial veins, caput medusa (liver failure)
NEURO	Argyll Robertson pupils, i.e., accommodate but do not react to light (syphilis) (Fig. 8–2) Cranial nerve palsies (Lyme disease) Asterixis, constructional apraxia (liver failure) (Fig. 8–3)
SKIN	Axillary fold, neck, upper chest petechiae (fat embolism syndrome)

Selective History and Chart Review

What drugs is the patient receiving?
Remember, even the "usual" doses of some drugs can cause confusion in the elderly because of alterations in intestinal, renal,

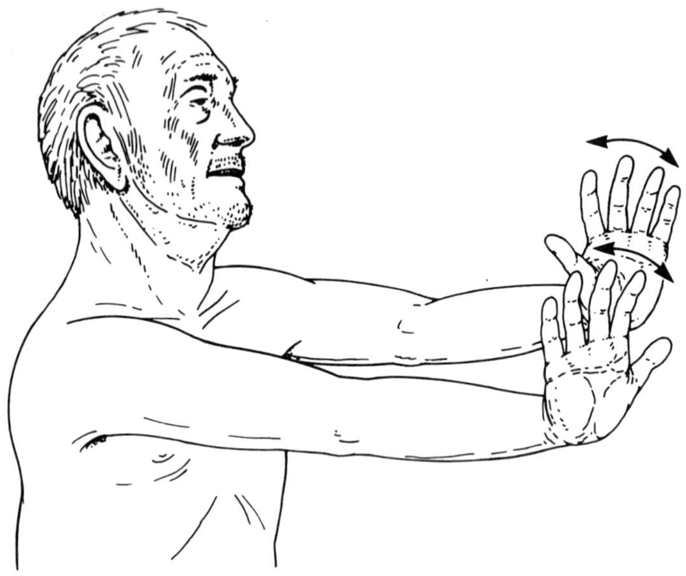

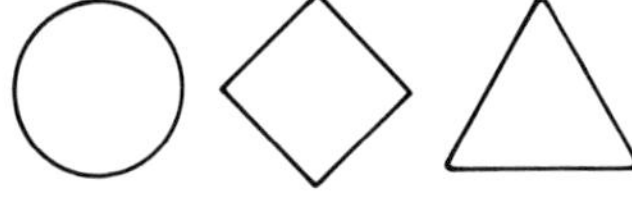

Figure 8–3 □ *Top*, Asterixis. Wrist flapping seen when the arms are outstretched. *Bottom*, Tests of constructional apraxia.

or hepatic blood flow, drug protein binding, or changes in body fluid compartments.

Is there a history of alcohol abuse?

It is important to establish when alcohol was last taken, since withdrawal symptoms are unlikely after 1 week of abstinence.

Is the patient postoperative?

Postoperative patients are predisposed to confusion because of CNS effects of anesthetic and analgesic medications, nutritional deficiencies (e.g., thiamine), and fluid and electrolyte disturbances. These physiological abnormalities may be exacerbated in the elderly patient because of sensory impairment (reduced visual or auditory acuity), psychological factors, and cultural expectations.

If there is a decreased level of consciousness, has the change been gradual or sudden?

A sudden decrease in the level of consciousness is usually due to drug ingestion or an acute intracranial catastrophe (hemorrhage, trauma). Gradually developing unresponsiveness (over days or weeks) is usually due to a preceding systemic medical disorder (e.g., metabolic or endocrine disorders, hepatic or renal failure).

Does the patient have AIDS?

HIV infection may result in cognitive impairment in the otherwise asymptomatic patient with AIDS. Patients in the more advanced stages of AIDS may suffer a wide variety of neurological problems associated with confusion, including HIV dementia, CNS opportunistic infections (e.g., toxoplasmosis, cryptococcal meningitis), and neoplasms (e.g., primary lymphoma of the brain).

Examine the most recent laboratory test results for those that may indicate the reason for confusion in the patient. Not all of the tests listed will be available or pertinent.

- Blood glucose (hypoglycemia, hyperglycemia)
- Urea, creatinine (renal failure)
- Liver function (liver failure)
- Sodium (hyponatremia, hypernatremia)
- Calcium (hypercalcemia)
- Hb, MCV, RBC morphology (anemia with oval macrocytes suggests vitamin B_{12} or folate deficiency)
- WBC and differential (infection)
- ABG (hypoxia or CO_2 retention)
- T_4, T_3, TSH (hyperthyroidism, hypothyroidism)
- ANA, rheumatoid factor, ESR, C3, C4 (vasculitis)
- Drug levels (digoxin, lithium, aspirin, antiepileptic drugs)

Management II

Drugs. If the confusion is secondary to drugs, stop the medication. If reversal of postoperative narcotic depression is indicated, give *naloxone* (Narcan) 0.2 to 2.0 mg IV, IM, or SC q5min (maximum total dose 10 mg) until the desired improved level of consciousness is achieved. Maintenance doses q1–2h may be required to maintain reversal of the CNS depression. Naloxone should be used with caution in patients known to be physically dependent on opiates.

Dementia.   Dementia is a diagnosis of exclusion. The following investigations are required to rule out a treatable cause of dementia.

- CBC, electrolytes, urea, creatinine
- Calcium, phosphorus
- Liver function tests
- Serum vitamin B_{12}, folate
- T_4, T_3, TSH
- STS
- CT or MRI head scan

Renal and Hepatic Failure.   In *end-stage* renal and liver failure, ensure that the problem has not been compounded by hepatotoxic or nephrotoxic medications. Aggressive treatment of the renal failure (dialysis if necessary) or the liver failure (lactulose, neomycin) should be undertaken when indicated.

Hyponatremia or Hypernatremia.   For the management of hyponatremia or hypernatremia, refer to Chapter 34.

Hypercalcemia.   For the management of hypercalcemia, see Chapter 30.

Vitamin B_{12} Deficiency.   Suspected vitamin B_{12} deficiency needs to be confirmed by a serum vitamin B_{12} level.

Mania, Depression, or Schizophrenia.   Suspected mania, depression, or schizophrenia requires psychiatric consultation for confirmation of diagnosis. Agitation in a confused patient may require *haloperidol* 1 to 5 mg PO or IM q4–6h.

Cerebral Vasculitis.   Cerebral vasculitis is rare. High-dose steroid therapy is the currently accepted treatment.

Fat Embolism.   Fat embolism syndrome can have a mortality rate of up to 8%. The mainstay of treatment is oxygen therapy. If the patient requires an F_{IO_2} of > 0.5, transfer to the ICU/CCU for probable intubation and mechanical ventilation with PEEP is recommended.

□ **9** □

DECREASED URINE OUTPUT

Decreased urine output is a problem frequently seen on both medical and surgical services. Proper management of these patients calls on your skills in assessing volume status.

PHONE CALL
Questions

1 **How much urine has been passed in the last 24 hours?**
Urine output less than 400 ml/day (<20 ml/h) = oliguria. Anuria suggests a mechanical obstruction of the bladder outlet or a blocked Foley catheter.
2 **What are the vital signs?**
3 **What was the reason for admission?**
4 **Is the patient complaining of abdominal pain?**
Abdominal pain is a clue to the possible presence of a distended bladder, as may be seen with bladder outlet obstruction.
5 **Does the patient have a Foley catheter?**
If the patient has a Foley catheter in place, the urine output assessment usually can be assumed to be accurate. If not, you will have to ensure that the total volume of voided urine has been collected and measured.
6 **What is the most recent serum potassium level?**

Orders

1. If a Foley catheter is in place and the patient is anuric, ask the nurse to flush the catheter with 20 to 30 ml NS to ensure patency. A Foley catheter clogged with sediment is a common problem and a satisfying one to treat before beginning a more detailed investigation for decreased urine output.
2. Serum electrolytes, urea, creatinine. A serum potassium level of >5.5 mmol/L indicates that hyperkalemia is present. This is the most serious complication of renal insufficiency. A serum HCO_3 measurement <20 mmol/L suggests metabolic acidosis due to renal insufficiency. A serum HCO_3 <15 mmol/L should prompt you to determine the arterial pH. Elevations in serum urea and creatinine levels can be used as guidelines to assess the degree of renal insufficiency present.

Inform RN

"Will arrive at bedside in . . . minutes."

Provided the patient is not in pain and a recent serum potassium level is not elevated, assessment of decreased urine output can wait 1 or 2 hours if other problems of higher priority exist.

ELEVATOR THOUGHTS (What causes decreased urine output?)

Prerenal causes (underperfusion of kidney)	Volume depletion Reduced cardiac output (CHF, constrictive pericarditis, cardiac tamponade) Hepatorenal syndrome
Renal causes	Nephritic syndromes (acute glomerulonephritis, SBE, SLE, other vasculitides) Tubulointerstitial problems 　Acute tubular necrosis due to 　　Hypotension 　　Nephrotoxins 　　　Exogenous (aminoglycosides, amphotericin B, IV contrast materials, chemotherapy) 　　　Endogenous (myoglobin, uric acid, oxalate, amyloid, Bence Jones protein) 　Acute interstitial nephritis due to penicillin, other beta-lactam antibiotics, NSAIDs, or diuretics Vascular problems 　Emboli (from aortic atheromas, SBE, or left heart thrombi) 　Renal artery thrombosis
Postrenal causes (obstruction)	Bilateral ureteric obstruction (e.g., stones, clots, sloughed papillae, retroperitoneal fibrosis, retroperitoneal tumors) Bladder outlet obstruction (e.g., prostatic hypertrophy, carcinoma of the cervix, stones, clots, urethral strictures) Blocked Foley catheter

MAJOR THREAT TO LIFE

- Renal failure
- Hyperkalemia

Decreased urine output from any cause may result in or may be a manifestation of progressive renal insufficiency, leading to renal failure. Of the complications of renal failure, hyperkalemia is the most immediately life threatening, as it may lead to potentially fatal cardiac dysrhythmias.

BEDSIDE
Quick Look Test

Does the patient look well (comfortable), sick (uncomfortable or distressed), or critical (about to die)?

A sick or critical looking patient suggests advanced renal insufficiency. A restless patient suggests pain from a distended bladder. However, both of these conditions can be present in a patient who appears deceptively well.

Airway and Vital Signs

Check for postural changes. A postural rise in HR > 15 beats/min, a fall is systolic BP > 15 mm Hg, or any fall in diastolic BP suggests significant hypovolemia. *Caution:* A resting tachycardia alone may indicate decreased intravascular volume. *Fever* suggests concomitant urinary tract infection.

Selective Physical Examination I

Examine for *prerenal* (volume status), *renal*, or *postrenal* (obstructive) causes of decreased urine output. *Caution:* More than one cause may be present at any time.

HEENT	Jaundice (hepatorenal syndrome)
	Facial purpura ⎫
	Enlarged tongue ⎭ Amyloidosis
RESP	Crackles, pleural effusions (CHF)
CVS	Pulse volume, JVP
	Skin temperature, color
ABD	Enlarged kidneys (hydronephrosis secondary to obstruction, polycystic kidney disease)
	Enlarged bladder (bladder outlet obstruction, neurogenic bladder, blocked Foley catheter)
RECTAL	Enlarged prostate gland (bladder outlet obstruction)
PELVIC	Cervical or adnexal masses (ureteric obstruction secondary to cervical or ovarian cancer)
SKIN	Morbilliform rash (acute interstitial nephritis)
	Livedo reticularis on lower extremities (atheromatous embolic renal failure)

Selective Chart Review

Review the patient's history and hospital course, looking specifically for factors that may predispose to prerenal, renal, or postrenal causes of decreased urine output (see ELEVATOR THOUGHTS.)

Look for recent blood urea and creatinine values. A Cr/urea ratio < 12 suggests a prerenal cause. A urine specific gravity > 1.020 or urine Na concentration < 20 mmol/L also suggests a prerenal cause.

Management I

Your job becomes simpler when you can find a *prerenal* or *postrenal* cause for decreased urine output.

Prerenal.   First ensure that the intravascular volume is normal. If in CHF, initiate diuresis as discussed in Chapter 24, p. 239. If volume depleted, replenish the intravascular volume with NS. Add *no* potassium supplement to the IV solution until the patient passes urine. Ringer's lactate should not be given, since it contains potassium.

Postrenal.   Lower urinary tract obstruction can be adequately excluded by passage of a Foley catheter into the bladder.
1. If there has been bladder outlet obstruction, the initial urine volume on catheterization usually will be greater than 400 ml, and the patient will experience immediate relief. Remember to listen carefully for heart murmurs before catheterizing the patient. If there is documented evidence of a cardiac valvular abnormality requiring SBE prophylaxis, refer to Chapter 21, p. 213. Following catheterization, watch for the development of postobstructive diuresis by monitoring urine volume status carefully for the next few days.
2. If a Foley catheter is already in place, ensure that flushing the catheter with 20 to 30 ml of NS allows free flow of fluid from the bladder. This maneuver will exclude an intraluminal blockage of the Foley catheter as a cause of postrenal obstruction.
3. The presence of a Foley catheter in the bladder only rules out lower urinary tract obstruction. If the preceding two steps fail to restore urine output, a *renal ultrasound* examination should be ordered first thing in the morning to exclude upper urinary tract obstruction. Additional useful information, such as documentation of the presence of both kidneys and an estimate of renal size, also may be obtained.

Renal.   If prerenal and postrenal factors are not operative in causing the patient's decreased urine output, you are left in the murky waters of renal causes of decreased urine output. A search for the *renal causes* of decreased urine output can wait until some more important questions are answered (see Management II).

Management II

Regardless of the causes of decreased urine output (prerenal, renal, or postrenal), you must now answer the following four questions.

1. Are any of the following five life-threatening complications of decreased urine output present?

- Hyperkalemia
- CHF
- Severe metabolic acidemia (pH < 7.2)
- Uremic encephalopathy
- Uremic pericarditis

Of these, *hyperkalemia* is the most immediately serious problem.

- Order a stat serum potassium level, if not already done.
- Review the chart for a recent serum potassium level.
- Order a stat ECG if suspicion of hyperkalemia exists. Peaked T waves are early signs of hyperkalemia (Fig. 9–1). More advanced ECG manifestations include depressed ST segments, prolonged PR intervals, loss of P waves, and wide QRS complexes.

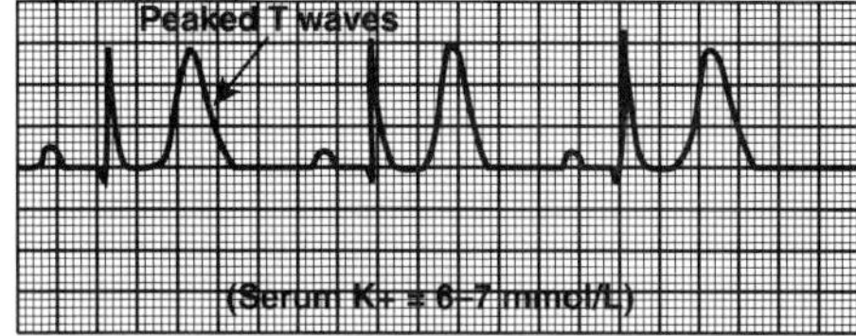

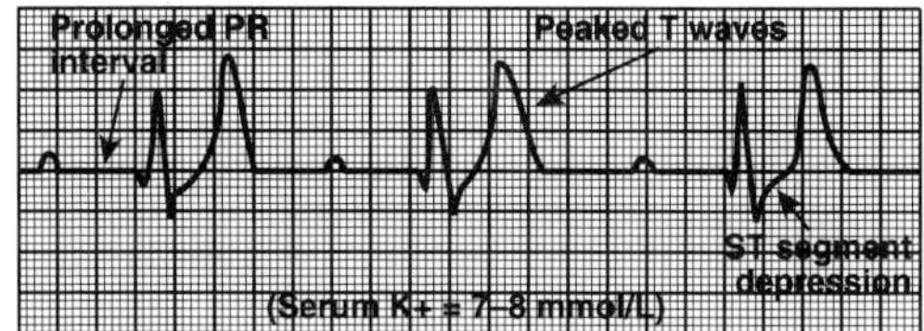

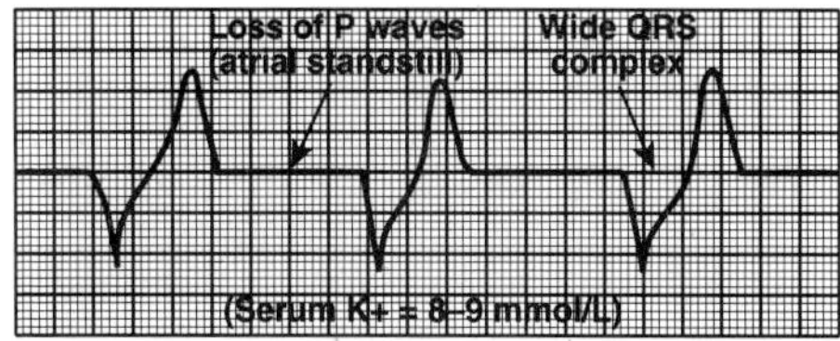

Figure 9–1 □ Progressive electrocardiographic features of hyperkalemia.

- Discontinue any potassium supplements.
- Treat as outlined in Chapter 33, p. 310.

CHF is suggested by tachypnea, elevated JVP, crackles on pulmonary auscultation, an S_3, and sacral or pedal edema. Refer to Chapter 24, p. 238, for management of CHF.

Metabolic acidemia is suggested by the presence of (compensatory) hyperventilation and confirmed by ABG measurement. Investigation should take place as outlined in Chapter 28, p. 275.

Uremic encephalopathy manifests itself as confusion, stupor, or seizures and is managed by dialysis. If seizures occur, they should be managed as outlined in Chapter 23 until dialysis can be initiated.

Uremic pericarditis is suggested by the presence of pleuritic chest pain, pericardial friction rub, or diffuse ST segment elevation on the ECG. It is managed best by dialysis.

2. Is the patient on any drugs that may worsen the situation?

- Potassium supplements
- Potassium sparing diuretics (spironolactone, triamterene, amiloride)
- Nephrotoxic drugs (NSAIDs, aminoglycosides). Review the need for these agents and discontinue immediately if possible. If aminoglycosides are required, doses will need to be adjusted based on serum levels.

3. Is the patient in oliguric renal failure?

If the patient has produced < 400 ml/d of urine (< 20 ml/h), the patient has oliguric renal failure. A favor you can do for your patient is to convert this from oliguric to nonoliguric renal failure, which portends a better prognosis.

- Correct prerenal and postrenal factors
- Give diuretics to increase urine output. *Furosemide* (Lasix) 40 mg IV given over 2 to 5 minutes. If no response, double the dose q1h (i.e., 40 to 80 to 160 mg) to a total of about 400 mg. Doses of furosemide > 100 mg should be infused at a rate not exceeding 4 mg/min to avoid ototoxicity. Smaller initial doses (e.g., 10 mg) may suffice for the patient who is frail and very elderly.
- If furosemide is ineffective, try *ethacrynic acid* (Edecrin) 50 mg IV q60min × 2 doses or *bumetanide* (Bumex) 1 to 10 mg IV over 1 to 2 minutes. Administering *hydroclorothiazide* 25 to 50 mg PO or *metolazone* (Zaroxolyn) 5 to 10 mg PO along with one of the loop diuretics may help potentiate their effects. An indwelling Foley catheter may be required to monitor urine output in these situations.

4. Does the patient need dialysis?

If the patient does not pass urine despite high doses of diuretics, the indications for urgent dialysis are as follows.

- Hyperkalemia
- CHF
- Metabolic acidemia (pH < 7.2)
- Severe uremia (urea level > 35 mmol/L; creatinine level > 800 mmol/L) ± uremic seizures
- Uremic pericarditis

If the patient is in renal failure and if one or more of these conditions is present, request an urgent nephrology consultation to dialyze the patient. While awaiting the nephrologist's arrival, all of the following problems can be temporarily treated with nondialysis measures.

- *Hyperkalemia:* Glucose with insulin infusion, $NaHCO_3$, calcium, sodium polystyrene sulfonate. (Refer to Chapter 33 for treatment of hyperkalemia.)
- *CHF:* Preload measures (sit the patient up, morphine, nitroglycerin ointment). Give O_2. (Refer to Chapter 24, p. 237 for management of CHF.)
- *Metabolic acidemia:* $NaHCO_3$. (Refer to Chapter 28, p. 275 for assessment of metabolic acidosis.)
- Patients with *uremic encephalopathy* should be kept calm and at bedrest until dialysis can be initiated.
- Patients with *uremic pericarditis* may be treated symptomatically for pain with an NSAID until dialysis can be initiated.

Once these tasks have been addressed, you can sit down and think about possible *renal causes* of decreased urine output. The majority of renal causes are diagnosed by history, physical examination, and laboratory findings. Occasionally, a renal biopsy is required. A simple urinalysis can often provide valuable clues to the diagnosis.

- *Urine dipstick.* Hematuria and proteinuria together suggest *glomerulonephritis.* A positive orthotoluidine test result for blood may represent red blood cells, free hemoglobin, or myoglobin. Suspect *rhabdomyolysis* if there is a positive orthotoluidine test result on dipstick but few or no RBCs on urine microscopy. (In this case, order tests of serum for CPK, Ca, and PO_4 and of urine for myoglobin.)

  A positive test result for urinary protein alone should prompt you to do a serum albumin and 24 hour urine collection for protein and creatinine clearance to identify the *nephrotic syndrome,* if present.
- *Urine microscopy.* RBC casts are diagnostic of *glomerulonephritis.* Oval fat bodies are suggestive of *nephrotic syndrome.*
- *Urine for eosinophils.* Ask for this test if there is a suspicion of *acute interstitial nephritis.*

In most cases, beyond these simple tests, no further investigation is required at night. Ensure, however, that for any suspected *renal* cause of decreased urine output, prerenal and postrenal factors are not additionally contributing to the poor urine output.

REMEMBER

All medications that the oliguric or anuric patient is receiving should be reviewed, and any potential nephrotoxins should be discontinued if possible. Drugs that depend on renal excretion (e.g., digoxin, aminoglycosides) also may require dosage adjustment.

10

DIARRHEA

Avoid treating diarrhea as a diagnosis. Diarrhea is always a symptom of another underlying disorder and seldom warrants nonspecific antimotility therapy. Your job at night is to determine what the likely cause of diarrhea is, whether additional investigations should be performed, and whether complications have arisen that require treatment.

PHONE CALL

Questions

1 **What are the vital signs?**
2 **What was the reason for admission?**
3 **Is this a new problem? If not, has a diagnosis of the reason for diarrhea been made?**
4 **Has the patient had recent surgery?**
5 **Is the patient HIV positive?**
6 **Is there blood in the stool?**
   Bloody stools suggest inflammation, as may be seen with infection, inflammatory bowel disease, or ischemic colitis.
7 **Does the patient have significant pain?**
   Significant associated abdominal pain suggests ischemic colitis, diverticulitis, or inflammatory bowel disease.

Orders

None.

Inform RN

"Will arrive at the bedside in . . . minutes."

A single episode of diarrhea in an otherwise well patient does not usually require bedside assessment. If the diarrhea is frequent, severe, or associated with passage of blood, the patient should be evaluated at the bedside as soon as possible. If the patient is hypotensive, tachycardic, or febrile, he or she should be assessed immediately.

ELEVATOR THOUGHTS (What causes diarrhea?)

Acute Diarrhea (Diarrhea of Less Than 2 Weeks Duration)

The 4 I's
- Infection   Inflammation and toxins (see Table 10–1)
- Iatrogenic   Drugs (Mg-containing antacids, laxatives, antibiotics, digoxin, quinidine, colchicine, anticholinergic agents) and surgery (postgastrectomy)

Table 10-1 □ ETIOLOGIC AGENTS IN INFECTIOUS DIARRHEA

Inflammatory

Bacterial

Salmonella sp.
Shigella sp.
Campylobacter sp.
Yersinia enterocolitica
Vibrio sp.
*Mycobacterium avium-intracellulare**
*Chlamydia**

Protozoal

*Entamoeba histolytica**
*Giardia lamblia**
Cryptosporidium sp.*
*Isospora belli**

Viral

Norwalk virus
Rota virus
Cytomegalovirus*
Herpes simplex*

Nematodes

*Strongyloides stercoralis**

Toxins

Toxins Produced in Vivo

Clostridium difficile (after antibiotic administration)
Clostridium perfringens (beef, poultry)
Bacillus cereus (fried rice)
Cytotoxic *Escherichia coli* (hamburger)

Preformed Toxins

Staphylococcus aureus (potato salads, mayonnaise, puddings)
Bacillus cereus (fried rice)

*Indicates prevalence in HIV-positive patients.

- ■ Ischemia   Ischemic bowel
- ■ Impactions   Fecal impaction

Chronic Diarrhea (Diarrhea Lasting Longer Than 2 Weeks)
The 3 Is and 2 Ms
- Inflammatory bowel disease
- Infiltrative disorders (amyloid, lymphoma)
- Irritable bowel syndrome
- Malabsorption (celiac disease)
- Metabolic/hormonal
  - Enzyme deficiencies (lactase deficiency, pancreatic deficiency)
  - Hormone production (gastrinoma, carcinoid, VIPoma, villous adenoma, medullary carcinoma of the thyroid)
  - Endocrinopathies (diabetic diarrhea, hyperthyroidism, Addison's disease)

Any of the causes of acute diarrhea, if left untreated, may also cause chronic diarrhea.

MAJOR THREAT TO LIFE

- Intravascular volume depletion, electrolyte imbalance
- Systemic infection

Volume depletion and *electrolyte disturbances* are the reasons that many children in underdeveloped countries die from diarrhea. This, of course, is seldom seen in the hospitalized adult patient, but if left untreated, diarrhea may certainly progress to serious volume depletion and electrolyte imbalance. Some bacterial causes of diarrhea, if left untreated, may become *systemic*, life-threatening disorders.

BEDSIDE

Quick Look Test

Does the patient look well (comfortable), sick (uncomfortable or distressed), or critical (about to die)?

Most patients with acute diarrhea do not look unwell. However, if the diarrhea is due to an invasive organism (e.g., *Salmonella, Shigella*), the patient may look sick and complain of headaches, diffuse myalgias, chills, and fevers.

Airway and Vital Signs

What is the BP?

Resting hypotension suggests significant volume depletion. If the resting BP is normal, examine for postural changes. A postural rise in HR > 15 beats/min, a fall in systolic BP > 15 mm Hg, or any fall in diastolic BP indicates significant hypovolemia.

What is the HR?

Intravascular volume depletion usually results in tachycardia unless the patient has a coexisting disorder (e.g., autonomic dysfunction due to beta blockade, SSS, or autonomic neuropathy), which may prevent the generation of a tachycardia. However, in diarrheal diseases, a tachycardia may also be seen due to anxiety, pain, or fever. A relative bradycardia despite fever raises the suspicion of *Salmonella* infection.

What is the temperature?

A fever in the patient with diarrhea is nonspecific but suggests the presence of inflammation, as may be seen with infectious diarrhea, diverticulitis, and inflammatory bowel disease. Some organisms (*Shigella* and *Salmonella* sp.) may cause systemic sepsis. However, remember that sepsis may occur in the absence of fever, especially in the elderly.

Selective Physical Examination

Is the patient volume depleted? Is there evidence of systemic sepsis?

        VITALS   (See above)
        CVS   Pulse volume, JVP (flat neck veins)
                      Skin temperature, color

Management I

1. **What immediate measures need to be taken to correct intra-vascular volume depletion?** Normalize the intravascular volume. This can be achieved quickly by administration of an IV fluid that will at least temporarily stay in the intravascular space, e.g., NS or Ringer's lactate. Give NS 250 to 500 ml IV over 1 to 2 hours, titrating the IV fluid to the patient's vital signs and JVP. Reassess the volume status after each bolus of IV fluid, aiming for a JVP of 2 to 3 cm H_2O above the sternal angle and concomitant normalization of HR and BP.
2. Check the chart for a recent electrolyte determination. If the patient has not had electrolytes checked within the last 24 hours, order serum electrolytes, urea, and creatinine levels now.
3. In the patient with fever > 38.5°C, two sets of blood cultures should be drawn. If the patient is also hypotensive, volume replacement should be instituted with NS, and consideration should be given to empiric antibiotic coverage (see Chapter 12, p. 84).
4. A rectal examination should be performed, and stool samples should be sent for culture, ova and parasite determination, *Clostridium difficile* toxin, and WBC stain. If unusual organisms are suspected (e.g., in the AIDS patient), the laboratory should be alerted so that appropriate culture technique and media can be employed.

Selective Chart Review (Are there potential causes of diarrhea apparent from the chart?)

Is the patient on any medications that may cause diarrhea?
Medications are the commonest cause of diarrhea in the hospital. Frequent offenders include laxatives, stool softeners, magnesium-containing antacids, digoxin, quinidine, colchicine, and xanthines. Laxatives and stool softeners should be discontinued. Mg-containing antacids may be withheld or switched to aluminum-containing preparations. Other medications should not be discontinued without first asking your resident or attending physician. Remember, also, in the celiac patient, that some medications (e.g., Anacin, Dristan, Dyazide) contain gluten.

Has the patient received antibiotics recently?
Many antibiotics cause transient diarrhea through alteration of the intestinal flora. In addition, *pseudomembranous colitis* due to *Clostridium difficile* enterotoxin may result in persistent diarrhea during or after antibiotic use. A *Clostridium difficile* toxin titer

should be ordered, but the diagnosis can be made immediately by sigmoidoscopy and the finding of yellowish white pseudomembranes. Treatment includes discontinuing the offending antibiotic and administering *vancomycin* 125 to 500 mg PO QID for 7 days. *Metronidazole* or *bacitracin* may be used as alternative therapies.

Does the patient have AIDS?

Immuncompromised patients and patients with AIDS may develop diarrhea for many reasons. In addition to the usual causes of diarrhea, homosexual men should be tested for sexually transmitted anorectal conditions, including infection with *Treponema pallidum, Neisseria gonorrhoeae, Chlamydia,* and herpes simplex. Other nonvenereal agents include CMV, *Cryptosporidium,* and *Mycobacterium avium-intracellulare.* If this is the first documented episode of diarrhea, stool samples should be sent for Gram's stain, acid-fast stain, WBC stain, bacterial, mycobacterial, and fungal culture, and ova and parasite determination. Diagnosis of anorectal infections may require proctoscopy or sigmoidoscopy, with specimens taken for gonorrhea, herpes simplex viral culture, and darkfield examination for syphilis, and can be arranged in the morning.

Has the patient had recent surgery?

Postgastrectomy dumping of hypertonic boluses of stomach contents into the jejunum is associated with vasomotor symptoms of flushing, anxiety, palpitations, sweating, and dizziness, and there may be associated diarrhea.

Does the patient have known inflammatory bowel disease, celiac disease, lactase deficiency, or other conditions known to cause chronic diarrhea?

Has there been recent travel abroad?

E. coli enterotoxin is a common cause of acute, self-limiting traveller's diarrhea. Giardiasis, amebiasis, and tropical sprue may cause a more chronic condition.

Has the patient been admitted for the investigation of diarrhea?

In these cases, a plan of investigation is usually already outlined. If the patient is not volume depleted and is otherwise comfortable, no additional measures are required at night.

Selective Physical Examination II (Look for Clues for Specific Causes of Diarrhea)

VITALS	Repeat now
ABD	Hepatosplenomegaly (*Salmonella* infection)

	RLQ mass or tenderness (Crohn's disease, ischemic colitis)
	LLQ mass or tenderness (diverticulitis, tumor, inflammatory bowel disease, ischemic colitis, fecal impaction)
RECTAL	Rectal fissure (Crohn's disease)
	Hard mass (fecal impaction, tumor)
	Fresh blood or stool positive for occult blood (inflammatory bowel disease, infection, tumor)
SKIN	Rose spots (*Salmonella* infection)

Management II

It is unusual to be able to pinpoint the specific cause of diarrhea when seeing a patient for the first time at night. Occasionally, a patient will tell you, "I'm sure it's my Crohn's disease acting up," or "I have lactose intolerance, and the kitchen gave me yoghurt for dinner," and most often in these cases the patient turns out to be right. When the diagnosis is not obvious at night, the goal is to make sure that the patient is adequately hydrated and that he or she is not suffering from a systemic infection. Additional specialized investigations for diarrhea can, in most cases, wait until the morning to be arranged.

Remember, in many cases of infectious diarrhea, frequent loose stools is the body's way of expelling the offending organism or toxin. Do not compound the problem by inhibiting the body's ability to do this. Diarrhea is always best treated by addressing the underlying cause, and this may take a few days (and sometimes weeks) to identify. Unless the diarrhea is profuse or disabling, nonspecific antidiarrheal agents are best avoided. Explain this to the patient and to the nurses caring for them, so that everyone is clear about the treatment approach.

If the patient's diarrhea is severe and disabling, it is occasionally warranted to use *one* of the nonspecific antidiarrheal agents listed below. However, none of these agents should be prescribed before examining the patient (including rectal examination and possibly sigmoidoscopy), and deciding on an appropriate plan of investigation.

- *Kaopectate* 60 to 90 ml PO QID PRN
- *Diphenoxylate hydrochloride* (Lomotil) 5 mg PO TID or QID until the diarrhea is controlled, then 2.5 mg PO BID or TID for maintenance. Diphenoxylate hydrochloride is contraindicated in patients with hepatic failure or cirrhosis. Respiratory depression may occur when it is used in combination with phenothiazines, tricyclic antidepressants, or barbiturates.
- *Codeine* 30 to 60 mg PO QID PRN

11

FALL-OUT-OF-BED

Patients always seem to be falling out of bed, but they fall while in other places too. You will find the content of this chapter applicable to any fall occurring in the patient's room or elsewhere in the hospital.

PHONE CALL

Questions

1 **Was the fall witnessed?**
2 **Is there an obvious injury?**
3 **What are the vital signs?**
4 **Has there been a change in the level of consciousness?**
5 **Is the patient receiving anticoagulants or antiepileptic medications?**
6 **What was the reason for admission?**

Orders

Ask the RN to phone immediately if the level of consciousness changes before you are able to assess the patient.

Inform RN

"Will arrive at the bedside in . . . minutes."

When other sick patients are in need of assessment, they take priority over a patient who has had an uncomplicated fall. However, a change in the level of consciousness, a fracture, or a coagulation disorder requires you to see the patient immediately.

ELEVATOR THOUGHTS (Why does a patient fall?)

CARDIAC	MI, dysrhythmias Postural hypotension (volume depletion, drugs, or autonomic failure) Vasovagal attack

NEURO	Confusion (particularly in the elderly)
	    Drugs (narcotics, sedatives, antidepressants, tranquilizers, cimetidine, antihypertensive agents)
	    Metabolic disorders (electrolyte abnormalities, renal failure, hepatic failure)
	    Dementia (Parkinson's disease, Alzheimer's disease, multiinfarction, normal-pressure hydrocephalus)
	TIA, stroke
	Seizure

77

ENVIRONMENTAL   Disorientation at night
Call bell not accessible
There are many potential environmental hazards within the hospital setting, e.g., a fall on a wet floor, a fall during an unassisted transfer from bed to chair, and a fall while walking in a patient who requires assistance. The elderly are particularly prone to accidental falls due to a combination of environmental hazards, poor vision, diminished muscular strength, and impaired righting reflexes.

MAJOR THREAT TO LIFE

- Head injury

Any patient who may have hit his or her head during a fall requires a complete neurological examination now. Even seemingly minor trauma can result in a serious intracranial bleed in an anticoagulated patient. If a new neurological problem is identified, an immediate CT scan of the head can be helpful. The consideration of immediate reversal of anticoagulation should be discussed in consultation with your resident and hematologist (see Chapter 31, p. 299 for reversal of anticoagulation). If no neurological deficit is identified at this time, observation by frequent assessment of the neurovital signs is required.

BEDSIDE
Quick Look Test

Does the patient look well (comfortable), sick (uncomfortable or distressed), or critical (about to die)?

Most patients do not have life-threatening problems to account for falling. Usually, they look well, and the vital signs are normal.

Airway and Vital Signs

What are the heart rate and rhythm?

A tachycardia, bradycardia, or irregular rhythm may indicate a dysrhythmia as the cause of the fall.

Are there postural (lying and standing) changes in BP and HR?

A postural fall in BP together with a postural rise in HR (> 15 beats/min) suggests volume depletion. A drop in BP without a change in HR suggests autonomic dysfunction. An initial drop in BP that corrects on standing also suggests autonomic dysfunction. Drugs are common causes of postural hypotension in elderly patients.

Selective History

Ask the patient why he or she fell—after all, they may know the answer!

What was the patient doing just before the fall?
Coughing, micturating, or straining are examples of maneuvers that may result in vasovagal syncope. **Question any witnesses who observed the fall.**

Were there any warning symptoms before the fall?
Lightheadedness and visual disturbances on standing may indicate postural hypotension. Palpitations suggest a dysrhythmia. Auras are rare but, if present, are highly suggestive of a seizure disorder.

Is there a history of previous falls?
Recurrent falls suggest an underlying disorder that has gone unrecognized. Here is your chance to shine!

Is the patient diabetic?
Hyperglycemia or hypoglycemia may cause confusion, and the patient may, as a consequence, fall. Order a Chemstrip or Glucometer reading. Check the diabetic record for the past 3 days.

Is the patient aware of any injury sustained during the fall?
Patients may fracture a hip as a result of falling. However, it is not uncommon for an elderly patient to sustain a fracture of the femoral neck while walking and subsequently fall.

Selective Physical Examination (Look for Both Cause and Consequence of the Fall.)

VITALS	Repeat now. Only supine BP and HR are necessary, providing both supine and standing measurements were already taken.
HEENT	Tongue or cheek lacerations (seizure) Hemotympanum (basal skull fracture)
CVS	Pulse rate and rhythm (dysrhythmia) Decreased JVP (volume depletion)
MSS	Palpate skull and face Palpate spine and ribs } Fractures, hematomas, lacerations Passive ROM of all four limbs
NEURO	Complete neurological examination. Pay particular attention to the level of consciousness and to any asymmetric neurological findings. New findings of asymmetry suggest structural brain disease.

Selective Chart Review (Search for the cause of the fall.)
1. **What was the reason for admission?**
2. **Is there a past history of cardiac dysrhythmia, seizure disorder, autonomic neuropathy, disorientation at night, or diabetes mellitus?**
3. **What drugs is the patient receiving?**

- Antihypertensives
- Diuretics (volume depletion)
- Antidysrhythmics
- Antiepileptics
- Narcotics
- Sedatives, tranquilizers
- Antidepressants
- Insulin, oral hypoglycemics

4. **Check the most recent laboratory results.**
   - Glucose ⎫
   - Na   ⎬ ↑ or ↓ may cause confusion.
   - ↑ K can cause AV blocks; ↓ K can cause weakness or tachy-dysrhythmias.
   - ↑ Ca causes confusion; ↓ Ca may cause seizures.
   - Urea, creatinine (uremia can result in confusion and sei-zures.)
   - Antiepileptic drug concentrations (subtherapeutic concen-trations may result in seizure breakthrough; toxic concen-trations may be associated with ataxia).

Management

Provisional Diagnosis.   Establish the reason for the fall (pro-visional diagnosis). The etiology is often multifactorial. For ex-ample, diuretic-induced nocturia forces an elderly patient, under the influence of nighttime sedation, to struggle to the bathroom in an unfamiliar, dimly lit hospital room.

Complications.   Are there any complications resulting from the fall, giving rise to a second diagnosis? For example, the stroke victim may have unknowingly dislocated or subluxated his or her shoulder on the paralyzed side during the fall. The anticoagulated patient may develop a serious, delayed hemorrhage at any site of trauma. Reexamine these patients frequently.

Treat the Cause.   Investigate and treat the suspected cause. A fall is a symptom, not a diagnosis!

Reversible Factors.   Reversible factors must be corrected, es-pecially volume depletion and inappropriate drug therapy in the elderly.

Nocturia.   The majority of elderly patients who fall-out-of-bed at night are on their way to the bathroom because of nocturia. Make sure the nocturia is not iatrogenic (e.g., an evening diuretic order or an unnecessary IV)!

Elderly Patient.   If the patient is disoriented at night, ensure that the call bell is easily accessible, a night light is left on, and the evening's fluid intake is limited. The use of side rails has been shown consistently to increase morbidity. It is best to leave the side rails down or lower the mattress to the floor.

12

FEVER

It is unusual to spend an entire night on call without being phoned about a febrile patient. The majority of fevers seen in hospitalized patients are due to infections. Locating the source of a fever usually requires some detective work. Whether the cause of the fever needs specific immediate treatment will depend both on the clinical status of the patient and on the suspected diagnosis.

PHONE CALL

Questions

1 **How high is the temperature and by what route was it taken? (37°C oral = 37.5°C rectal or 36.5°C axillary)**
2 **What are the other vital signs?**
3 **Are there any associated symptoms?**
4 **Is this a "new" fever?**
5 **What was the reason for admission?**
6 **Is this a postoperative patient?**

Fever occurring 24 to 48 hours after an operation is often due to atelectasis, fever occurring 5 days after an operation is often due to pneumonia, and fever occurring 10 days after an operation may be due to pulmonary embolism. Wound infection may result in fever as early as 24 to 48 hours postoperatively.

Orders

1. If febrile and hypotensive, give IV 500 ml NS as rapidly as possible.
2. If febrile with meningitis symptoms (headache, seizure, or change in sensorium), order an LP tray to the bedside now.

Inform RN

"Will arrive at bedside in . . . minutes."

An elevated temperature alone is seldom life threatening. However, fever in association with hypotension or meningitis symptoms requires you to see the patient immediately.

ELEVATOR THOUGHTS (What causes fever?)

1. *Infection* is by far the most common cause of fever in the hospitalized patient. Common sites of infection are the lung and urinary tract. Less common sites include skin (IV sites, surgical wounds), CNS, abdomen, and pelvis.

The *immunocompromised patient* is not only predisposed to infection but also more susceptible to serious complications of infection.

2. Pulmonary embolism
3. Drug-induced fever
4. Neoplasm
5. Connective tissue diseases
6. Postoperative atelectasis.

MAJOR THREAT TO LIFE

- Septic shock
- Meningitis

Fever is most commonly a manifestation of infection in the hospitalized patient. Most infections can be brought under control by a combination of the body's natural defense mechanisms and judicious antibiotic use. Infection at any site, if progressive, may lead to septicemia with attendant *septic shock. Meningitis,* by virtue of its location, can result in permanent neurological deficit or death if allowed to go untreated.

BEDSIDE
Quick Look Test

Does the patient look well (comfortable), sick (uncomfortable or distressed), or critical (about to die)?

Toxic signs, such as apprehension, agitation, or lethargy, suggest serious infection.

Airway and Vital Signs

What is the heart rate?

Tachycardia, proportionate to the temperature elevation, is an expected finding in the febrile patient. Normally, the heart rate rises by 16 beats/min for each degree Celsius of temperature rise. A relative bradycardia in the febrile patient has been observed in *Legionella* pneumonia, *Mycoplasma pneumoniae* pneumonia, ascending cholangitis, typhoid fever, and *Plasmodium falciparum* malaria with profound hemolysis.

What is the blood pressure?

Fever in association with supine or postural hypotension indicates relative hypovolemia and can be the forerunner of septic shock. Ensure that an IV is in place. Infuse NS or Ringer's lactate to correct the intravascular volume deficit.

Selective Physical Examination I

What is the volume status? Is the patient in septic shock? Are there signs of meningitis?

VITALS	Repeat now
HEENT	Photophobia, neck stiffness
CVS	Pulse volume, JVP, skin temperature and color
NEURO	Change in sensorium
SPECIAL MANEUVERS	*Brudzinski's sign:* With the patient supine, passively flex the neck forward. Flexion of the patient's hips and knees in response to this maneuver constitutes a positive test result (see Fig. 11–3a).
	Kernig's sign: With the patient supine, flex one hip and knee to 90 degrees, then straighten the knee. Pain or resistance in the ipsilateral hamstrings constitutes a positive test result (see Fig. 11–3b).

Septic shock is a clinical diagnosis consisting of two stages. Serious delays in treatment are made through failure to recognize the first stage. Early in the development of septic shock, the patient may be warm, dry, and flushed because of peripheral vasodilation and increased cardiac output (warm shock). As septic shock progresses, the patient becomes hypotensive, and the skin becomes cool and clammy (cold shock) as a result of peripheral vasoconstriction.

Fever in the elderly patient, regardless of cause, can produce changes in sensorium ranging from lethargy to agitation. If a specific site of infection is not obvious, an LP should be performed to rule out meningitis (see p. 85).

Management I

What immediate measures need to be taken to prevent septic shock or to recognize meningitis?

Septic Shock. If the patient is febrile and hypotensive, determine the volume status and give IV fluids (NS or Ringer's lactate) promptly until the volume status returns to normal. Aggressive volume repletion in a patient with a history of CHF may compromise cardiac function. Do not overshoot the mark!

While IV fluid resuscitation is taking place, obtain samples for necessary cultures, usually including blood from two different sites, urine (for gram stain and culture), and any other potentially infected body fluid.

Septic shock is a major threat to life, and once culture samples are taken, antibiotics must be given to cover both gram-positive and gram-negative organisms. A common, empiric broad-spectrum regimen includes a cephalosporin and an aminoglycoside, e.g., *cefazolin* (Ancef) 1 to 2 g IV q8h and *gentamicin* 2 to 3 mg/kg IV as a loading dose. Further maintenance doses of gentamicin should be 1.5 to 1.7 mg/kg IV given at an interval that is adjusted for creatinine clearance.

Some patients are allergic to penicillin. Ensure that the patient is *not* allergic before ordering penicillin or cephalosporin.

Aminoglycosides are common causes of nephrotoxicity and oto-toxicity. Select maintenance dosing intervals according to the patient's calculated CrCl (see Appendix, pp. 339 and 340). Follow the serum aminoglycoside concentrations, usually after the third or fourth dose, and the serum creatinine concentration.

If the volume status is normal and the patient is still hypotensive, transfer to the ICU/CCU for inotropic or vasopressor support. (Refer to Chapter 18 for further discussion of septic shock.)

A Foley catheter should be placed in a patient with septic shock to monitor urine output.

Meningitis. Fever plus headache, seizure, stiff neck, or change in sensorium is meningitis until proved otherwise.

Ideally, an LP should be performed without delay to confirm the diagnosis and guide antimicrobial therapy. If, on fundoscopic examination, there is no evidence of raised intracranial pressure (see Fig. 14–2) and if a CT scan of the head is not immediately available, perform an LP without delay. (An exception here is the patient with a severe coagulopathy, in whom the risk of intrathecal hematoma formation may result in cord compression.)

If you are unable to visualize the fundi or if there is papilledema or focal neurological signs (suggesting a mass lesion), give the first dose of antibiotics and arrange for an urgent CT scan of the head to exclude a space-occupying lesion before performing the LP. An LP done in the presence of an intracranial space-occupying lesion can result in uncal herniation and brainstem compression (coning).

Selective Chart Review

If the patient is not in septic shock and does not have symptoms or signs of meningitis, perform a selective chart review—looking for *localizing clues* (Table 12–1). Also check the chart for the following.

- Temperature pattern during hospital stay
- Recent WBC count and differential, CD4 lymphocyte count
- Evidence of immunodeficiency, e.g., cancer chemotherapy, hematological malignancy, HIV infection
- Allergies to antibiotics
- Other possible reasons for fever, e.g., connective tissue disease, neoplasm
- Antipyretics, antibiotics, or steroids that may modify the fever pattern

Selective Physical Examination II

Confirm localizing symptoms or signs already documented in chart review.

Table 12–1 □ SELECTIVE CHART REVIEW—LOOKING FOR LOCALIZING CLUES

Localizing Clues	Diagnostic Considerations	Comments
Recent surgery	Atelectasis	Postoperative fever due to atelectasis is a diagnosis to be made after exclusion of infection
	Pneumonia	Characteristically occurs 5 days postoperatively
	Pulmonary embolism	Characteristically occurs 7–10 days postoperatively
	Infected surgical wound, biopsy site, or deeper infection of biopsy organ	Despite modern surgical techniques, *any* incision or puncture site may serve as a portal for bacteria
Blood transfusion	Transfusion reaction	See Chapter 27
Headache, seizure, stiff neck, changes in sensorium	Meningitis Intracranial abscess Encephalitis	Delirium tremens can mimic meningitis in some patients; is the patient withdrawing from alcohol?
Sinus discomfort	Sinusitis	
Dental caries, toothache	Periodontal abscess	
Sore throat	Pharyngitis Tonsillitis	
Dysphagia	Retropharyngeal abscess Epiglottitis	Either of these diagnoses is a medical emergency; consult ENT or anesthesia immediately
SOB, cough, or chest pain	Pneumonia Lung abscess Pulmonary embolus	
Murmur, CHF, or peripheral embolic lesions	Infective endocarditis	
Pleuritic chest pain	Pneumonia Empyema Pulmonary embolus Pericarditis	

Table 12–1 □ SELECTIVE CHART REVIEW—LOOKING FOR LOCALIZING CLUES—*Continued*

Localizing Clues	Diagnostic Considerations	Comments
Costovertebral angle (CVA) tenderness	Pyelonephritis Perinephric abscess	
Foley catheter, dysuria, hematuria, or pyuria	Cystitis Pyelonephritis	Condom catheters and Foley catheters predispose patients to urinary tract infections
Abdominal pain		If there are peritoneal signs, consider surgical consultation
RUQ	Subphrenic abscess Hepatic abscess Hepatitis RLL pneumonia Ascending cholangitis	Does the patient have Charcot's triad (fever + RUQ pain + jaundice)? If so, consider surgical consultation
RLQ	Crohn's disease Appendicitis Salpingitis	
LUQ	Splenic abscess Infected pancreatic pseudocyst LLL pneumonia	
LLQ	Diverticular abscess Salpingitis	
Ascites	Peritonitis	Perform abdominal paracentesis to exclude spontaneous bacterial peritonitis in any ascitic patient who becomes unwell
Diarrhea	Enteritis Colitis	
Swollen red tender joint	Septic arthritis Gout or pseudogout	A monoarticular effusion *must be* tapped to exclude infection

Continued.

Table 12–1 □ SELECTIVE CHART REVIEW—LOOKING FOR LOCALIZING CLUES—*Continued*

Localizing Clues	Diagnostic Considerations	Comments
Prosthetic joint	Infected prosthesis	
Vaginal discharge	Endometritis	
	Salpingitis	
Red or tender IV site	Septic phlebitis	
TPN line	Catheter sepsis	Fever may be the only symptom

VITALS	Repeat now	
HEENT	Fundi—papilledema (intracranial abscess), Roth's spots (infective endocarditis) (Fig. 12–1).	
	Conjunctival or scleral petechiae (infective endocarditis)	
	Ears—red tympanic membranes (otitis media, a complication of the intubated patient)	
	Sinuses—tenderness, inability to transilluminate (sinusitis)	
	Oral cavity—dental caries, tender tooth on tongue blade percussion (periodontal abscess)	
	Pharynx—erythema, pharyngeal exudate (pharyngitis, thrush)	
	Neck—stiff (meningitis)	
RESP	Crackles, friction rub, signs of consolidation (pneumonia, pulmonary embolism)	
CVS	New murmurs (infective endocarditis)	
ABD	Localized tenderness (see p. 28)	
RECTAL	Tenderness or mass (rectal abscess)	
MSS	Joint erythema or effusion (septic arthritis)	
SKIN	Decubitus ulcers (cellulitis)	
	Osler's nodes and Janeway's lesions	
	Petechiae (infective endocarditis)	
	IV sites (phlebitis, cellulitis)	

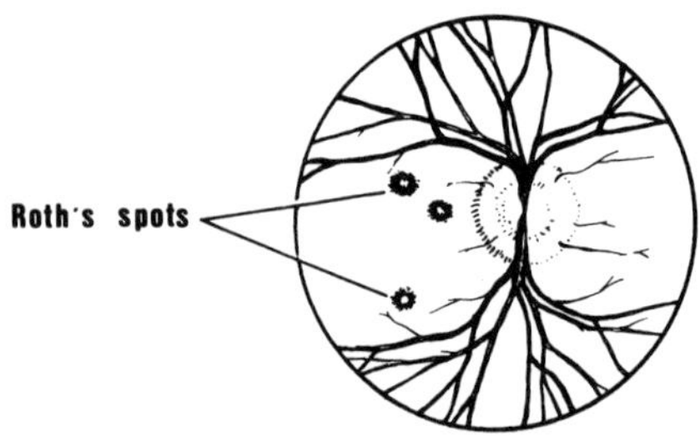

Figure 12–1 □ Roth's spots. Round or oval hemorrhagic retinal lesions with central pallor.

All surgical wounds *must* be examined (that means taking the dressings off)

PELVIC A pelvic examination should be done if a pelvic source of fever is possible

Management II

Any patient with an unexplained oral temperature >38.5°C that has developed in hospital should have the following.

- Blood cultures immediately from two different sites
- Urinalysis (routine and microscopic) and urine culture (immediately)
- WBC count and differential

Other more *selective tests* depend on the *localizing clues* you have been able to elicit with your chart review, history, and physical examination.

- Throat swab for Gram's stain and culture
- Sputum for Gram's stain and culture
- CXR
- LP
- Blood culture for infective endocarditis (refer to your institution's protocol)
- Cervical culture (also obtain specific medium for gonococcal isolation before performing the pelvic examination)
- Joint aspiration
- Swab decubitus ulcers or infected/draining wounds for Gram's stain and culture (aerobic and anaerobic)
- Retrograde milking of IV sites for purulent exudate for Gram's stain and culture

Fluid from any source should be examined microscopically immediately to help in your choice of antibiotics.

Remove *suspected IVs* and replace if necessary at a new site. Central TPN lines that may be infected should be replaced in consultation with your resident or TPN service. Catheter tips should be sent to the laboratory for culture.

Remove a Foley catheter in a patient suspected of having *urinary tract infection*. A few days of incontinence in the patient is an annoyance for the nursing staff but will not harm the patient if there is no perineal skin breakdown. An exception to this occurs when a Foley catheter is placed to treat urinary retention, since urinary stasis predisposes the patient to infection.

In regard to* antibiotic selection, *which patient needs* broad-spectrum antibiotics *now?

1. The patient with *fever and hypotension* requires broad-spectrum antibiotics (see p. 84).
2. The patient (e.g., on chemotherapy) with *fever and neutropenia* (<1000/mm³), or the patient with acute leukemia may not have enough functioning WBCs to produce the localizing

signs seen in an immunocompetent host. A minimum workup includes the following.

- Blood cultures
- Urinalysis and urine culture
- Sputum for Gram's stain and culture
- CXR

Anticipate this event in the immunocompromised patient and agree on an appropriate broad-spectrum antibiotic regimen with the hematologist or oncologist well ahead of time. Your institution may have special protocols to follow.

3. A patient who is febrile, appears toxic and acutely ill, and is suspected of having an infection despite no evidence of a clear-cut source also should receive broad-spectrum antibiotics.

Which patient needs specific antibiotics now?

1. The patient with *fever and meningitis symptoms* requires antibiotics immediately after the LP is done. However, do not delay initial antibiotic treatment if a CT scan of the head must be done before the LP (see p. 85).
2. The patient with *fever and a clear localizing clue* should be given specific antibiotics following procurement of culture specimens. Antibiotic therapy should be considered an urgent requirement in the diabetic patient.

Which patient needs no antibiotics until a specific microbiological diagnosis is made?

1. A patient who does not look sick or critical, who is immunologically competent, and in whom the source of fever is not readily apparent (e.g., a patient admitted for workup of FUO).
2. Low-grade fever (<38.5°C) in a patient who does not look sick.

Which antibiotic should you choose?

The common infecting organisms change much more slowly than the antibiotics synthesized to inhibit them. Specific antibiotic choices depend on knowledge of your hospital's local microbial flora and their antibiotic sensitivities. Current guidelines may be found in Appendix, pp. 362 and 363).

What about fever in the HIV-positive patient?

Patients with HIV disease may have a fever as a direct effect of HIV infection, as a result of opportunistic infections, or as a result of a variety of malignancies. In the HIV-positive patient, one should assume that fever is due to infection until proven otherwise. Although HIV patients are susceptible to any of the common conditions, a number of opportunistic pathogens should be considered. The organ system involved in such a patient may suggest the offending organism (see Table 12–2). More than in any other common condition, multiple infections are often present at the same time in the HIV-positive patient.

Table 12–2 □ COMMON INFECTING ORGANISMS RESPONSIBLE FOR FEVER IN PATIENTS WITH HIV DISEASE, ACCORDING TO ORGAN SYSTEM INVOLVED

Organ System	Organism	Diagnostic Test
Lungs (cough, SOB)	*Pneumocystis carinii*	Induced sputum or bronchoscopy specimens for toluidine blue or silver stain
	Bacteria (pneumococcus, *Haemophilus influenzae, Staphylococcus aureus*)	Sputum culture and Gram's stain, blood cultures
	Mycobacterium (M. tuberculosis, M. avium-intracellulare)	Sputum smears for AFB × 3; sputum and blood for culture
	Occasionally fungi (cryptococcosis, histoplasmosis, aspergillosis)	Sputum and blood for fungal culture
	Occasionally CMV	Diagnosis difficult without lung biopsy, which is rarely indicated. CMV is often recovered on bronchoscopy specimens, but does not indicate CMV pneumonia
CNS (meningitis)	*Cryptococcus neoformans*	Serum cryptococcal antigen; CSF: cryptococcal antigen, India ink stain, fungal culture
	Bacteria (pneumococcus, meningococcus, *Listeria*)	CSF Gram's stain, culture, and bacterial antigens
	Mycobacterium (M. tuberculosis)	CSF smears and culture for TB
	Treponema pallidum (syphilis)	Serum and CSF VDRL, serum MHA-TP or FTA-ABS
	HIV	By exclusion

Continued.

Table 12–2 □ COMMON INFECTING ORGANISMS RESPONSIBLE FOR FEVER IN PATIENTS WITH HIV DISEASE, ACCORDING TO ORGAN SYSTEM INVOLVED—*Continued*

Organ System	Organism	Diagnostic Test
CNS (mass lesion)	*Toxoplasma gondii*	CT scan head (with contrast); serum serology (IgG ± IgM) usually positive but not diagnostic—if serology negative, argues against diagnosis. Brain biopsy may be required if no response to empiric treatment
	Occasional tuberculoma, cryptococcoma, histoplasmoma	Brain biopsy
CNS (diffuse disease)	JC virus (progressive multifocal leukoencephalopathy)	CT scan head ± brain biopsy
	Herpes simplex encephalitis	CT scan head ± brain biopsy
	CMV encephalitis	CT scan head ± brain biopsy
	HIV dementia complex	Clinical diagnosis plus exclusion of other causes
GI tract		
Esophagitis (dysphagia, odynophagia)	*Candida albicans*	Empiric antifungal treatment (ketoconazole or fluconazole)—if no response, endoscopy brushings and biopsy; smears/cultures
	CMV	Endoscopy for biopsy and viral culture
	Herpes simplex	Endoscopy for biopsy and viral culture
Diarrhea	Bacteria *(Salmonella, Shigella, Campylobacter, Yersinia, Clostridium difficile)*	Stool culture for bacterial pathogens, stool toxin assay and culture for *C. difficile*
	Parasites *(Giardia, Entamoeba histolytica, Cryptosporidium, Isospora belli)*	Stools for ova and parasites × 3; stools for cryptosporidia (modified AFB smear or fluorescent stain)

Table 12–2 □ COMMON INFECTING ORGANISMS RESPONSIBLE FOR FEVER IN PATIENTS WITH HIV DISEASE, ACCORDING TO ORGAN SYSTEM INVOLVED—*Continued*

Organ System	Organism	Diagnostic Test
	CMV	Sigmoidoscopy ± colonoscopy and biopsy
	M. avium-intracellulare	Stool smear for AFB, culture, ± endoscopy and biopsy, blood cultures for mycobacteria
Disseminated Infection	*Mycobacterium (M avium-intracellulare, M. tuberculosis)*	Blood, sputum, urine, stool for smears and mycobacterial culture
	CMV	Blood (buffy coat) and urine viral cultures; ± biopsies
	Cryptococcosis	Blood, CSF, and urine fungal cultures; serum and CSF for cryptococcal antigen
	Histoplasmosis	Blood, sputum, and bone marrow biopsy for fungal culture; buffy coat smear for yeast forms in WBCs
	Herpes zoster	Tzanck smear, viral culture of skin lesions
	Coccidioidomycosis	Sputum, blood, and CSF for fungal culture; serology
	Bacillary angiomatosis	Biopsy of skin lesion

REMEMBER

1. The immunocomprised patient is especially susceptible to infection and liable to complications. You should not hesitate to call for the help of your resident or attending physician.
2. The definition of FUO is a temperature >38.3°C for 3 weeks with no cause found despite thorough in-hospital investigation for 1 week.
3. Fever due to neoplasm, connective tissue disorder, or drug reaction is a diagnosis to be made *after* exclusion of fever due to infection.
4. Drug-induced fever is uncommon and usually occurs within 7 days of beginning the offending drug.
5. Treating a fever with antipyretics is only treating a symptom. It is useful to observe the fever pattern, and if the patient is

not uncomfortable, it is not necessary to treat with aspirin or acetaminophen.

6. If antipyretics are ordered, ask the RN to indicate with an arrow the time of administration on the bedside temperature chart. In addition, assessment of therapeutic response is made easier by charting the antibiotics given as well (Fig. 12–2).

7. Steroids may elevate the WBC count and suppress fever response regardless of the cause. Defervescence with steroids should be interpreted cautiously.

8. Microorganisms love foreign bodies. Look for foreign bodies as sites of infection—IVs, Foley catheters, VP shunts, prosthetic joints, peritoneal dialysis catheters, and porcine or mechanical heart valves.

9. Fever occurring while the patient is already on antibiotics may mean the following.
   a. You are not giving the right dose.
   b. You are not treating the right organism, or resistance or superinfection has developed.
   c. The antibiotic is not getting to the right place (e.g., thick-walled abscess).
   d. The fever may not be due to an infection.

10. Delirium tremens is a serious cause of fever occasionally seen in patients withdrawing from alcohol. It is associated with confusion, including delusions and hallucinations, agitation,

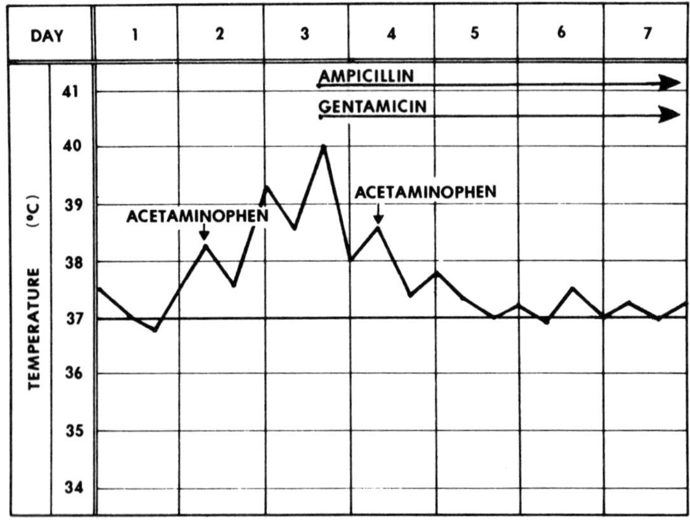

Figure 12–2 □ Bedside temperature chart.

seizures, and signs of autonomic hyperactivity, including fever, tachycardia, and sweating. This condition is often fatal and requires high doses of benzodiazepines to stabilize the patient (see p. 57).

13

GASTROINTESTINAL BLEEDING

GI bleeding is common in hospitalized patients. Whether the bleeding is from minor gastric stress ulceration or from life-threatening exsanguination of aortoduodenal fistula, the initial principles of assessment and management are the same.

PHONE CALL
Questions

1. **Clarify the situation. Is the blood old or new and from where is it coming?**
   Vomiting of bright red blood or "coffee grounds" and most cases of melena indicate an upper GI bleed. Bright red blood passed rectally usually indicates a lower GI bleed.
2. **How much blood has been lost?**
3. **What are the vital signs?**
   This information helps determine the urgency of the situation.
4. **What was the admitting diagnosis?**
   Recurrent bleeding from duodenal ulcer or esophageal varices carries a high mortality rate.
5. **Is the patient receiving anticoagulants (heparin, warfarin) or thrombolytic therapy (streptokinase, tissue plasminogen activator)?**
   Anticoagulants or thrombolytic agents may require immediate discontinuation or reversal in an actively bleeding patient.

Orders

1. Large-bore IV (size 16 if possible) immediately, if not already in place. IV access is a priority in the bleeding patient.
2. Hb stat. *Caution:* The Hb level may be normal during an acute bleed and drops only with correction of the intravascular volume by a shift of fluid from the extravascular space.
3. Crossmatch: Is there blood on hold? If not, order stat crossmatch of 2, 4, or 6 units of packed RBCs, depending on your estimate of blood loss.
4. If the admitting diagnosis is bleeding esophageal varices and the patient is hypotensive, order a Minnesota (Sengstaken-Blakemore) tube to be at the bedside immediately. If not familiar with the use of this tube, call your resident for assistance now. Also, commence an IV *vasopressin* infusion (0.4 units/ml) if not contraindicated (unstable angina or arrhythmias).
5. Ask the RN to take the patient's chart to the bedside.

Inform RN

"Will arrive at bedside in . . . minutes."

Hypotension or tachycardia requires you to see the patient immediately.

ELEVATOR THOUGHTS (What causes GI bleeding?)

Upper GI Bleed
1. Esophagitis
2. Esophageal varices
3. Mallory-Weiss syndrome (tear)
4. Gastric ulcer, gastritis
5. Duodenal ulcer, duodenitis
6. Neoplasm (esophageal Ca, gastric Ca)

Lower GI Bleed
1. Neoplasm
2. Angiodysplasia
3. Diverticulosis
4. Colitis (ulcerative, ischemic, infectious)
5. Mesenteric thrombosis
6. Meckel's diverticulum
7. Hemorrhoids

GI bleeding in the HIV-positive patient may result from any of the conditions listed, which are unrelated to the HIV-positive state. However, additional etiologies should be considered—upper GI bleeding may result from Kaposi's sarcoma, gastric lymphoma, CMV infection of the esophagus or duodenum, or herpes simplex infection of the esophagus. Lower GI bleeding also may result from Kaposi's sarcoma or from colitis caused by CMV, bacterial pathogens (including atypical mycobacteria), or herpes simplex.

MAJOR THREAT TO LIFE

- Hypovolemic shock

The major concern with GI bleeding is the progressive loss of intravascular volume in the patient whose bleeding lesion is not identified and managed correctly. If allowed to progress, even minor intermittent or continuous bleeding eventually may result in hypovolemic shock, with hypoperfusion of vital organs.

Initially, lost blood volume may be corrected by infusion of NS or Ringer's lactate, but if bleeding continues, replacement of lost RBCs will also be required in the form of packed RBC transfusion. Hence, your initial assessment should be directed toward determining the patient's volume status to ascertain whether a significant amount of intravascular volume has been lost.

BEDSIDE
Quick Look Test

Does the patient look well (comfortable), sick (uncomfortable or distressed), or critical (about to die?)

The patient in hypovolemic shock due to blood loss appears pale and apprehensive and may have other symptoms and signs, including cold and clammy skin, due to stimulation of the sympathetic nervous system.

Airway and Vital Signs

Are there any postural changes in blood pressure or heart rate?

First check for changes with the patient in the lying and sitting (with legs dangling) positions. If there are no changes, the BP and HR should then be checked with the patient standing. A rise in heart rate > 15 beats/min, a fall in systolic BP > 15 mm Hg, or any fall in diastolic BP indicates significant hypovolemia. *Caution:* A resting tachycardia alone may indicate decreased intravascular volume. If the resting systolic BP is < 90 mm Hg, order a second large-bore IV immediately.

Selective Physical Examination I

What is the patient's volume status? Is the patient in shock?

VITALS	Repeat now
CVS	Pulse volume, JVP
	Skin temperature and color
NEURO	Mental status

Shock is a clinical diagnosis as follows: systolic BP < 90 mm Hg with evidence of inadequate tissue perfusion, e.g., skin (cold and clammy) and CNS (agitation or confusion). In fact, the kidney is a sensitive indicator of shock (i.e., urine output < 20 ml/h). The urine output of a patient who is hypovolemic ordinarily correlates with the renal blood flow, which, in turn, is dependent on cardiac output and is an extremely important measurement. However, placement of a Foley catheter should not take priority over resuscitation measures.

Management I

What immediate measures need to be taken to correct or prevent shock from occurring?

Replenish the intravascular volume by giving IV fluids. The best immediate choice is a crystalloid (NS or Ringer's lactate), which will at least temporarily stay in the intravascular space. Albumin or banked plasma can be given but is expensive, carries a risk of hepatitis, and is not readily available.

Blood has been lost from the intravascular space, and ideally blood is what needs to be replaced. If there is no blood on hold for the patient, a stat crossmatch will usually take 50 minutes. If blood is on hold, it should be available at the bedside in 30 minutes. In an emergency, O-negative blood may be given, though this practice is usually reserved for the acute trauma victim. Transfusion-associated hepatitis can be minimized by transfusing only when necessary. *Rule of thumb:* Maintain a Hb level of 90 to 100 g/L.

Order the appropriate IV rate, which will depend on the patient's volume status. *Shock* will require running IV fluid wide open through at least two large-bore IV sites. Elevating the IV bag, squeezing the IV bag, or using IV pressure cuffs may help increase the rate of delivery of the solution. *Moderate volume depletion* can be treated with 500 to 1000 ml of NS given as rapidly as possible, with serial measurements of volume status and assessment of cardiac status. If blood is not at the bedside within 30 minutes, delegate someone to find out why there is a delay.

Aggressive volume repletion in a patient with a history of CHF may compromise cardiac function. Do not overshoot the mark!

What can you do at this time to stop the source of bleeding?
Treat the underlying cause. Treating hypovolemia is treating a symptom.

Upper GI Bleed (Hematemesis and Most Cases of Melena). *Cimetidine* (Tagamet) 300 mg IV q6h (300 mg IV q12h in renal failure) or *ranitidine* (Zantac) 50 mg IV q8h (50 mg IV q12h in renal failure) will help promote healing in four of the six causes listed, i.e., all except Mallory-Weiss syndrome (tear) and esophageal varices. Studies have failed to show that H_2 blockers decrease the incidence of rebleeding while patients are in the hospital. Most specialists still would begin one until the specific site of bleeding is known. Antacids are contraindicated if endoscopy or surgery is anticipated. They obscure the field in endoscopy and increase the risk of aspiration in surgery.

Lower GI Bleed (Usually Bright Red Blood per Rectum and, Occasionally, Melena). No other treatment is immediately required until the specific site of bleeding is identified, but continue to monitor the volume status.

Abnormal Coagulation. If the PT or aPTT is prolonged or if the patient is thrombocytopenic, fresh frozen plasma (2 units) and platelet infusion (6 to 8 units), respectively, may be required. If the patient has recently received thrombolytic therapy, additional agents, such as *antagosan* (Trasylol), may be required but should be initiated only after consultation with your resident or attending physician.

Selective Chart Review

What was the reason for admission?

Has the cause of this GI bleed already been identified during this admission?

Is the patient on any medication that may worsen the situation?

NSAIDs	Counteract the protective effect of prostaglandins on gastric mucosa and may result in gastric erosions or peptic ulcers.
Steroids	Increased frequency of ulcer disease in patients on steroids. Most disease processes for which the patient is receiving steroids will not allow their immediate discontinuation.
Heparin	Prevents clot formation by enhancing the action of antithrombin III.
Warfarin	Prevents activation of vitamin K-dependent clotting factors.
Streptokinase	Converts free plasminogen to plasmin, which then causes lysis of fibrin.
Tissue Plasminogen Activator	Binds specifically to fibrin, becoming active, and then converts plasminogen to plasmin on the tissue surface.

Laboratory Data

- Most recent Hb value
- PT, aPTT, platelets. Are there any platelet or coagulation abnormalities that may predispose the patient to bleeding?
- Bleeding time (if a platelet disorder is suspected)
- Urea, creatinine levels. (Uremia prolongs bleeding time.) Remember, in prerenal failure, urea level may be more markedly elevated than creatinine level. This difference may be further accentuated in a GI bleed by absorption of urea from the breakdown of blood in the GI tract.

Selective Physical Examination II

Where is the site of bleeding?

VITALS	Repeat now
HEENT	Nosebleed
ABD	Epigastric tenderness (peptic ulcer disease)
	RLQ tenderness or mass (cecal cancer)
	LLQ tenderness (sigmoid cancer, diverticulitis, or ischemic colitis)
RECTAL	Bright red blood, melena, hemorrhoids, or mass (rectal cancer)

Also, look for signs of chronic liver disease (hepatosplenomegaly, ascites, parotid gland hypertrophy, spider angiomata, gynecomastia, palmar erythema, testicular atrophy, dilated abdominal veins), which may suggest the presence of esophageal varices.

Management II

Once hypovolemia is corrected, ongoing management includes maintaining adequate intravascular volume while trying to determine the specific site of bleeding.

What procedures are available to determine the site of bleeding?
- Esophagogastroduodenoscopy
- Tagged RBC scan
- Angiography
- Sigmoidoscopy
- Colonoscopy

In a patient with an *upper GI bleed* that has stopped and who is stable hemodynamically, elective endoscopy can be performed within the next 24 hours. Urgent endoscopy may be required if bleeding continues or the patient is hemodynamically unstable. Some conditions can be temporarily stabilized at the time of endoscopy, e.g., sclerosis for esophageal or gastric varices, electrocoagulation or epinephrine injection in ulcers with a visible vessel at the base.

Esophageal varices can be treated with sclerotherapy, an IV vasopressin infusion (100 units in 250 ml D5W beginning at a rate of 0.4 units/min = 60 ml/h), or a Minnesota (Sengstaken-Blakemore) tube (Fig. 13–1). In most cases, the presence of bleeding varices should be documented endoscopically before initiating any treatment. Sclerotherapy is the preferred emergency treatment, as vasopressin may precipitate angina or MI in the atherosclerotic patient. A Minnesota tube is a temporizing measure reserved for a life-threatening bleed.

Patients with *lower GI bleeds* who are hemodynamically stable should be scheduled for colonoscopy. If unstable, an urgent tagged RBC scan should be arranged and, if possible, be followed by angiography. Tagged RBC scans and mesenteric angiography are most sensitive if performed while there is still active bleeding but should not take priority over resuscitation measures.

When is early surgical consultation appropriate?
- Exsanguinating hemorrhage
- Continued bleeding with transfusion requirements > 5 units/ day
- A second bleed from an ulcer, requiring transfusion during the same hospital stay
- Ulcer with a visible vessel at the base on endoscopy

Order an ECG and cardiac enzyme tests if there are any risk factors for coronary artery disease. A hypotensive episode in a patient with atherosclerosis may result in myocardial infarction.

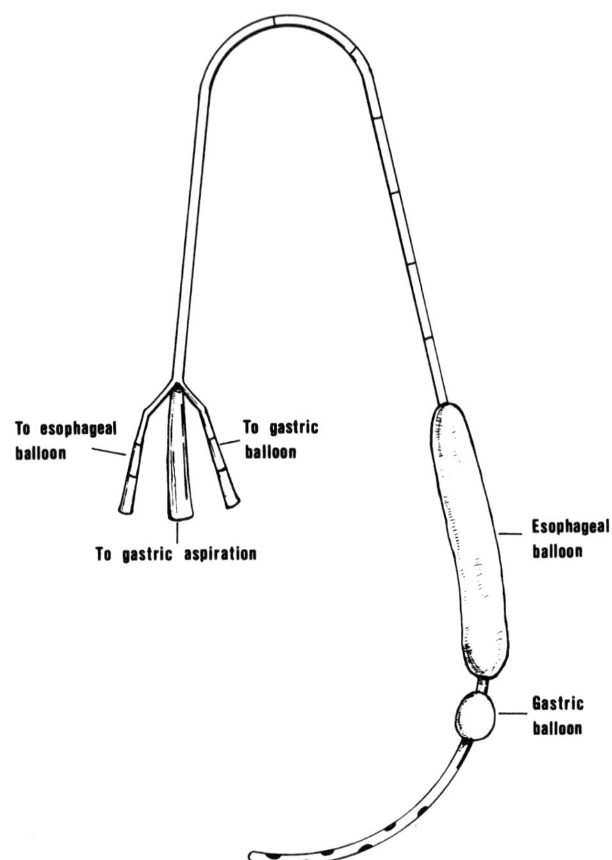

Figure 13–1 □ The Sengstaken-Blakemore tube. The Minnesota tube is similar; it has an additional port for esophageal aspiration.

REMEMBER

1. Keep the patient NPO for endoscopy or possible surgery.
2. Insertion of an NG tube to look for bright red blood may help identify an upper GI source of bleeding. However, negative NG returns do not rule out an upper GI bleed. Do not leave the NG tube in to monitor bleeding. The patient's volume status is the best indicator of further blood loss, and an NG tube may cause mucosal artifacts, hampering interpretation of endoscopic findings.
3. Bismuth compounds (e.g., Pepto-Bismol) and iron supplements can turn stools black. True melena is pitch black, sticky, and tarlike, with an odor that is hard to forget.

4. An aortoduodenal fistula can appear as a sentinel (minor) bleed that can be followed by rapid exsanguination. Consider this possibility in any patient with abdominal vascular surgery or in any patient with a midline abdominal scar who is unable to give a history.
5. Never attribute a GI bleed to hemorrhoids before thorough exclusion of other sources of bleeding.

14

HEADACHE

Patients in hospital often complain of headache. You must decide whether the headache is chronic and of no urgent concern or whether it is a symptom of more serious concern.

PHONE CALL
Questions

1 **How severe is the headache?**
Most headaches are mild and not of major concern unless associated with other symptoms.
2 **Was the onset sudden or gradual?**
The sudden onset of a severe headache is suggestive of a subarachnoid hemorrhage.
3 **What are the vital signs?**
4 **Has there been a change in the level of consciousness?**
5 **Is there a past history of chronic or recurrent headaches?**
6 **What was the reason for admission?**

Orders

1. Ask the RN to measure the patient's temperature if it has not been recorded within the past hour. Bacterial meningitis may present with only fever and headache.
2. If you are confident that the headache represents a chronic or previously diagnosed, recurrent problem, the patient can be given medication that has previously relieved the headache or a nonnarcotic analgesic agent (e.g., acetaminophen). Ask the RN to phone back in 2 hours if the headache has not been relieved by the medication.

Inform RN

"Will arrive at the bedside in . . . minutes."

Headaches associated with a fever, vomiting, or a decreased level of consciousness and severe headaches of acute onset require you to see the patient immediately. Assessment at the bedside of chronic recurrent headaches is necessary if the headache is more severe than usual or if the character of the pain is different. This assessment can wait an hour or two if other problems of higher priority exist.

ELEVATOR THOUGHTS (What causes headaches?)

Chronic (recurrent) Headaches
1. Muscle contraction

   a. Psychogenic—depression, anxiety, stress (tension headaches)
   b. Cervical osteoarthritis
   c. Temporomandibular joint disease
2. Vascular
   a. Migraine
   b. Cluster
3. Drugs
   a. Nitrates
   b. Calcium channel blockers
   c. NSAIDs

Acute Headaches
1. Infectious
   a. Meningitis
   b. Encephalitis
2. Posttrauma
   a. Concussion
   b. Cerebral contusion
   c. Subdural or epidural hematoma
3. Vascular
   a. Subarachnoid hemorrhage
   b. Intracerebral hemorrhage
4. Increased intracranial pressure
   a. Space-occupying lesions
   b. Malignant hypertension
   c. Benign intracranial hypertension
5. Local causes
   a. Temporal arteritis
   b. Acute angle-closure glaucoma

MAJOR THREAT TO LIFE

- Subarachnoid hemorrhage
- Bacterial meningitis
- Herniation (transtentorial, cerebellar, central)

Subarachnoid hemorrhage is associated with a very high mortality if left untreated. *Bacterial meningitis* must be recognized early if antibiotic treatment is to be successful. *Herniation* may occur as a result of a tumor, subdural or epidural hematoma, or any other mass lesion (Fig. 14–1).

BEDSIDE
Quick Look Test

Does the patient look well (comfortable), sick (uncomfortable or distressed), or critical (about to die)?

Most patients with chronic headaches look well. Those with severe migraines, subarachnoid hemorrhage, or meningitis look sick.

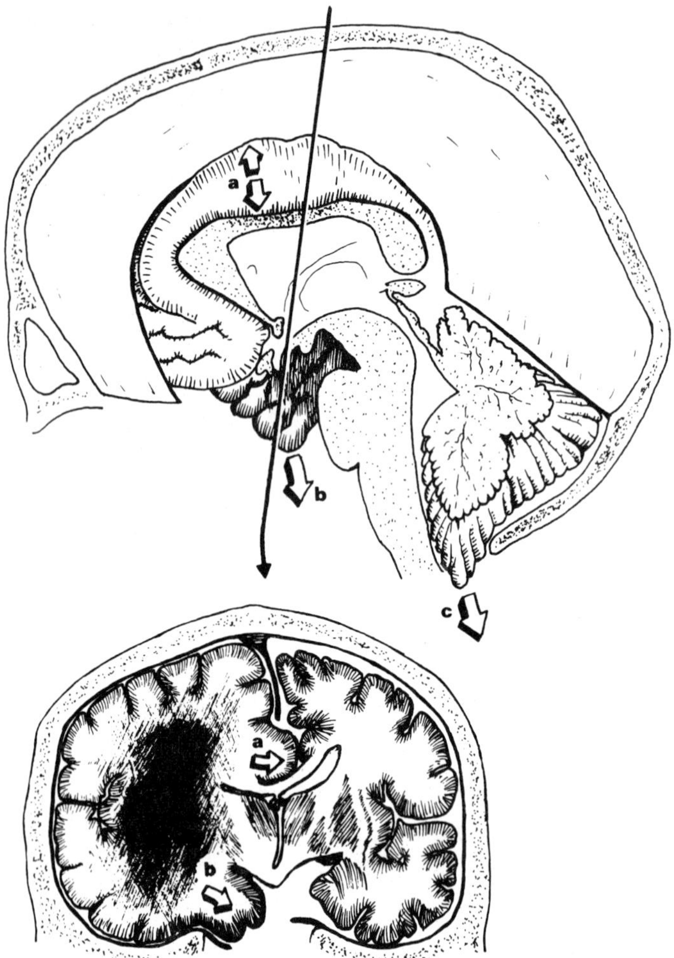

Figure 14–1 □ CNS herniation. *a.* Cingulate herniation. *b.* Uncal herniation. *c.* Cerebellar herniation.

Airway and Vital Signs

What is the temperature?
Fever associated with a headache requires you to decide soon whether an LP should be performed.

What is the BP?
Malignant hypertension (hypertension with papilledema) is usually associated with a systolic BP > 190 mm Hg and a diastolic

BP > 120 mm Hg. Headache usually is not a symptom of hypertension unless there has been a recent increase in pressure and the diastolic BP is > 120 mm Hg.

What is the HR?

Hypertension in association with bradycardia may be a manifestation of increasing intracranial pressure.

Selective Physical Examination I (Does the Patient Have Meningitis or Increased Intracranial Pressure?)

HEENT	Nuchal rigidity (meningitis or subarachnoid hemorrhage) Papilledema (increased intracranial pressure) See Figure 14–2 for the fundoscopic features of papilledema. An early sign of increased intracranial pressure is absence of venous pulsations.
NEURO	Mental status Pupil symmetry Asymmetrical pupils associated with a rapidly decreasing

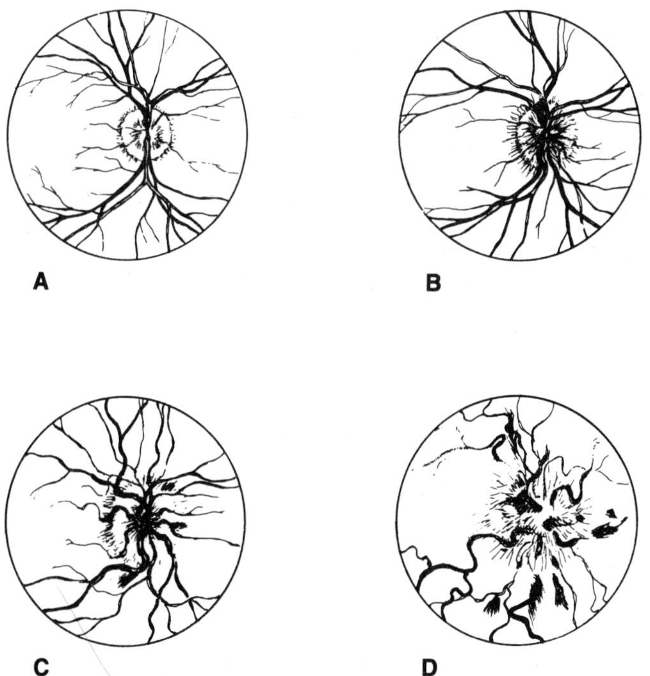

Figure 14–2 □ Disc changes seen in papilledema. **A.** Normal. **B.** Early papilledema. **C.** Moderate papilledema with early hemorrhage. **D.** Severe papilledema with extensive hemorrhage.

level of consciousness represent a life-threatening situation. Call neurosurgery immediately for assessment and treatment of probable uncal herniation.

Kernig's sign and Brudzinski's sign (meningitis or subarachnoid hemorrhage) (Fig. 14–3).

A full neurological examination is required, if there is nuchal rigidity, pupillary asymmetry, or papilledema.

Management I

If there is **nuchal rigidity** *without papilledema, order*
- Immediate CT scan of the head
- LP tray

Note the time. If bacterial meningitis is suspected, you should be able to complete the CT scan of the head followed by the LP with the patient receiving the first dose of antibiotics within 1 hour.

When bacterial meningitis is suspected but the CT scan of the head is not available within the hour, use one of two alternatives as follows: (1) perform an LP to be followed by IV antibiotics or (2) give appropriate, empiric IV antibiotics now (see subsequent discussion), performing an LP after the CT scan of the head is available.

If there is *nuchal rigidity with papilledema,* an LP is contraindicated because of the risk of brain herniation. Meningitis, a subdural empyema, and a brain abscess each can cause nuchal rigidity and papilledema. The CT scan of the head may help differentiate among the three. The empiric antibiotic coverage is as follows.

Bacterial Meningitis

Adult	Penicillin G 2 million units IV over 30 minutes q2h or 4 million units IV q4h
Immunosuppressed, alcoholic, or >60 years old	A third-generation cephalosporin that crosses the blood–brain barrier plus penicillin or ampicillin
Postcraniotomy, spinal trauma	Vancomycin 1 g IV q12–16h and ceftazidime 2 g IV q8h

Subdural Empyema and Brain Abscess

Secondary to frontoethmoid sinusitis, otitis media, mastoiditis, or lung abscess	Cloxacillin plus a third-generation cephalosporin plus metronidazole (60%–90% of subdural empyemas are caused by extension of a sinusitis or an otitis media)
Posttraumatic	Cloxacillin or nafcillin plus a third-generation cephalosporin

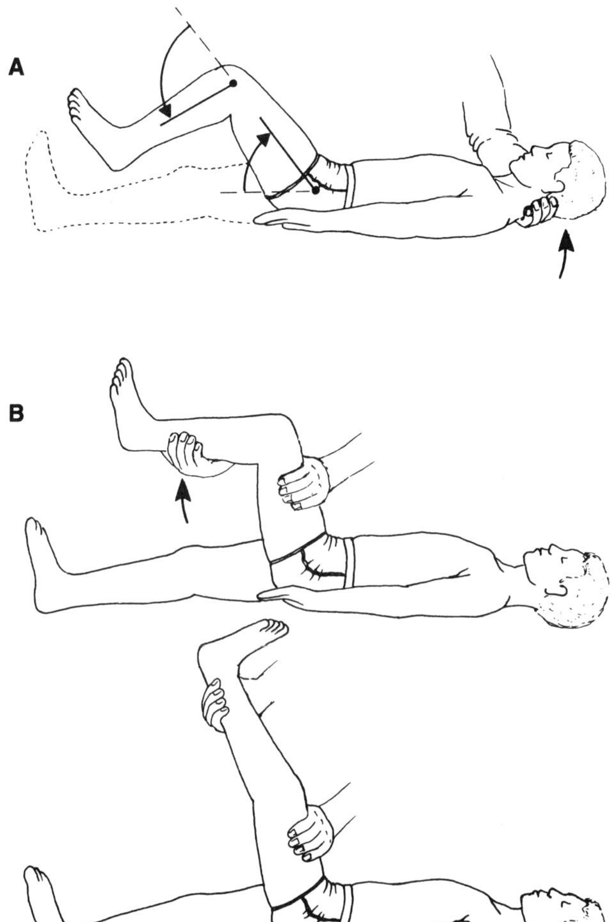

Figure 14–3 □ **A.** Brudzinski's sign. The test result is positive when the patient actively flexes his or her hips and knees in response to passive neck flexion by the examiner. **B.** Kernig's sign. The test result is positive when pain or resistance is elicited by passive knee extension, from the 90-degree hip/knee flexion position.

In addition to beginning antibiotics, a patient with a subdural empyema or a brain abscess should be referred for neurosurgical assessment. Also, prophylactic antiepileptic therapy should be administered routinely as follows: *phenytoin* (Dilantin) loading dose 18 mg/kg IV at a rate no faster than 25 to 50 mg/min IV followed by a maintenance dosage of 100 mg IV q8h or 300 mg PO daily. Steroid treatment or surgery or both may be required to relieve increased intracranial pressure due to cerebral edema.

Selective History and Chart Review

Was the onset of the headache sudden or insidious?
The abrupt onset of severe headache suggests a vascular cause, the most serious being subarachnoid or intracerebral hemorrhage.

How severe is the headache?
Most muscle contraction headaches are mild and not incapacitating. However, when migraine headaches are associated with severe pain, the patient may look sick.

Is the headache improved or worsened in the supine position?
Most muscle contraction headaches are improved by lying down. Headaches made worse by lying down suggest increasing intracranial pressure, and an intracranial mass should be considered.

Were there any prodromal symptoms?
Nausea and vomiting are associated with increased intracranial pressure but may also occur with migraine or angle-closure glaucoma. *Photophobia and neck stiffness* are associated with meningitis. The classic *visual aura* (scintillations, migratory scotomata, and blurred vision) that precedes a migraine headache is helpful in making the diagnosis, but the absence of an aura does not rule out migraine headache.

Is there a past history of chronic, recurring headaches?
Migraine and muscle contraction headaches follow a pattern. Ask the patient whether this headache is the same as their "usual headache." The patient will probably make the diagnosis for you!

Is there a history of recent head trauma?
An epidural hematoma may occur after even a relatively minor head injury, particularly in teenagers or young adults. Subdural hematomas can appear insidiously 6 to 8 weeks after seemingly minor trauma and are not uncommonly seen in the alcoholic patient.

Does the patient have joint disease in the neck or upper back?
Muscle contraction headaches in the elderly often are caused by cervical osteoarthritis. These headaches characteristically start in the neck region and radiate to the temple or forehead.

Does the patient have clicking or popping when opening or closing the jaw?

These symptoms are a clue to the presence of temporomandibular joint dysfunction. In addition, the pain may be located predominantly in the ear or face.

Has an ophthalmologist or another MD dilated the patient's pupils within the past 24 hours?
Acute angle-closure glaucoma can be precipitated by pupillary dilatation. The patient complains of a severe unilateral headache located over the brow and may experience nausea, vomiting, and abdominal pain.

Is there any decrease or loss in vision? Is there a history of jaw claudication?
Temporal arteritis is a systemic illness (fever, malaise, weight loss, anorexia, weakness, myalgia) seen in patients over 50 years of age. If this condition is suspected, order a stat ESR. Visual loss in temporal arteritis is a medical emergency and should be managed in consultation with a neurologist or rheumatologist (for treatment, see p. 113).

What drugs is the patient receiving?
Drugs such as nitrates, calcium entry blockers, and NSAIDs can cause headaches.

Selective Physical Examination II

VITALS	Repeat now
HEENT	Red eye (acute angle-closure glaucoma)
	Hemotympanum or blood in the ear canal (basal skull fracture)
	Tender, enlarged temporal arteries (temporal arteritis)
	Retinal hemorrhages (hypertension)
	Lid ptosis, dilated pupil, eye deviated down and out (posterior communicating cerebral artery aneurysm)
	Tenderness on palpation or failure of transillumination of the frontal and maxillary sinuses (sinusitis or subdural empyema)
	Inability to fully open the jaw (temporomandibular joint dysfunction)
	Cranial bruit (arteriovenous malformation)
NEURO	Complete neurological examination
	What is the level of consciousness?
	Drowsiness, yawning, and inattentiveness associated with headache all are ominous signs. In a patient with a small subarachnoid hemorrhage, these may be the only signs.
	Is there any asymmetry of pupils, visual fields, eye movements, limbs, tone, reflexes, or plantar responses? Asymmetry suggests structural brain disease. If this is a new finding, a CT scan of the head will be required.

MSS   Palpate skull and face looking for fractures, hematomas, and lacerations.
Evidence of recent head trauma suggests the possibility of a subdural or an epidural hematoma.

Management II

Muscle Contraction Headaches.   Chronic muscle contraction headaches may temporarily be treated with non-narcotic analgesics. These are the commonest types of headaches you will see in the hospital. A long-term treatment plan, if not already established, may be discussed in the morning.

Mild Migraine Headaches.   Mild migraine headaches can be treated adequately with aspirin or acetaminophen.

Severe Migraine Headaches.   Severe migraine headaches are best treated immediately during the prodromal stage, but it is unlikely you will be called until the headache is well established. Ask the patient what they usually take for their migraine headache. It will probably be the most effective agent you can prescribe immediately. A severe migraine often requires a narcotic analgesic agent, such as *codeine* 30 to 60 mg PO or IM q3–4h PRN or *meperidine* (Demerol) 50 to 100 mg IM q3–4h PRN.

Vasoconstrictors, such as *ergotamine* or *sumatriptan succinate* (Imitrex), are most effective if administered in the early prodromal stage of a migraine. However, such agents are contraindicated in uncontrolled hypertension, unstable coronary artery disease, coronary spasm, pregnancy, and in the presence of hemiplegic migraine.

Cluster Headaches.   Cluster headaches are difficult to treat. Most last less than 45 minutes, and oral treatment has minimal effect. If a cluster headache develops in hospital and is severe, a parenteral narcotic, such as *codeine* 30 to 60 mg IM or *meperidine* (Demerol) 50 to 100 mg IM may be tried. Alternatively, *dihydroergotamine* 0.75 mg IV now and repeat in 30 minutes may be effective.

Postconcussion Headaches.   Postconcussion headaches (provided subdural and epidural hemorrhages have been ruled out by physical examination or by a CT scan of the head) should be treated with an analgesic agent that is unlikely to cause sedation, e.g., acetaminophen or codeine. Aspirin is contraindicated in the posttrauma patient, since the inhibition of platelet aggregation may predispose the patient to bleeding complications.

Hemorrhages and Space-Occupying Lesions.   Patients with *subdural, epidural, and subarachnoid* hemorrhages and space-occupying lesions (brain abscess, tumor) causing raised intracranial pressure should be referred to a neurosurgeon as soon as possible.

Malignant Hypertension. Malignant hypertension (hypertension and papilledema) should be managed by careful reduction of BP (see Chapter 16, p. 140).

Benign Intracranial Hypertension. Benign intracranial hypertension (pseudotumor cerebri) is a syndrome of unknown etiology, with increased intracranial pressure (headache and papilledema) and no evidence of a mass lesion or hydrocephalus. Refer the patient to a neurologist in the morning for further investigation and management.

Temporal Arteritis.   Temporal arteritis should be treated immediately to prevent irreversible blindness. *Prednisone* 60 mg PO daily can be started immediately when this diagnosis is suspected and supported by an ESR of > 60 mm/h (Westergren's method). Confirmation by temporal artery biopsy should be arranged within the next 3 days.

Glaucoma.   A patient with *acute angle-closure glaucoma* should be referred to an ophthalmologist immediately.

15

HEART RATE AND RHYTHM DISORDERS

There are only three abnormalities in heart rate or rhythm that you will be called to assess at night—*too fast, too slow, and irregular.* Remember that the main purpose of one's heart rate is to keep cardiac output high enough to perfuse the following three vital organs: (1) the heart, (2) the brain, and (3) the kidney. Your task is to find out why the heart is beating too quickly, too slowly, or irregularly before it results in hypoperfusion of the patient's vital organs. Begin by asking whether the heart rate is too fast or too slow. (Rapid heart rates are discussed subsequently; slow heart rates are addressed on p. 128 of this chapter.) Next, decide whether the rhythm is regular or irregular.

■ RAPID HEART RATES
PHONE CALL
Questions

1 **What is the heart rate?**
2 **Is the rhythm regular or irregular?**
3 **Is this a new problem since admission?**
4 **What is the BP?**
   Remember that hypotension may be a *cause* of tachycardia (i.e., compensatory) or a *result* of tachycardia that does not allow adequate diastolic filling of the left ventricle to maintain BP.
5 **Is the patient having chest pain or SOB?**
   Dysrhythmias are common in patients with underlying coronary artery diseases. A rapid heart rate may be the result of angina or CHF or may precipitate angina or CHF in such a patient.
6 **What is the respiratory rate?**
   Any illness causing hypoxia may result in tachycardia.
7 **What is the temperature?**
   Tachycardia, proportional to the temperature elevation, is an expected finding in a febrile patient. However, you must still examine the patient to make sure there is no other cause for the rapid heart rate.

Orders

1. If the patient is experiencing tachycardia and *hypotension,* order a large-bore (size 16 if possible) IV immediately.
2. If the patient is having *chest pain,* ask the RN to put the cardiac arrest cart in the room and attach the patient to the ECG monitor.
3. Order a stat 12-lead ECG and rhythm strip.

Inform RN

"Will arrive at bedside in . . . minutes."

A rapid heart rate in association with chest pain (angina), shortness of breath (CHF), or hypotension requires you to see the patient immediately.

ELEVATOR THOUGHTS (What causes rapid heart rates?)

Rapid Irregular Heart Rate	Atrial fibrillation
	Atrial flutter with variable block
	Multifocal atrial tachycardia
	Sinus tachycardia with PACs
	Sinus tachycardia with PVCs
Rapid Regular Heart Rates	Sinus tachycardia
	Supraventricular tachycardia
	Atrial flutter
	AV nodal reentry
	WPW
	Ectopic atrial tachycardia
	Ventricular tachycardia

MAJOR THREAT TO LIFE

- *Hypotension*, leading to shock
- *Angina*, progressing to myocardial infarction
- *CHF*, leading to hypoxia

It is useful to recall the determinants of BP as expressed in the following two formulas:

$$\text{Blood pressure (BP)} = \text{cardiac output (CO)} \times \text{total peripheral resistance (TPR)}$$

$$\text{Cardiac output (CO)} = \text{heart rate (HR)} \times \text{stroke volume (SV)}$$

As evidenced by the first formula, any fall in CO will result in a fall in BP, unless it is accompanied by a compensatory increase in TPR. Although in most instances a rapid heart rate serves to increase CO, many of the rapid heart rates do not allow adequate time for diastolic filling of the ventricles, resulting in a low SV and, hence, a decreased CO. The low CO may result in *hypotension*, in *angina* in the patient with underlying coronary artery disease, or in *CHF* in the patient with inadequate left ventricular reserve.

BEDSIDE
Quick Look Test

Does the patient look well (comfortable), sick (uncomfortable or distressed), or critical (about to die)?

Patients with tachycardia severe enough to cause hypotension usually look sick or critical. However, a patient with supraventricular or ventricular tachycardia may look deceptively well if adequate BP is maintained.

Airway and Vital Signs

What is the HR? Is it regular or irregular?
Read the ECG and rhythm strip.

What is the BP?
If hypotensive (systolic BP < 90 mm Hg), you must decide the following quickly.

- Whether the tachycardia is a result of the hypotension (i.e., a compensatory tachycardia),

OR

- Whether the hypotension is a result of the tachycardia (i.e., inadequate diastolic filling leading to low CO with low BP). Three rapid heart rhythms occasionally can cause hypotension due to decreased diastolic filling, resulting in hypoperfusion of vital organs. These rhythms are atrial fibrillation with rapid ventricular response, supraventricular tachycardia, and ventricular tachycardia (Figs. 15–1, 15–2, and 15–3). If the patient is hypotensive, it is important to recognize these three rhythms immediately because prompt treatment is required to restore adequate cardiac output.

Management I

If the patient is *hypotensive* and has atrial fibrillation with rapid ventricular response, supraventricular tachycardia, or ventricular tachycardia, emergency cardioversion may be required.

- Ask the RN to call for your resident immediately.
- Ask the RN to bring the cardiac arrest cart into the room. Attach the patient to the ECG monitor.
- Give the patient 100% O_2 by mask (28% if COPD).
- Ask the RN to draw *diazepam* (Valium) 10 mg IV into a syringe.
- Ensure that an IV is in place.

If the patient is *hypotensive* and none of these three rhythms is present, the tachycardia is most likely *secondary* to hypotension. You must perform a selective physical examination to decide

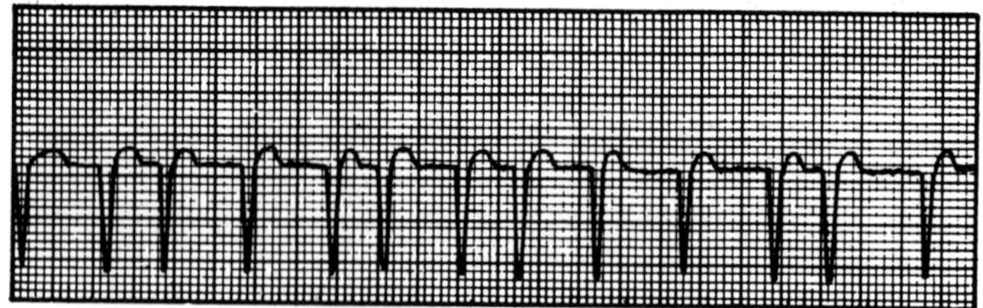

Figure 15–1 □ Atrial fibrillation with rapid ventricular response.

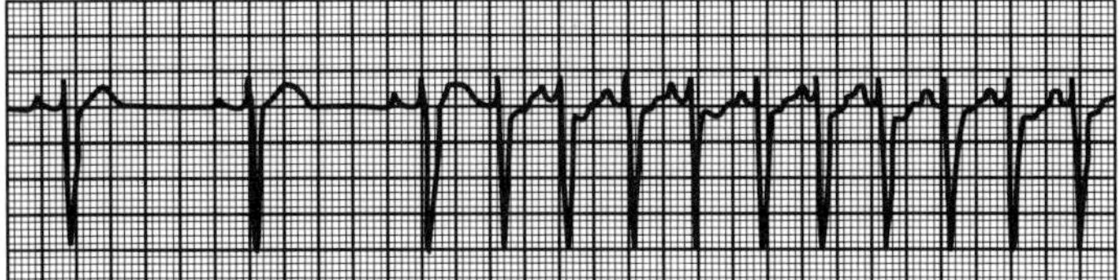

Figure 15–2 □ Supraventricular tachycardia.

which of the four major causes of hypotension is resulting in compensatory tachycardia: (1) cardiogenic causes, (2) hypovolemic causes, (3) sepsis, or (4) anaphylaxis. (Refer to Chapter 18 for investigation and management of hypotension.)

Fortunately, most of the patients you will see with rapid heart rates will not be hypotensive. In these cases, you may relax for a minute. Look at the ECG and rhythm strip and decide which rapid rhythm the patient is experiencing.

Rapid Irregular Rhythms
- Atrial fibrillation (Fig. 15–4)
- Atrial flutter with variable block (Fig. 15–4a)
- Multifocal atrial tachycardia (Fig. 15–5)
- Sinus tachycardia with PACs (Fig. 15–6)
- Sinus tachycardia with PVCs (Fig. 15–7)

Rapid Regular Rhythms
- Sinus tachycardia (Fig. 15–8)
- SVT: atrial flutter (Fig. 15–9)
- SVT: ectopic atrial tachycardia (Fig. 15–10)
- SVT: AV nodal reentry or WPW tachycardia (Fig. 15–11)
- Ventricular tachycardia (Fig. 15–12)

Management of Rapid Irregular Rhythms

Management of Atrial Fibrillation.   If *unstable*—hypotensive, chest pain (angina), or SOB (CHF)—and if atrial fibrillation is of recent onset (less than 3 days), the treatment of choice is cardioversion, beginning with 100 J.

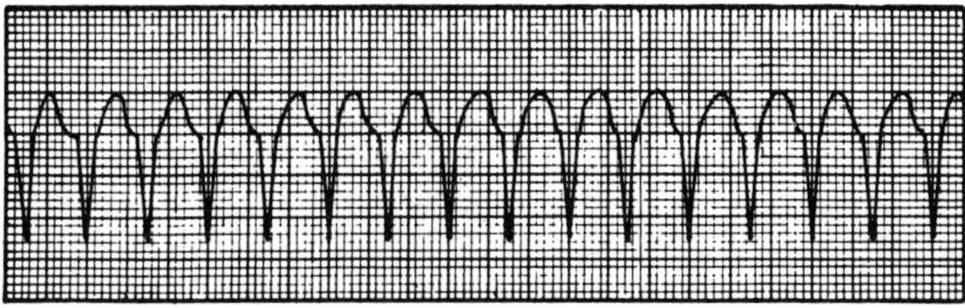

Figure 15–3 □ Ventricular tachycardia.

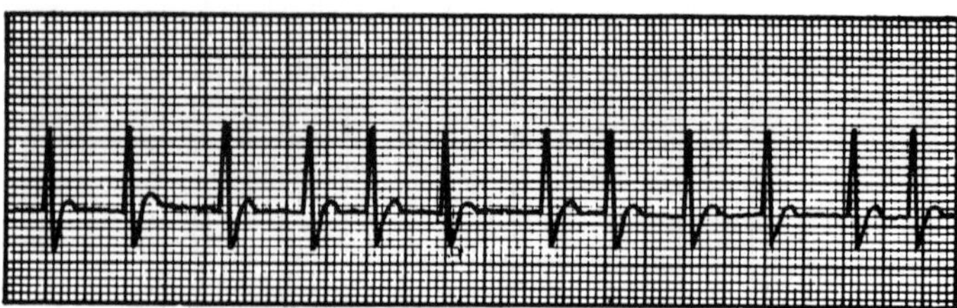

Figure 15–4 □ Rapid irregular rhythms. Atrial fibrillation.

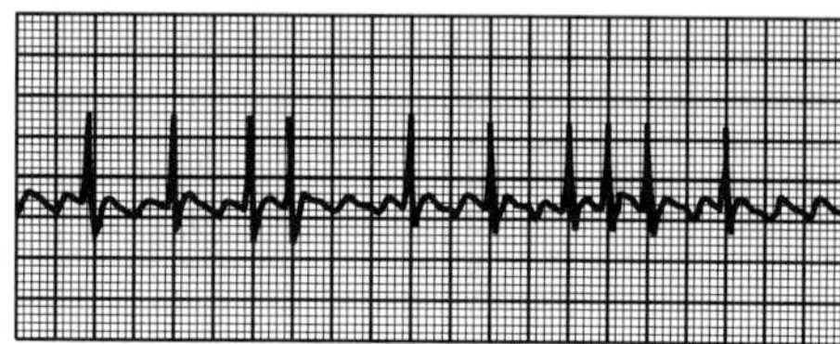

Figure 15–4a □ Atrial flutter with variable block.

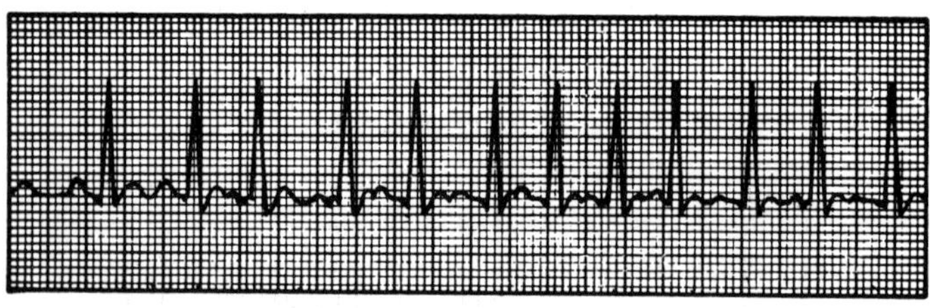

Figure 15–5 □ Rapid irregular rhythms. Multifocal atrial tachycardia.

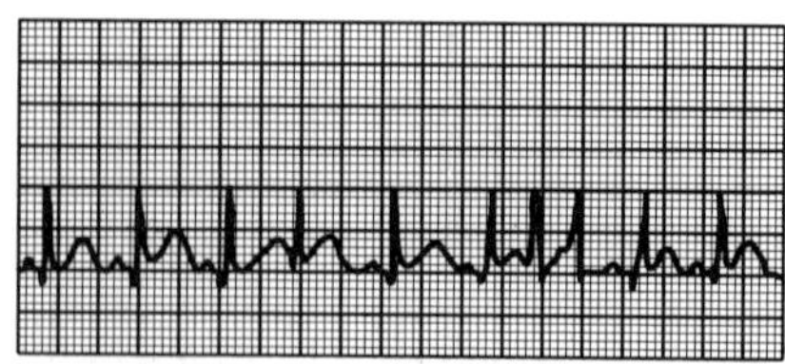

Figure 15–6 □ Rapid irregular rhythms. Sinus tachycardia with PACs.

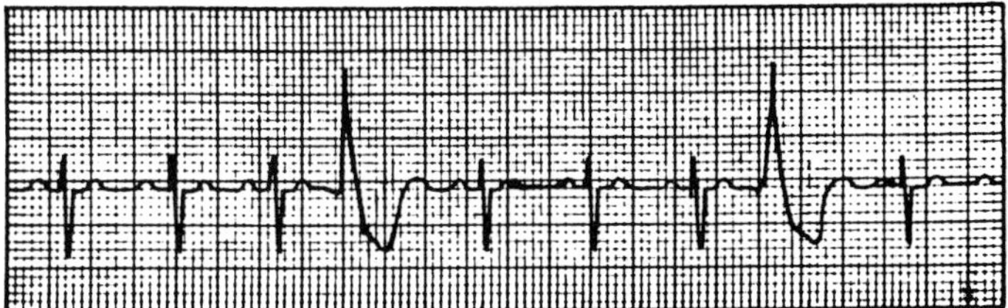

Figure 15–7 □ Rapid irregular rhythms. Sinus tachycardia with PVCs.

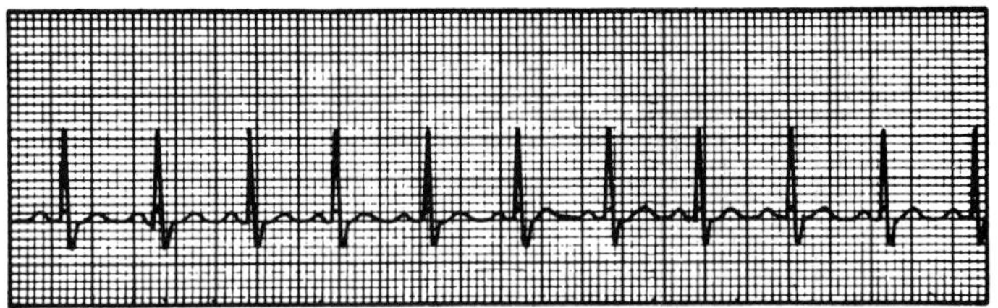

Figure 15–8 □ Rapid regular rhythms. Sinus tachycardia.

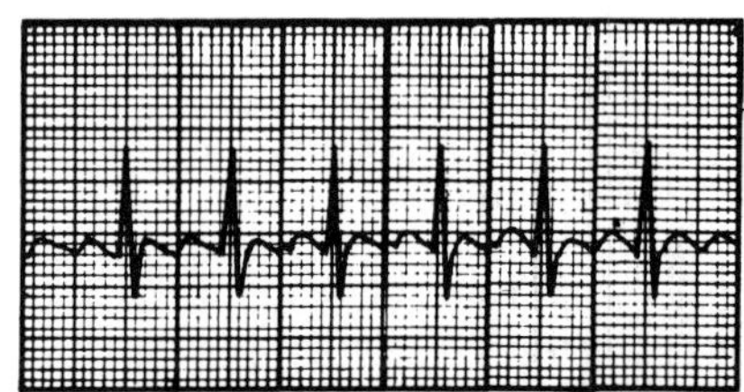

Figure 15–9 □ Rapid regular rhythms. Atrial flutter.

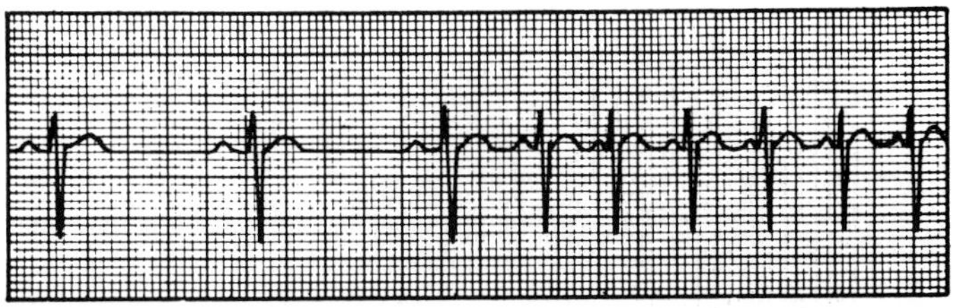

Figure 15–10 □ Rapid regular rhythms. SVT. Ectopic atrial tachycardia.

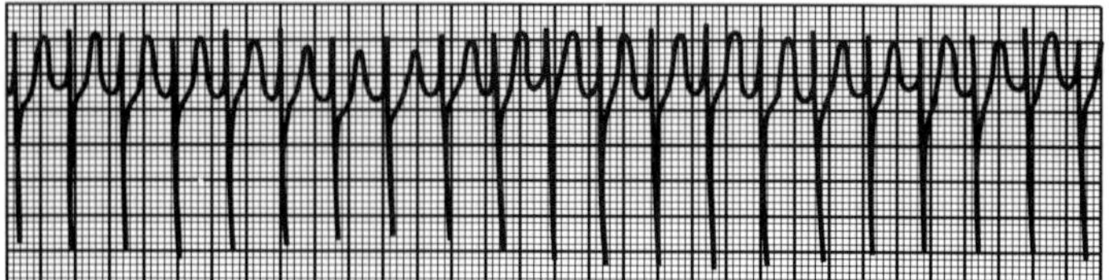

Figure 15–11 □ Rapid regular rhythms. SVT. AV nodal reentry or WPW tachycardia.

Atrial fibrillation with ventricular rates greater than 100/min and without evidence of hemodynamic compromise (no hypotension, angina, or CHF) can be treated with oral digoxin tablets. If the patient is not already receiving digoxin, give *digoxin* 0.25 mg PO q4h × 4 doses. Then, give 0.125 to 0.25 mg PO daily thereafter in a patient with normal renal function. Since digoxin is predominantly excreted by glomerular filtration, smaller maintenance doses are required in the presence of renal dysfunction.

In a patient already receiving digoxin, additional doses should be given with caution and careful observation.

Digoxin overdose is a common cause of morbidity in both community and hospital settings. Common side effects include dysrhythmias, heart blocks, anorexia, nausea, vomiting, and neuropsychiatric symptoms, such as hallucinations. It is unusual for these side effects to develop acutely when digoxin is prescribed in the regimen previously outlined. The subsequent development of these side effects can be minimized by adjusting maintenance digoxin doses according to renal function. The risk of digoxin-induced ventricular dysrhythmias can be reduced by avoiding hypokalemia.

Atrial fibrillation with ventricular rates less than 100/min in the untreated patient suggests underlying AV nodal dysfunction. These patients do not require immediate treatment unless hemodynamically compromised (e.g., hypotension, angina, or CHF).

Once the ventricular rate is controlled, perform a *selective history*

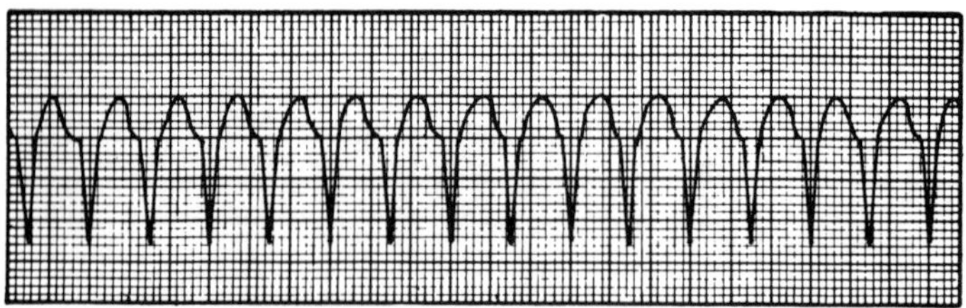

Figure 15–12 □ Rapid regular rhythms. Ventricular tachycardia.

and chart review looking for the following causes of atrial fibrillation.

- Coronary artery disease
- Hypertension
- Hyperthyroidism (check T_4)
- Pulmonary embolism (check for risk factors, see p. 240)
- Mitral or tricuspid valve disease (stenosis or regurgitation)
- Cardiomyopathy
- Congenital heart disease (e.g., atrial septal defect)
- Pericarditis, recent cardiac surgery
- Recent alcohol ingestion (holiday heart syndrome)
- Wolff-Parkinson-White syndrome (Fig. 15–13)
- Sick sinus syndrome
- Hypoxia
- Idiopathic (lone fibrillator)

SELECTIVE PHYSICAL EXAMINATION.   Look for specific causes of atrial fibrillation. Note that this process takes place *after* you have already begun to treat the patient.

VITALS	Repeat now
HEENT	Exophthalmos, lid lag, lid retraction (hyperthyroidism)
RESP	Tachypnea, cyanosis, wheezing, pleural effusion (pulmonary embolus)
CVS	Murmur of mitral regurgitation or mitral stenosis (mitral valve disease)
EXT	Swelling, erythema, calf tenderness (DVT)

Management of Multifocal Atrial Tachycardia.   This rhythm does not always require specific management. One should treat the underlying cause, which is usually pulmonary disease and usually already being treated. Check for the following underlying causes.

- Pulmonary disease (especially COPD)
- Hypoxia, hypercapnea

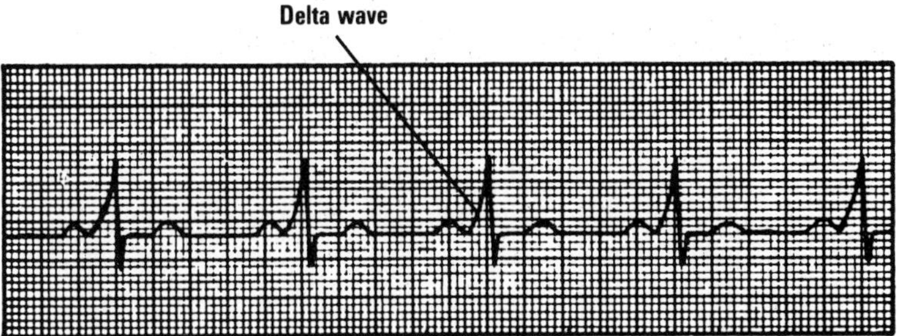

Figure 15–13 □ Wolff-Parkinson-White syndrome. This condition is characterized by a regular rhythm, a PR interval < 0.12 second, a QRS complex > 0.11 second, and a delta wave (i.e., slurred beginning of the QRS).

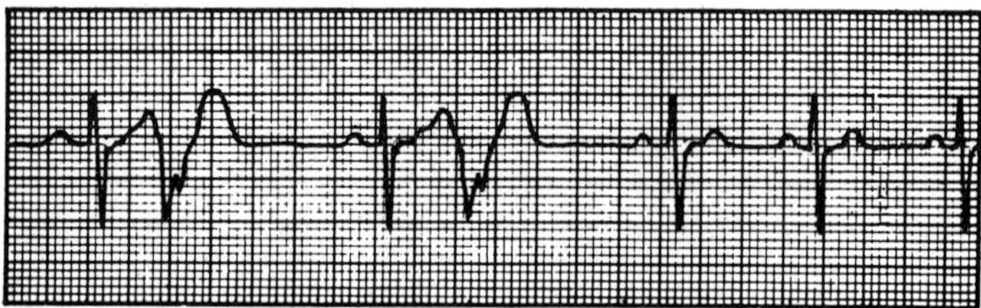

Figure 15–14 □ PVCs. R on T phenomenon.

- Hypokalemia
- CHF
- Drugs: theophylline toxicity
- Caffeine, tobacco, alcohol use

Multifocal atrial tachycardia can be a forerunner of atrial fibrillation. If no remediable causes can be found, *verapamil* 80 mg PO TID or *diltiazem* 30–60 mg PO QID may provide rate control and diminish the frequency of ectopics.

Management of Sinus Tachycardia with PACs. Treatment is the same as that for multifocal atrial tachycardia. Again, PACs may be forerunners of multifocal atrial tachycardia or of atrial fibrillation, but PACs do not need to be treated unless atrial fibrillation develops.

Management of Sinus Tachycardia with PVCs. Look carefully at the ECG and rhythm strip and decide whether the PVCs are malignant. The following features *suggest* a more ominous, malignant arrhythmia: *R on T phenomenon* (Fig. 15–14), *multifocal PVCs* (Fig. 15–15), *couplets or salvos* (three or more PVCs in a row) (Fig. 15–16), and *more than 5 PVCs/min* (Fig. 15–17).

Unless you can be certain that (1) the patient has not had an MI, (2) the patient is hemodynamically stable, and (3) the patient has had PVCs chronically, the patient with very frequent PVCs or runs of nonsustained ventricular tachycardia should be transferred to the ICU/CCU for further investigation and continuous ECG monitoring.

Look for the following common causes of PVCs in the hospital.

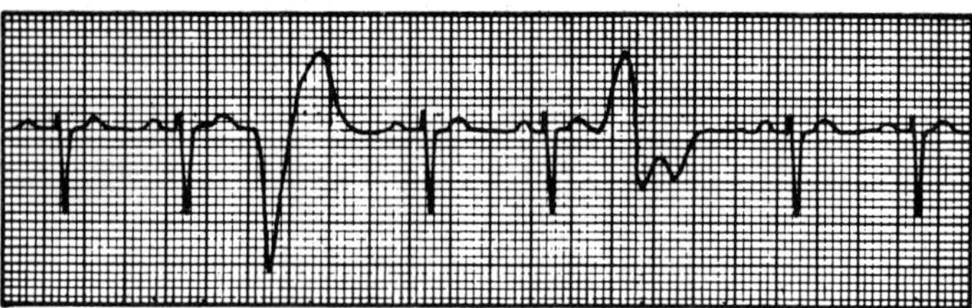

Figure 15–15 □ PVCs. Multifocal.

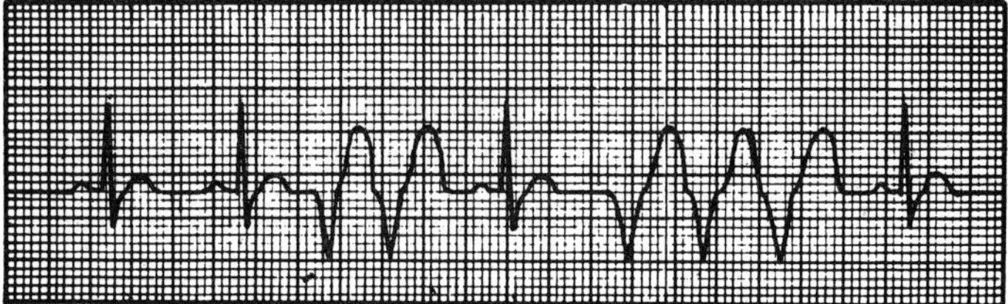

Figure 15–16 □ PVCs. Couplets or salvos.

- *Myocardial ischemia* (symptoms or signs of angina or MI). This is the most important cause of PVCs to identify, if present. PVCs are not generally associated with an increased risk of death unless they occur in the setting of myocardial ischemia or infarction.
- *Hypokalemia.* Look for a recent serum potassium value in the chart, and order a repeat measurement if a recent one is not available. Check the 12-lead ECG for evidence of hypokalemia (Fig. 15–18). Ascertain whether the patient is on diuretics that may cause hypokalemia (refer to Chapter 33 for treatment).
- *Hypoxia.* Obtain ABGs if hypoxia is suspected clinically.
- *Acid-base imbalance.* Check the chart for a recent HCO_3 determination. Obtain ABGs if acidosis or alkalosis is suspected.
- *Cardiomyopathy.* Patients with cardiomyopathy severe enough to cause PVCs almost always have a cardiologist and an established diagnosis of cardiomyopathy before you see them. Consult the patient's cardiologist for guidance in treating cardiomyopathy-related PVCs.
- *Mitral valve prolapse.* Mitral valve prolapse may be associated with PVCs. Listen carefully for a systolic click and murmur. Diagnosis can usually await confirmation by echocardiography in the morning.
- *Drugs.* Drugs, such as digoxin and other antiarrhythmics, may actually *cause* PVCs.
- *Hyperthyroidism.* Look for signs of hypermetabolism, such as diaphoresis, tremor, heat intolerance, diarrhea, and ocular

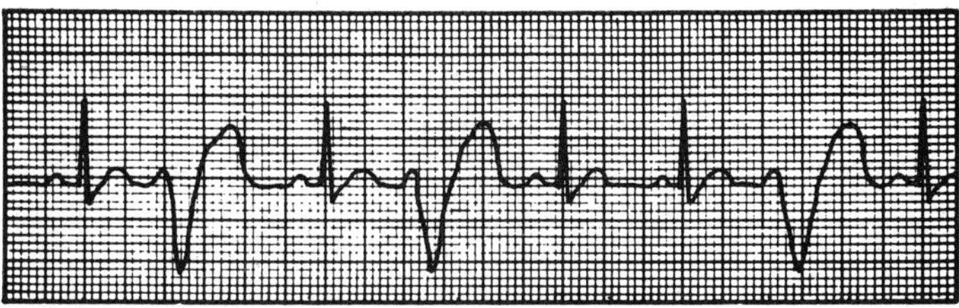

Figure 15–17 □ PVCs. More than 5/min.

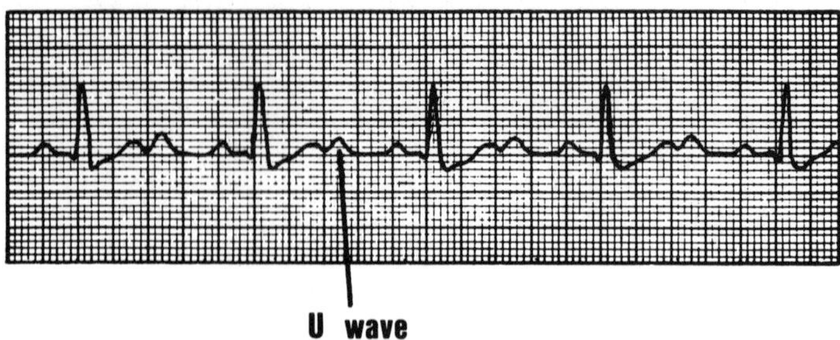

Figure 15–18 □ Electrocardiographic features of hypokalemia.

manifestations of hyperthyroidism, including lid lag, lid retraction, and exophthalmos. Order a serum T_4 if hyperthyroidism is suspected.

Try to identify whether any of the preceding eight factors is responsible for the PVCs and correct them if possible. Hypokalemia, hypoxia, and acid-base disturbances usually can be identified and corrected in the patient's room. However, if there is suspicion of myocardial ischemia, cardiomyopathy, digoxin toxicity, or hyperthyroidism, the patient should be transferred to the ICU/CCU for continuous electrocardiographic monitoring and initiation of antiarrhythmics if indicated.

After the PVCs have been treated, the patient may still be left with *sinus tachycardia*. Investigation and management of the underlying sinus tachycardia should be undertaken as subsequently outlined.

Management of Rapid Regular Rhythms

Management of Sinus Tachycardia.   There is no specific drug for the treatment of sinus tachycardia. The key is to find the *underlying cause* of this dysrhythmia. The most common causes in hospitalized patients of persistent sinus tachycardia are as follows.

- *Hypovolemia*
- *Hypotension* (cardiogenic, hypovolemic, sepsis, anaphylaxis). (Refer to Chapter 18 for investigation and management of hypotension.)
- *Hypoxia* of any cause (CHF, pulmonary embolism, pneumonia, bronchospasm of COPD and asthma). (Refer to Chapter 24 for investigation and management of SOB.)
- *Fever*
- *Anxiety or pain*
- *Hyperthyroidism*
- *Drugs*

The treatment for sinus tachycardia is *always* treatment of the underlying causes.

Management of Supraventricular Tachycardias: Atrial Flutter. The treatment of atrial flutter is similar to that of atrial fibrillation. If *unstable*, the patient requires cardioversion; if *stable*, the patient may be treated with verapamil or digoxin IV (see p. 126). Often, atrial flutter requires higher doses of digoxin than atrial fibrillation to slow the ventricular rate. Ironically, treatment of atrial flutter often produces atrial fibrillation. Look for causes in the chart that may predispose the patient to atrial flutter. For the most part, these are the same diseases that can cause atrial fibrillation (see p. 121).

Management of Supraventricular Tachycardia: AV Nodal Reentry and Ectopic Atrial Tachycardias. You will undoubtedly be anxious if called to see a patient with PAT who is unstable because you know that may mean *cardioversion,* a technique with which you may not be familiar. Stay calm; there is still much you can do. If the patient is *unstable,* i.e., hypotensive, chest pain (angina), or SOB (CHF), prepare for immediate cardioversion as follows:

- Ask the RN to call your resident immediately.
- Ask the RN to bring the cardiac arrest cart into the room. Attach the patient to the ECG monitor. Set the defibrillator to 25 J, in the Synchronize mode.
- Give the patient 100% O_2 by mask (28% for COPD).
- Ask the RN to draw *diazepam* (Valium) 10 mg IV into a syringe. Double check that an IV is in place. While waiting for the resident to arrive, try nonelectrical means to convert the rhythm, e.g., Valsalva's maneuver, carotid sinus massage (see next section).

If the patient is hemodynamically stable, you may try one or more of the following measures to break the tachycardia.

- *Valsalva maneuver.* Ask the patient to hold his or her breath and to "bear down as if you are going to have a bowel movement." This maneuver increases vagal tone and may terminate an SVT.
- *Carotid sinus massage.* This maneuver is an effective form of vagal stimulation and may thereby terminate PAT. It should always be performed with IV atropine available and with continuous ECG monitoring both for safety (some patients have developed asystole) and for documentation of results.

Listen over the carotid arteries for bruits, and if they are present, do not perform carotid sinus massage. If no bruit is heard, proceed as follows: Turn the patient's head to the left. Locate the carotid sinus just anterior to the sternocleidomastoid muscle at the level of the top of the thyroid cartilage (Fig. 15–19). Feel the carotid pulsation at this point and apply steady pressure to the carotid artery with two fingers for 10 to 15 seconds. Try the right side and, if not effective, try the left side. Simultaneous bilateral

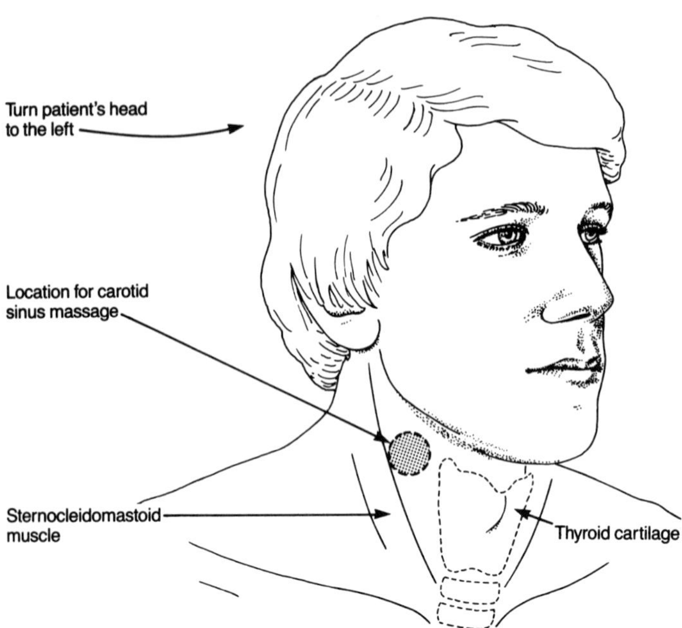

Figure 15–19 □ Carotid sinus massage.

massage of the carotid sinus should never be done, as you will effectively cut off cerebral blood flow!

Carotid sinus massage has resulted, on several occasions, in cerebral embolization of an atherosclerotic plaque from carotid artery compression. Although this is a rare complication, it can be minimized by first listening over the carotid artery for a bruit. If a bruit is heard, forego carotid sinus massage on that side.

- *Verapamil.* Begin with 2.5 to 5.0 mg IV over 2 minutes. If there has been no effect, the dose may be repeated in 5 to 10 minutes. Verapamil increases AV conduction time and may slow ventricular rate. Verapamil may cause hypotension if injected too rapidly. It is essential to give the dose slowly over 2 minutes. Verapamil is also a negative inotropic agent and may precipitate pulmonary edema in the patient with a predisposition to CHF.
- *Adenosine.* IV adenosine may be given at 6 mg as a rapid IV bolus followed by a saline flush. If ineffective, increase to 12 mg IV push. A third dose of 18 mg IV push may be given if the first two lower doses were ineffective but well tolerated. Because of the very short half-life of adenosine, the three incremental doses may be administered at intervals of 60 seconds, if required. IV adenosine should be used with caution

in patients with asthma and COPD. Lower doses may be required in patients on dipyridamole and in patients who have undergone cardiac transplantation, because of supersensitivity to the drug.

- *Digoxin.* Provided the SVT is not due to digoxin toxicity (i.e., PAT with block), you may use *digoxin* 0.25 to 0.5 mg IV, followed by 0.125 to 0.25 mg q4–6h until a full loading dose of 1 mg is given instead of verapamil. Then, a daily maintenance dose of 0.125 to 0.25 mg PO daily may be given if the patient has normal renal function. Digoxin slows AV nodal conduction and may terminate SVT. The common side effects of digoxin (dysrhythmias, heart blocks, GI upsets, neuropsychiatric symptoms) are seldom seen acutely when digoxin is prescribed in the regimen as outlined.

If the patient is known to have Wolff-Parkinson-White syndrome and is having SVT, *procainamide* is the drug of choice.

If hemodynamically stable and the aforementioned measures have not worked, the patient should be transferred immediately to the ICU/CCU for semielective cardioversion.

The underlying causes of SVT are, for the most part, the same as those of atrial fibrillation and flutter (see p. 121).

Management of Ventricular Tachycardia.   If the patient has no BP or pulse, call for a cardiac arrest and proceed with resuscitation as described on pages 334 and 335.

If the patient is *unstable* (hypotensive, angina, or CHF), do the following.

- Call for the cardiac arrest cart, your resident, and a 12-lead ECG immediately.
- Attach the patient to the ECG monitor.
- Make sure that an IV is in place.
- Give the patient 100% O_2 by mask (28% for COPDs).
- Order *lidocaine* 1 mg/kg IV to be given by syringe as rapidly as possible. At the same time, begin a maintenance infusion of lidocaine at a rate of 1 to 4 mg/min. In elderly patients and in patients with liver disease, CHF, or hypotension, give half the maintenance dose. In 5 to 15 minutes after the initial loading dose, give a second bolus of lidocaine, 0.5 to 1 mg/kg IV. Lidocaine may cause drowsiness, confusion, slurred speech, and seizures, especially in the elderly and in patients with heart failure or liver disease. Once your patient has been transferred to the ICU/CCU, the staff there will need to watch carefully for these signs of lidocaine toxicity.
- *Procainamide* 750 to 1000 mg IV given at a rate of 50 mg/min may also be tried. Although it is often more effective than lidocaine in breaking ventricular tachycardia, the patient will need to be monitored carefully for hypotension.
- *Cardioversion,* beginning at 50 J. Ventricular tachycardia with

hemodynamic compromise or without prompt response to lidocaine or procainamide requires cardioversion. A patient with an episode of ventricular tachycardia should be transferred to the ICU/CCU for continuous ECG monitoring.

After immediate resuscitation, look for the following precipitating or potentiating causes of ventricular tachycardia.

- Myocardial ischemia or infarction
- Hypoxia
- Electrolyte imbalance (hypokalemia, hypomagnesemia, hypocalcemia)
- Hypovolemia
- Valvular heart disease (MVP)
- Acidemia
- Cardiomyopathy, CHF
- Drugs

Digoxin
Quinidine
Procainamide
Disopyramide
Phenothiazines
Tricyclic antidepressants
Amiodarone
Sotalol

These drugs may prolong the QT interval to produce a characteristic type of ventricular tachycardia known as torsades de pointes, which resembles a corkscrew pattern in the ECG rhythm strip, with complexes rotating above and below the baseline (Fig. 15–20). The drugs listed should be discontinued if such a rhythm develops, and lidocaine should be started as previously outlined.

■ SLOW HEART RATES
PHONE CALL
Questions

1 **What is the heart rate?**
2 **What is the blood pressure?**
3 **Is the patient on digoxin, a beta blocker, or a calcium entry blocker?**

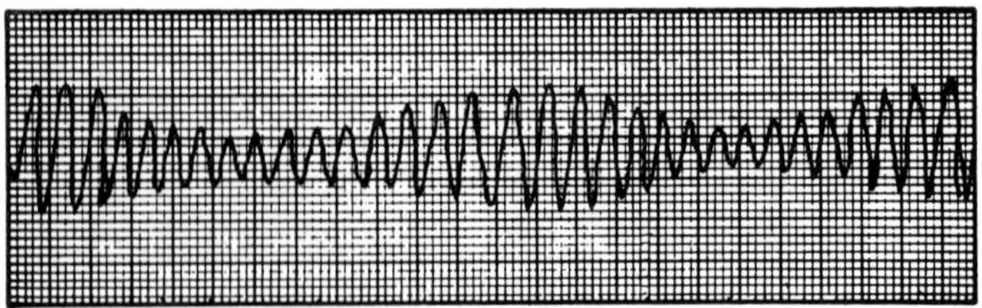

Figure 15–20 □ Torsades de pointes.

Each drug may prolong AV nodal conduction and result in bradycardia due to heart block. The beta blockers and calcium antagonists may also profoundly decrease the sinus node rate.

Orders

1. If the patient is hypotensive (systolic BP < 90 mm Hg), order an IV to be started immediately and ask the RN to place the patient in the Trendelenburg position (foot of the bed up). IV access is essential to deliver medications to increase the heart rate. Placing the patient in Trendelenburg position achieves an autotransfusion of 200 to 300 ml of blood.
2. If the heart rate is less than 40/min, ask the RN to have a premixed syringe of *atropine* 1 mg ready at the bedside.
3. Stat ECG and rhythm strip.
4. Ask the RN to bring the cardiac arrest cart into the room and to attach the patient to the ECG monitor.

Inform RN

"Will arrive at bedside in . . . minutes."

"Bradycardia + hypotension" or any heart rate less than 50/min requires you to see the patient immediately.

ELEVATOR THOUGHTS (What causes slow heart rates?)

Sinus Bradycardia (Fig. 15–21)

Drugs	Beta blockers
	Calcium entry blockers
	Digoxin
Cardiac	Sick sinus syndrome
	Acute MI (usually of inferior wall)
	Vasovagal attack
Misc	Hypothyroidism
	Healthy young athletes
	Increased intracranial pressure in association with hypertension.

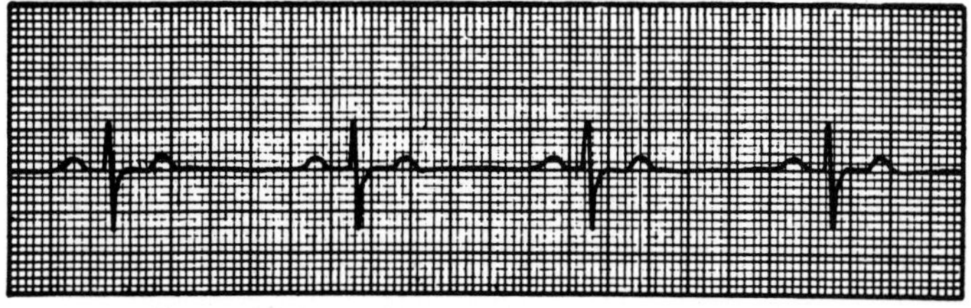

Figure 15–21 □ Slow heart rate. Sinus bradycardia.

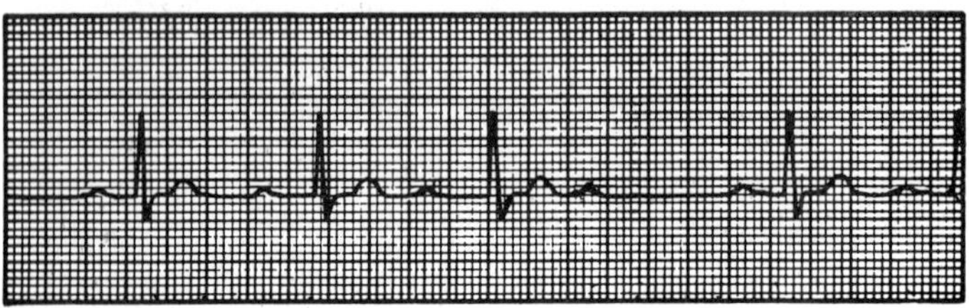

Figure 15–22 □ Slow heart rate. Second-degree AV block (type I).

Second-Degree AV Block: Type I (Wenckenbach's) (Fig. 15–22) and Type II (Fig. 15–23)

Drugs	Beta blockers
	Digoxin
	Calicum entry blockers
Cardiac	Acute MI
	Sick sinus syndrome

Third-Degree AV Block (Fig. 15–24)

Drugs	Beta blockers
	Calcium entry blockers
	Digoxin
Cardiac	Acute MI
	Sick sinus syndrome

Atrial Fibrillation with Slow Ventricular Rate (Fig. 15–25)

Drugs	Digoxin
	Beta blockers
	Calcium entry blockers
Cardiac	Sick sinus syndrome

Notice that no matter which bradycardia is present, the most common causes are drug-related and cardiac.

MAJOR THREAT TO LIFE

- Hypotension
- Myocardial infarction

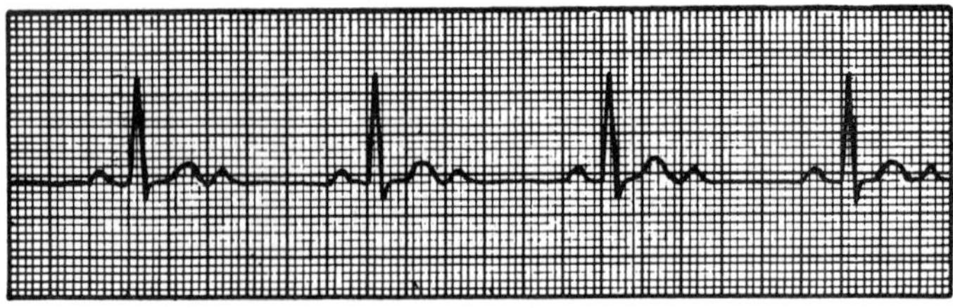

Figure 15–23 □ Slow heart rate. Second-degree AV block (type II).

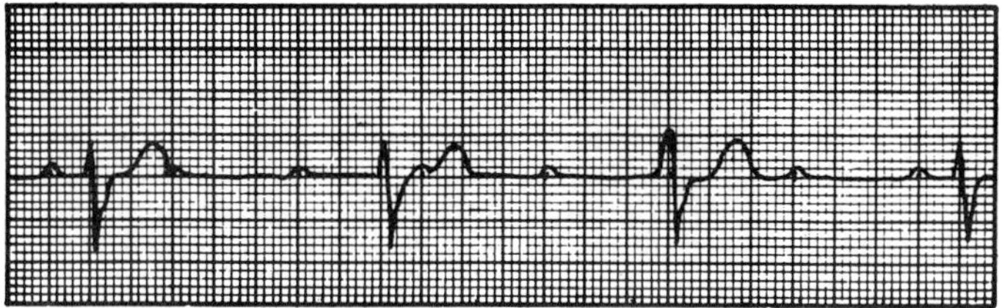

Figure 15–24 □ Slow heart rate. Third-degree AV block.

Two major threats to life exist in the patient with bradycardia as follows. First, if the heart rate is low enough, it will result in hypotension due to inadequate CO, resulting in hypoperfusion of vital organs. A second concern is that if the bradycardia is due to MI, the patient will be prone to even more ominous dysrhythmias, such as ventricular tachycardia or fibrillation or asystole.

BEDSIDE
Quick Look Test
Does the patient look well (comfortable), sick (uncomfortable or distressed), or critical (about to die?)
If the patient looks sick or critical, ask the RN to bring the cardiac arrest cart to the bedside and attach the patient to the ECG monitor. This may give instant diagnosis of the patient's rhythm, allow continuous monitoring, and provide instant feedback of the effects of your interventions.

Airways and Vital Signs
What is the HR?
Read the ECG to identify which slow rhythm is occurring.

What is the BP?
Most causes of hypotension are accompanied by a compensatory reflex *tachycardia*. If hypotension exists with any of the bradycardias, proceed as follows.
- Notify your resident as soon as possible.

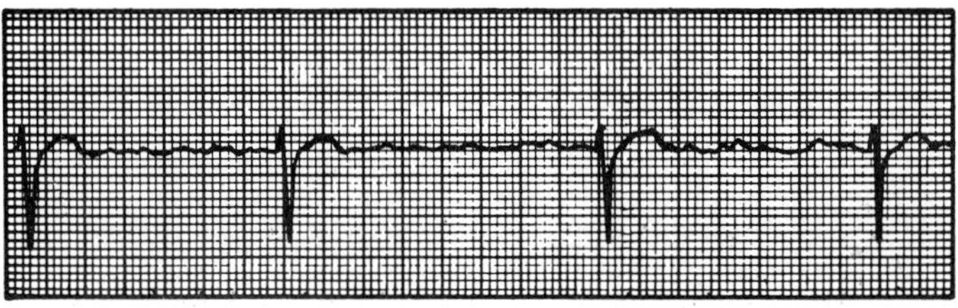

Figure 15–25 □ Atrial fibrillation with slow ventricular rate.

- Elevate the legs. This is a temporary measure serving to shift blood volume from the legs to the central circulation.
- *Atropine* 0.5 mg IV as rapidly as possible. If no response after 5 minutes, give an additional 0.5 mg atropine IV q5min up to a total dose of 2.0 mg IV. If still no improvement, begin an IV *isoproterenol* (Isuprel) infusion by adding 2 mg of isoproterenol to 500 ml D5W, running at 1 to 10 µg/min (15 to 150 ml/h). Any patient receiving an isoproterenol infusion should be transferred to the ICU/CCU for further monitoring and possible pacemaker placement.

Selective History and Chart Review

Look for the cause of bradycardia.

Drugs	Beta blockers Calcium entry blockers Digoxin
Cardiac ischemia	Does the patient have a history of angina or previous MI? Has there been any hint (chest pain, SOB, nausea, or vomiting) of a cardiac ischemic event occurring within the last few days? Does the patient have other evidence of atherosclerosis (previous stroke, TIAs, peripheral vascular disease) that may be a clue to the concomitant presence of coronary artery disease? Does the patient have current risk factors (hypertension, diabetes mellitus, smoking, hypercholesterolemia, family history of coronary artery disease) that may suggest that this is the first episode of cardiac ischemia? If there is any evidence that the bradycardia is due to an acute myocardial infarction, the patient should go to the ICU/CCU for ECG monitoring.
Vasovagal attack	Is there a history of pain, straining, or other Valsalva-like maneuver immediately before the occurrence of the bradycardia?

Selective Physical Examination

Look for a cause of bradycardia.

VITALS	Bradypnea (hypothyroidism) Hypothermia (hypothyroidism) Hypertension (risk factor for coronary artery disease)
HEENT	Coarse facial features (hypothyroidism) Loss of lateral third of eyebrows (hypothyroidism) Periorbital xanthomas (coronary artery disease) Fundi with hypertensive or diabetic changes (coronary artery disease) Carotid bruits (cerebrovascular disease with concomitant coronary artery disease)

CVS	New S_3, S_4, or mitral regurgitant murmur (nonspecific but common findings in acute MI)
ABD	Renal, aortic, or femoral bruits (concomitant coronary artery disease)
EXT	Poor peripheral pulses (peripheral vascular disease with concomitant coronary artery disease)
NEURO	Delayed return phase of deep tendon reflexes (hypothyroidism)

Management
Sinus Bradycardia
- No immediate treatment is required if the patient is not hypotensive.
- If on digoxin with an HR less than 60/min, further digoxin doses should be held until the HR is greater than 60/min.
- If the patient is on beta blockers or calcium entry blockers that depress conduction, no immediate treatment is required as long as the patient is not hypotensive. However, with very slow heart rates (less than 40/min), one should hold subsequent doses of these medications until the HR is greater than 60/min. Further maintenance doses can be determined in consultation with the attending physician.

Second-Degree AV Block (Type I and Type II) and Third-Degree Block
- Patients with either second- or third-degree AV block should be temporarily taken off any drugs that are known to prolong AV conduction and transferred to a bed where continuous ECG monitoring is available.

Atrial Fibrillation With Slow Ventricular Response
- This dysrhythmia does not require treatment unless the patient is hypotensive or has symptoms (syncope, confusion, angina, CHF) suggestive of vital organ hypoperfusion. Definitive treatment includes discontinuation of drugs that depress conduction, and in some cases, requires transfer to the ICU/CCU for pacemaker placement.

REMEMBER
1. Discontinuation of digoxin may mean that the original tachydysrhythmia or CHF for which the patient was being treated may return. Observe the patient closely over the next few days to ensure that tachydysrhythmia or CHF does not recur.
2. Abrupt discontinuation of some beta blockers may result in rebound hypertension, angina, or MI. Again, observe the patient closely over the next several days. When the heart rate rises to > 60/min, the beta blocker may be reinstituted

at a lower dosage. If treated in this manner, rebound hypertension or cardiac ischemia is seldom a problem.

3. Occasionally, digoxin overdose results in life-threatening arrhythmias that are unresponsive to conventional measures. In these instances, *digoxin-specific antibodies* may be effective in reversing the toxic effects of digoxin.

16

HIGH BLOOD PRESSURE

Calls concerning high blood pressure are frequent at night. They rarely require the use of drugs that rapidly reduce the pressure. The level of the BP itself is of less importance than the rate of the rise and the setting in which the high BP is occurring.

PHONE CALL
Questions

1 **Why is the patient in the hospital?**
2 **Is the patient pregnant?**
   Hypertension in the pregnant patient may indicate the development of preeclampsia or eclampsia and should be assessed immediately.
3 **Is the patient taking antidepressant drugs?**
   Hypertension occurring in a patient receiving MAO inhibitors or tricyclics suggests the possibility of a catecholamine crisis due to food or drug interaction.
4 **Is the patient in the emergency room?**
   Hypertension in young individuals appearing in the emergency room may be caused by catecholamine hypertension due to cocaine or amphetamine abuse.
5 **How high is the pressure, and what has the pressure been previously?**
6 **Does the patient have symptoms suggestive of a hypertensive emergency?**
   a. Back and chest pain (aortic dissection)
   b. Chest pain (myocardial ischemia)
   c. Shortness of breath (pulmonary edema)
   d. Headache, neck stiffness (subarachnoid hemorrhage)
   e. Headache, vomiting, confusion, seizures (hypertensive encephalopathy)
7 **What antihypertensive medication has the patient been taking?**

Orders

If the patient has any symptoms of a hypertensive emergency, order IV D5W TKVO immediately.

Inform RN

"Will be at bedside in . . . minutes."

Situations requiring immediate assessment and possibly prompt lowering of blood pressure include the following.

- Eclampsia
- Aortic dissection

- Pulmonary edema resistant to other emergency treatment (see Chapter 24, p. 237)
- Coronary ischemia
- Catecholamine crisis
- Hypertensive encephalopathy

ELEVATOR THOUGHTS

The diagnosis of *preeclampsia* can be made in the obstetric patient with hypertension, edema, and proteinuria. This syndrome usually occurs in the third trimester of pregnancy, at which stage hypertension is defined as a BP of 140/85 mm Hg or greater for more than 4 to 6 hours or as an increase of 30 mm Hg in systolic or 15 mm Hg in diastolic pressure, or more, from the pregestational values.

Aortic dissection is potentiated by high shearing forces determined by the rate of rise of the intraventricular pressure as well as the systolic pressure.

Elevation of afterload (increased systemic vascular resistance and elevated blood pressure) may be a readily correctable detrimental factor in *coronary ischemia* and *pulmonary edema.*

Catecholamine crises can be caused by the following.

Drug overdoses	Cocaine and amphetamines
Drug interactions	MAO inhibitors and indirect acting catechols (wine, cheese, ephedrine) Tricyclics and direct acting catechols (epinephrine, pseudoephedrine, norepinephrine)
Drug withdrawal	Abrupt withdrawal from antihypertensive agents, such as beta blockers, centrally acting alpha agonists, and ACE inhibitors, may result in a rebound hypertensive crisis.
Pheochromocytoma	This neoplasm may produce a hypertensive crisis through overproduction of epinephrine or norepinephrine.
Burns	Some patients with second- or third-degree burns will develop a transient hypertensive crises, usually resolving within 2 weeks, due to high circulating levels of catecholamines, renin, and angiotensin II.

Hypertensive encephalopathy is a rare complication of hypertension and even more unusual in hospitalized patients. Vomiting developing over several days, and headache, lethargy, and confusion are suggestive symptoms. Focal neurological deficits are uncommon in the early course of encephalopathy.

BP fluctuates in normal individuals and more so in hypertensive individuals. Excitement, fear, and anxiety from unrelated medical conditions or procedures can cause marked transient increases in BP. BP measurements require care in regard to proper cuff size and proper cuff placement and should be repeated to confirm the readings.

MAJOR THREAT TO LIFE

The major immediate threat to life is a marked increase in blood pressure with the following.

- Eclampsia
- Aortic dissection
- Pulmonary edema
- Myocardial infarction
- Hypertensive encephalopathy

BEDSIDE

Quick Look Test

Does the patient look well (comfortable), sick (uncomfortable or distressed), or critical (about to die)?

Unless the patient is having seizures (eclampsia, hypertensive encephalopathy) or is markedly SOB (pulmonary edema), the severity of the situation cannot be assessed by the initial appearance. The patient may be suffering from hypertensive encephalopathy yet look deceptively well.

Airway and Vital Signs

What is the BP?

Retake the BP in both arms.

Accompanying arteriosclerosis may unilaterally reduce brachial artery flow and may give an artifactually low BP reading. A lower pressure in the left arm may be a clue to aortic dissection. Too small a cuff on an obese patient or a patient with rigid arteriosclerotic peripheral vessels may give readings that are factitiously high in relationship to the intraarterial pressure.

What is the HR?

Bradycardia and hypertension in a patient not on beta blockers may indicate increasing intracranial pressure. Tachycardia and hypertension can be seen in catecholamine crisis.

Selective History

Can the patient further elucidate the duration of hypertension? Ask the patient about any symptoms suggestive of a hypertensive emergency.

- Headache (an occipital headache or a neckache, lethargy, or visual blurring suggests hypertensive encephalopathy)
- Chest pain (myocardial ischemia)
- SOB (pulmonary edema)
- Back or chest pain (aortic dissection)
- Unilateral weakness or sensory symptoms suggest a cerebrovascular accident. Such an episode in a previously hyperten-

sive patient may be associated with a transient increase in BP.

Selective Physical Examination

Does the patient have evidence of a hypertensive emergency?

HEENT   Assess the fundi for hypertensive changes (generalized or focal arteriolar narrowing, flame-shaped hemorrhages near the disc, dot and blot hemorrhages, exudates) Papilledema is an ominous finding in patients with hypertension and is a hallmark sign of malignant hypertension and hypertensive encephalopathy (Fig. 16–1).

RESP   Crackles, pleural effusion (CHF)

CVS   Elevated JVP, S_3 (CHF)

NEURO   Confusion, delirium, agitation, or lethargy (hypertensive encephalopathy)
Localized deficits (stroke)

Management

Most often, the elevated BP will be an isolated finding in an asymptomatic patient known to have hypertension. Although long-term control of hypertension in such patients is of proven benefit, acute lowering of BP is not. Remember the risk of overshooting the mark in acute reduction of BP in patients with long-standing high BP and high levels of autoregulation of cerebral blood flow. Do not treat a BP reading. Treat the condition associated with it!

True emergencies require special management. These include the following.

- Hypertensive encephalopathy

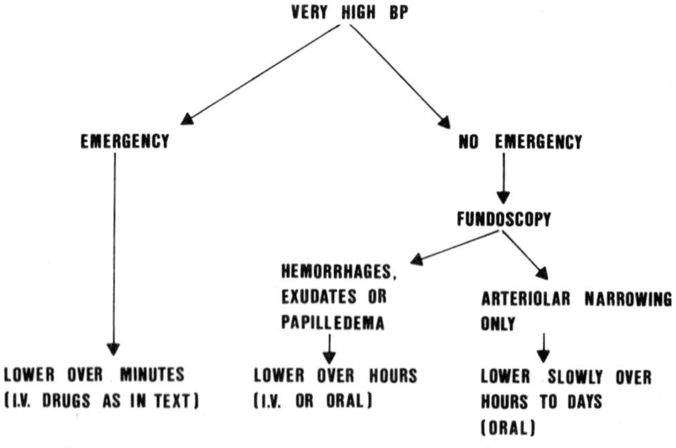

Figure 16–1 □ Approach to management of very high blood pressure.

- Malignant hypertension (marked elevation of diastolic pressure with fundal hemorrhages and exudates and usually some compromise in renal function)
- Eclampsia
- Subarachnoid or cerebral hemorrhage
- Aortic dissection
- Hypertension and pulmonary edema or myocardial ischemia
- Catecholamine crisis

Call your resident now for help if you are unfamiliar with the management of these conditions.

Hypertensive Encephalopathy. This is almost always accompanied by papilledema in addition to retinal exudates and hemorrhages. Focal neurological deficits are unusual early on and suggest that the elevated pressure is most likely associated with a stroke. Remember particularly the risk of lowering pressure too quickly in patients with atherothrombotic cerebrovascular disease; you can precipitate a stroke!

1. Transfer the patient to the ICU/CCU for ECG monitoring and intraarterial BP monitoring.

2. Since transfer to the ICU/CCU often takes longer than 30 minutes, you may temporarily achieve BP control by giving the patient *nifedipine* (Adalat) 5 to 10 mg PO × one dose. Patients with longstanding hypertension are at risk from abrupt reduction of BP, which may compromise coronary and cerebral blood flow. In the presence of atherosclerosis, this circumstance can result in MI or stroke. The risk can be reduced if nifedipine is given orally as the intact capsule in an initial dose of 5 to 10 mg. The effect of this dose usually is apparent in 30 minutes, and a repeat dose of 5 to 10 mg may be given if insufficient BP lowering has been achieved. Few situations require the more rapid but less predictable response that occurs after biting and swallowing the capsule or after its sublingual administration. Aim for diastolic BP levels of around 100 mm Hg.

3. *Diazoxide* may be given in the patient's room under your resident's guidance in an emergency, such as hypertensive encephalopathy. Diazoxide is a direct arterial vasodilator and may be administered in the following regimen: *diazoxide* (Hyperstat) 50 mg IV injected over 3 minutes q15min × two doses while monitoring the BP q5min. If ineffective, increase the dosage to 100 mg IV q15min × two doses until a total of 300 to 450 mg diazoxide has been given. A diazoxide infusion at a rate of 15 mg/min is another alternative that will usually effect a smooth reduction in blood pressure within 30 minutes. Because diazoxide causes reflex tachycardia and increases CO, it is contraindicated for the treatment of hypertension in the setting of acute MI, dissecting aortic aneurysm, or intracerebral hemorrhage. Because of its potent antidiuretic effect, it is also contraindicated in hyper-

tension complicated by CHF. Diazoxide has been observed to interrupt labor during treatment for preeclampsia. Side effects due to the too rapid lowering of the BP (reflex tachycardia, angina, cerebral ischemia) can be minimized by monitoring the BP closely and by discontinuing the IV bolus or infusion when the desired BP response is achieved.

4. *Labetalol* (Normodyne, Trandate) is a combined alpha and beta blocking agent that may be given IV without intraarterial monitoring. It may be given in repeated incremental doses, beginning at 20 mg IV q10–15min (e.g., 20 mg, 20 mg, 40 mg, 40 mg). Alternatively, a labetalol infusion beginning at 2 mg/min and titrating to a BP response may be given. Labetalol is not as useful in lowering BP if the patient is already on a beta blocker.

5. A *nitroprusside infusion* may be required. In most medical situations, IV nitroprusside cannot be given to patients in general medical units because of the requirement for intraarterial blood pressure monitoring. However, you may expedite treatment by informing the ICU/CCU staff in advance when patients will be requiring IV nitroprusside infusions.

6. Once BP control is achieved through parenteral means, the patient should be started on an appropriate oral regimen to maintain satisfactory BP control.

Malignant Hypertension.   Unless accompanied by another feature (e.g., encephalopathy, pulmonary edema), you have more time to gain control of the BP. Control may be achieved by using a combination of orally effective antihypertensive drugs. Review the patient's current antihypertensive treatment. Increase to their maximum effective dose or add other agents. More aggressive approaches can wait until morning.

Preeclampsia and Eclampsia.   Treatment in these patients is complicated by the risk from both the disorder and the treatment to the fetus and to the mother. The treatment of choice near term is magnesium sulfate until delivery of the baby can be effected. Treatment should be initiated only in consultation with the patient's obstetrician. *Magnesium sulfate* is given as an IV infusion: mix 16 g of magnesium sulfate in 1 L of D5W and give a loading dose of 250 ml (4 g) IV over 20 minutes. The maintenance dose is 1 to 21 g (62.5 to 125 ml)/h or more, as required. Order a serum magnesium level every 4 hours, aiming for serum magnesium level of 6 to 8 mmol/L.

Note that magnesium sulfate does not lower BP. Local practice may include other drug selections, such as *labetalol, hydralazine,* or *nitroprusside*. Diuretics should be avoided, since these patients are usually already volume depleted, with an activated renin-angiotensin system.

Subarachnoid or Cerebral Hemorrhage.   Although there is no proof that lowering of pressure alters outcome, many neurologists will administer drugs to control elevated pressures in these situations. Unless you are familiar with the local practice, a neurologist should be consulted.

Aortic Dissection
1. Transfer the patient to the ICU/CCU immediately for intra-arterial BP monitoring and control of BP with parenteral drugs.
2. *Nitroprusside* is useful in the management of aortic dissection but should not be used without an accompanying beta blocker, which will reduce the rate of rise of intraventricular pressure and, hence, the shearing force. These beta blockers should be given parenterally, and high doses may be required as follows: *propranolol* 0.5 mg IV followed by 1 mg IV q5min until the pulse pressure is reduced to 60 mm Hg or to a total dose of 0.15 mg/kg in any 4-hour period, with a maintenance dosage of q4–6h, or *labetalol* alone may be used for aortic dissection in the same regimen as for hypertensive encephalopathy (see p. 140).

Hypertension and Pulmonary Edema or Myocardial Ischemia
1. In addition to BP control, pulmonary edema should be treated with the measures outlined in Chapter 24, p. 238.
2. Transfer the patient to the ICU/CCU for continuous ECG and intraarterial BP monitoring.
3. Notify the ICU/CCU staff that the patient will require an IV *nitroglycerin infusion*. Experimental evidence suggests that IV nitroglycerin is preferable to IV nitroprusside for the control of BP in a patient with myocardial ischemia, as nitroprusside may cause a coronary steal phenomenon, resulting in extension of the ischemic zone. It is, therefore, preferable to attempt control of the BP in a cardiac patient with IV nitroglycerin and, if unsuccessful, nitroprusside.

Catecholamine Crisis.   Pheochromocytoma is the classic condition (pallor, palpitations, and perspiration) associated with intermittent and alarmingly high blood pressures. Other conditions associated with similar, sudden, and severe increase in BP include cocaine and amphetamine abuse, major second- or third-degree burns, abrupt antihypertensive drug withdrawal, and food (cheese), drug (ephedrine), and drink (wine) interactions with MAO inhibitors (antidepressants). Currently used MAO inhibitors include tranylcypromine sulfate (Parnate), phenelzine sulfate (Nardil), and isocarboxazid (Marplan). If sudden increases in pressure are observed in patients on these drugs, the most likely cause is an interaction with a substance that is releasing the stores of catecholamines, which are overabundant because of inhibition of one of the catecholamine metabolizing enzymes (MAO).

1. Transfer the patient to the ICU/CCU for ECG and intraarterial BP monitoring.

2. Notify the ICU/CCU staff that the patient will require special parenteral antihypertensive drugs.

3. *Phentolamine mesylate*, a direct alpha blocker, may be given IV for marked elevation of BP. This drug causes a decrease in peripheral resistance and an increase in venous capacity, owing to a direct action on vascular smooth muscle. This effect may be accompanied by cardiac stimulation with tachycardia that is more than can be explained as a reflex response to peripheral vasodilation. In an emergency, 2.5 to 5 mg may be given intravenously. However, if time permits and for continuous control, phentolamine mesylate should be given at an initial dosage of 5 to 10 μg/kg/min by continuous IV infusion.

4. In cocaine-induced hypertension, *propranolol* 1 to 3 mg q2–5min IV to a maximum of 8 mg is useful in reversing hypertension and tachycardia.

5. In amphetamine-induced hypertension, *chlorpromazine* 1 mg/kg IM can reverse hypertension and hyperactivity.

17

HYPNOTICS, LAXATIVES, ANALGESICS, AND ANTIPYRETICS

Phone calls regarding the reordering of hypnotic, laxative, analgesic, and antipyretic medications are frequent. The majority of these requests can be managed over the phone.

■ HYPNOTICS
PHONE CALL
Questions

1 **Why is a hypnotic being requested?**
   The majority of requests for nighttime sedation are because of insomnia. Sleeping pills should not be prescribed for restless or agitated patients who have not been examined.
2 **Has the patient received hypnotics before?**
3 **What are the vital signs?**
4 **What was the reason for admission?**
5 **Does the patient have any of the following conditions in which hypnotics are contraindicated?**
   a. Depression: An antidepressant is the drug of choice if insomnia is a manifestation of depression.
   b. Confusion
   c. Hepatic or respiratory failure
   d. Sleep apnea
   e. Myasthenia gravis
6 **Is the patient receiving other centrally active drugs that may interact, e.g., alcohol, antidepressants, antihistamines, narcotics?**
7 **Does the patient have any drug allergies?**
   The major contraindication to a specific hypnotic is a known allergy to the drug.

Orders

A benzodiazepine is the drug of choice for short-term treatment of insomnia. Sedative effects are comparable among all benzodiazepines. Only the onset and duration of the effects differ. Table 17–1 lists the drug doses of various benzodiazepines.

Inform RN

"Will arrive at the bedside in . . . minutes."

Agitated, restless patients should be assessed before hypnotics are prescribed.

Table 17-1 □ CHARACTERISTICS OF SOME BENZODIAZEPINES

Drug	Usual Adult Dose (mg)	Time of Peak Effect (h)	Biological Half-life (h)
Premedication			
Midazolam (Versed)	0.035–0.1/kg IV		
Hypnotic			
Temazepam (Restoril)	30 PO hs	0.8–1.4	8–10
Nitrazepam (Mogadon)	5–10 PO hs	2	26
Flurazepam (Dalmane)	15–30 PO hs	1	50–100
Antianxiety			
Oxazepam (Serax)	30–120/d	1–4	4–13
Bromazepam (Lectopam)	6–30/d	1–4	12
Alprazolam (Xanax)	0.5–1.5/d	1–2	6–20
Lorazepam (Ativan)	2/d	1–6	12–15
Chlordiazepoxide (Librium)	15–75/d	2–4	20–24
Clorazepam (Traxene)	30/d	1–2	48
Ketazolam (Loftran)	15–30/d	?	50
Diazepam (Valium)	4–40/d	2	50–100

REMEMBER

1. The biological half-lives of benzodiazepines vary from 4 hours for oxazepam to 50 to 100 hours for diazepam (Valium). Accumulation can occur if the second and subsequent doses of drugs are given before the previous dose has been metabolized and excreted. Diazepam (Valium) and flurazepam (Dalmane) have active metabolites; the half-lives stated in Table 17–1 include the active metabolites.

When the drugs are prescribed once or twice, the half-life of the drug is of no great concern, since diffusion out of the brain rather than the rate of elimination from the body is the major factor responsible for the duration of effect. However, with repeated use of benzodiazepines, the drug's half-life must be taken into account, since rates of metabolism then become more important in determining the duration of effects. Flurazepam (Dalmane) given repeatedly will cause a daytime hangover, whereas oxazepam (Serax) will not. However, the shortest-acting drugs may be associated with early morning insomnia and rebound daytime anxiety.

2. Benzodiazepines should not be prescribed on a continuous nightly basis but should be discontinued temporarily once one or two nights of acceptable sleep have been achieved. Using benzodiazepines for less than 14 consecutive nights helps to prevent development of drug tolerance and dependence.

3. Be aware of the adverse effects of any drug you prescribe. The *adverse effects of benzodiazepines* are CNS depression (tiredness, drowsiness, detached feeling); headache, dizziness, ataxia, confusion, disorientation in the elderly; and psychological dependence.

4. Barbiturates and nonbarbiturate hypnotics, other than benzodiazepines, usually carry more risks than advantages as hypnotics and should be avoided.

■ LAXATIVES

Laxatives are overused by the public at large. However, hospitalized patients require laxatives in certain circumstances as follows: after acute MI to limit straining, during the administration of narcotics, during prolonged bedrest, and during evacuation of the bowels before abdominal surgery and some GI diagnostic procedures. The solutions employed in *enemas* have either hypertonic properties to stimulate rectal peristalsis or surfactant properties to achieve softening of impacted feces.

PHONE CALL
Questions

1 **Why is a laxative being requested?**
   The frequency of bowel movements is highly variable in the normal population, ranging from twice daily to once every 3 days. Make certain you know what this patient's normal bowel pattern is before prescribing a laxative.

2 **Has the patient received laxatives before? If so, which ones have been tried so far?**

3 **What are the vital signs?**

4 **What was the reason for admission?**

5 **When was a rectal examination last performed?**
   Fecal impaction, which requires a rectal examination for diagnosis (and sometimes for treatment!) is a relative contraindication to oral laxative use.

6 **Does the patient have nausea, vomiting, or abdominal pain?**
   These symptoms suggest an acute GI disorder.

Orders

Table 17–2 lists the drug doses of selective laxatives and Table 17–3 those of enemas. Bowel movements can be increased in frequency by liquefying the stool. Both bulk and osmotic laxatives increase the water content in the intestine. An increase in the frequency of bowel movements can also be induced by stool softeners and colon-irritating drugs that increase peristalsis.

Inform RN

"Will arrive at the bedside in . . . minutes."

The only time you need to assess a patient when a laxative has been requested is when the patient has associated nausea, vomiting, or abdominal pain or when fecal impaction is suspected. (See Chapter 5 for the assessment and management of abdominal pain.)

REMEMBER

1. When a patient is constipated (unless there is fecal impaction), an oral laxative is the treatment of choice. If the oral

Table 17–2 □ SOME CHARACTERISTICS OF LAXATIVES

Drug	Dose	Comments
Bulk Forming		
Psyllium hydrophilic mucilloid (Metamucil and others)	3–6.5 g PO once to TID	Cellulose binds drugs e.g., digoxin
Surface Active		
Docusate (dioctyl sodium sulfosuccinate, Colace)	100 mg PO TID 50 mg/90 ml enema fluid	See p. 347
Lubricant		
Mineral oil	Emulsion 15 ml BID	Impairs the absorption of fat-soluble vitamins
Osmotic		
Glycerin	2.67 g suppository	Onset in 30 min
Magnesium citrate oral solution (Sorbitol)	75–100 ml of a 15 g/300 ml solution 7–21 ml of a 70% solution	Do not use in renal impairment; often used with cation exchange resins
Stimulant		
Anthraquinones (cascara, senna)	Variable	Onset in 6 h; urine may be brown
Diphenylmethanes (e.g., Bisacodyl)	5–15 mg PO 10 mg PR	See p. 343
Castor oil	15–60 ml	May give profound evacuation

Table 17–3 □ EXAMPLES OF ENEMAS

Sodium Phosphate and Sodium Biphosphate (Fleet enema)

Onset: Immediate

Caution: Do not use when nausea, vomiting, or abdominal pain is present.

Usual adult dose: 60 to 120 ml (6 gm sodium phosphate and 16 gm sodium biphosphate/100 ml). (Available in a disposable plastic container.)

Use: Acute evacuation of the bowel prior to diagnostic procedures; acute constipation.

Bisacodyl (Fleet Bisacodyl)

Onset: Immediate

Caution: Do not use when nausea, vomiting, or abdominal pain is present. Avoid in pregnancy and MI. May worsen orthostatic hypotension, weakness, and incoordination in the elderly.

Usual adult dose: 37.5 ml (10 mg/30 ml). (Available in disposable plastic containers.)

Use: Acute evacuation of the bowel prior to diagnostic procedures; acute constipation.

Mineral Oil (Fleet Mineral Oil Enema)

Onset: Immediate

Caution: Do not use when nausea, vomiting, or abdominal pain is present.

Usual adult dose: 60 to 120 ml. (Available in disposable plastic containers.)

Use: Impacted feces.

---

laxative fails, a stronger-acting laxative can be used, and, failing this, a suppository is prescribed next. Finally, enemas can be used as follows: first, a hypertonic enema solution (e.g., Fleet) and last, an oil retention enema.

2. When there is fecal impaction, an oil-based enema is the treatment of choice.

3. Soapsuds enemas are no longer used. They have been replaced by hypertonic enema solutions.

■ ANALGESICS

Most hospital pharmacies do not allow narcotic medication orders to stand indefinitely. Narcotic medications need to be reordered every 3 to 5 days, depending on the individual medical institution. Consequently, if the housestaff fail to reorder these medications during the day, you may be called to do so at night.

Table 17–4 □ CHARACTERISTICS OF SOME COMMONLY USED ANALGESICS IN MILD TO MODERATE PAIN

Drug	Usual Adult Dose (mg)	Comments
Aspirin (acetylsalicylic acid)	325–650 q4–6h PO	See p. 342
Diflunisal (Dolobid)	1000, then 500 q12h PO	Salicylate derivative
Ibuprofen (Motrin)	200 q6–8h PO	NSAID
Naproxen (Naprosyn)	200 q12h PO	NSAID
Fenoprofen (Nalfon)	300 q6–8h PO	NSAID
Acetaminophen (Paracetamol, Tylenol)	325–1000 q4–6h PO	See pp. 340–341
Codeine	30–60 SC/PO/IM q4–6h	More effective than propoxyphene and less addicting than oxycodone
Propoxyphene (Darvon)	100 q4–6h PO	Equipotent to 650 mg acetylsalicylic acid

PHONE CALL

Questions

1 **Why is an analgesic being requested?**
The majority of requests are for reordering of medications.

2 **How severe is the pain?**
This question will help to determine whether a nonnarcotic analgesic may be sufficient.

Table 17–5 □ CHARACTERISTICS OF SOME NARCOTIC DRUGS

	Usual Adult Dose		
Drug	Oral (mg)	SC/IM/IV (mg)	Duration of Effect (h)
Morphine (MS Contin)	20–30	10	4–5*
Anileridine (Leritine)	75	25	2–4
Hydromorphone (Dilaudid)	4	1.5	4–5
Meperidine (Demerol)	300	75–100	2–4
Pentazocine (Talwin)	180	60	2–4

*Modified release preparations are available that can be given every 12 hours.

3 Is this a new problem?
The new onset of undiagnosed pain requires you to assess the patient, at the bedside, before ordering an analgesic medication.
4 What are the vital signs?
The onset of fever in association with pain suggests a localized infectious process.
5 What was the reason for admission?
6 Does the patient have any drug allergies?

Orders

See Tables 17–4 and 17–5 for drug dosages of selected analgesics.

Inform RN

"Will arrive at bedside in . . . minutes."

Any undiagnosed pain, new onset of severe pain, or change in character of previous pain requires you to assess the patient at the bedside before ordering an analgesic.

REMEMBER

If reversal of a narcotic overdose is required, the following are recommended.

1. *Reversal of postoperative narcotic depression. Naloxone* (Narcan) 0.2 to 2.0 mg IV q5min until the desired improved level of consciousness is achieved (maximum total dose 10 mg). Doses q1–2h may be required to maintain reversal of CNS depression.
2. *Reversal of suspected narcotic overdose.* If the patient is comatose, intubation for airway protection should be undertaken before reversal. Abrupt reversal may induce nausea and vomiting with the attendant risk of aspiration pneumonia. Give *naloxone* (Narcan) 0.2 mg IV, SC, or IM q5min for several doses. If the initial dosages are ineffective, the dose may be increased incrementally to a maximum total dose of 10 mg.
3. *Adverse effects of abrupt narcotic reversal.* Nausea and vomiting, if provoked in the patient with an unprotected airway, may result in aspiration pneumonia. Hypertension and tachycardia can occur during narcotic reversal and may result in CHF in the patient with poor left ventricular function.

■ ANTIPYRETICS

Antipyretics should not be prescribed in the adult patient with fever unless the cause of the fever is known or the patient is symptomatic from the fever itself. (Refer to Chapter 12 for the approach to the febrile patient. Table 17–4 lists the dosages and side effects of acetaminophen and aspirin.)

18

HYPOTENSION AND SHOCK

Hypotension is a common call at night. Don't panic. Remember that hypotension does not become shock until there is evidence of inadequate tissue perfusion. An adequate BP is required to perfuse three vital organs—the *brain, heart* and *kidneys*. Some patients normally have systolic blood pressures in the range of 85 to 100 mm Hg. The BP is usually adequate as long as the patient is not confused, disoriented, or unconscious, is not having angina, and is passing urine. However, a BP of 105/70 mm Hg may result in serious hypoperfusion in a patient who is normally hypertensive.

PHONE CALL

Questions

1 **What is the BP?**
2 **What is the HR?**
3 **What is the temperature?**
   "Fever + hypotension" suggests impending septic shock.
4 **Is the patient conscious?**
5 **Is the patient having chest pain?**
6 **Is there evidence of bleeding?**
7 **Has the patient been given IV contrast material or an antibiotic within the last 6 hours?**
   If you are called to see a hypotensive patient in the x-ray department or a patient who has recently returned to the room from an x-ray procedure involving the administration of IV contrast material, your primary thought should be that the patient may be having an anaphylactic reaction.
8 **What was the admitting diagnosis?**

Orders

1. If the information provided over the telephone supports the possibility of impending or established shock, order the following.
   a. A large-bore (#16 if possible) IV immediately, if not already in place. IV access is a high priority in the hypotensive patient.
   b. Place the patient in reverse Trendelenburg position (i.e., head of the bed down and foot of the bed up). Although hypotension should be assessed immediately, if you are unable to get to the bedside for 10 to 15 minutes, also ask the nurse to give 500 ml NS IV as rapidly as possible.

   c. ABG tray at bedside. Identification and correction of hypoxia and acidemia are essential in the management of shock.

   d. Oxygen 4 to 10 L by face mask while awaiting ABG.

2. If there is a suspicion of *anaphylaxis*, ask the RN to have a premixed syringe of IV epinephrine from the cardiac arrest cart available.

3. If the admitting diagnosis is *GI bleed* or there is visible evidence of blood loss

   a. Ensure that the patient has blood on hold. If not, order a stat crossmatch for 2, 4, or 6 units of packed RBCs depending on your estimate of blood loss.

   b. Hb stat. *Caution:* The Hb may be normal during an acute hemorrhage and drop only with correction of the intravascular volume by a shift of fluid from the interstitial and intracellular spaces, or by fluid therapy. (Refer to Chapter 13 for further investigation and management of GI bleeds.)

4. If an arrhythmia or ischemic myocardial event is suspected, order a stat ECG and rhythm strip. These may help you identify a rapid heart rhythm or an acute MI, which may be responsible for hypotension.

Inform RN

"Will arrive at bedside in . . . minutes."

Hypotension requires you to see the patient immediately.

ELEVATOR THOUGHTS (What causes hypotension or shock?)

- Cardiogenic causes
- Hypovolemia
- Sepsis
- Anaphylaxis

Two formulas, as follows, are useful to remember when considering the causes of hypotension.

$$\text{Blood pressure (BP)} = \text{cardiac output (CO)} \times \text{total peripheral resistance (TPR)}$$

$$\text{Cardiac output (CO)} = \text{heart rate (HR)} \times \text{stroke volume (SV)}$$

From these formulas, it can be seen that hypotension results from a fall in either cardiac output or total peripheral resistance. *Cardiogenic causes* result from a fall in cardiac output due to either a fall in heart rate (e.g., heart block) or a fall in stroke volume (e.g., pump failure). *Hypovolemia* reduces stroke volume, and hence cardiac output falls. *Sepsis* and *anaphylaxis* cause hypotension by lowering TPR.

MAJOR THREAT TO LIFE

- Shock

Remember that hypotension does not become shock until there is evidence of inadequate tissue perfusion. As you will see, shock is a relatively easy diagnosis to make. Your goal is to identify and correct the cause of hypotension before it results in hypoperfusion of vital organs.

BEDSIDE

Quick Look Test

Does the patient look well (comfortable), sick (uncomfortable or distressed), or critical (about to die)?

A patient with hypotension but adequate tissue perfusion usually looks well. However, once perfusion of vital organs becomes compromised, the patient will look sick or critical.

Airway and Vital Signs

Is the airway clear?

If the patient is obtunded and cannot protect his or her airway, endotracheal intubation will be required. Ask the RN to notify the ICU/CCU immediately. Roll the patient onto the left side to avoid aspiration until intubation is achieved.

Is the patient breathing?

Assess respiration by checking the respiratory rate, position of the trachea, chest expansion, and auscultation. All patients in shock should receive high-flow oxygen. If acute respiratory distress and marked respiratory effort accompany shock, intubation and ventilation may be necessary.

Assess the circulation.

1. If hypotension is not severe, examine for postural changes. A postural rise on standing in HR >15 beats/min, a fall in systolic BP >15 mm Hg, or any fall in diastolic BP indicates significant hypovolemia.
2. Time the HR. Most causes of hypotension are accompanied by a compensatory reflex sinus tachycardia. If the patient is experiencing bradycardia or if you suspect a rhythm other than sinus tachycardia, refer to page 153 for further evaluation and management.
3. Is the patient in *shock?* This should take less than 20 seconds to determine.

VITALS	Repeat now
CVS	Pulse volume, JVP
	Skin temperature and color
	Capillary refill (normal <2 seconds)
NEURO	Mental status

Shock is a clinical diagnosis: systolic BP < 90 mm Hg with evidence of inadequate tissue perfusion, e.g., of the skin (cold, clammy, and cyanotic) and of the CNS (agitation, confusion, lethargy, coma). In fact, the kidney is a sensitive indicator of shock (urine output <20 ml/h), but immediate placement of a Foley catheter should not take priority over resuscitation measures.

What is the temperature?

An elevated temperature *or* hypothermia (<36°C) suggests sepsis. However, remember that sepsis may appear in some patients, especially the elderly, with a normal temperature. Hence, the absence of fever does not rule out the possibility of septic shock.

Look at the ECG and take the pulse.

Bradycardia.   If the resting HR is <*50/min* in the presence of hypotension, suspect one of three things as follows.

1. Vasovagal attack. If this is the case, the patient is usually normotensive by the time you arrive. Look for retrospective evidence of straining, Valsalva's maneuver, pain, or some other stimulus to vagal outflow. If vasovagal attack is suspected and there is persistent bradycardia despite leg elevation, give *atropine* 0.5 mg IV. If not effective, the same dose may be repeated q15min up to a total dose of 2 mg IV.
2. Autonomic dysfunction. The patient may be on a beta blocker or calcium channel blocker and has been given too much, resulting in hypotension, or is hypotensive for some other reason but is unable to generate a tachycardia because of beta blockade, calcium channel blockade, underlying sick sinus syndrome, or autonomic neuropathy. If the systolic BP is <90 mm Hg, administer *atropine* 0.5 mg IV. If not effective, the same dose may be repeated q5min up to a total dose of 2 mg IV.
3. Heart block. The patient may be suffering from a heart block (e.g., acute MI). Obtain a stat ECG to document the dysrhythmia. If systolic BP is <90 mm Hg, administer *atropine* 0.5 mg IV. If not effective, the same dose may be repeated q5min up to a total dose of 2 mg IV. Refer to Chapter 15 for further investigation and management of heart block.

Tachycardia.   A compensatory sinus tachycardia is an expected appropriate response in the hypotensive patient. Ensure by looking at the ECG that the patient does not have one of the following three rapid heart rhythms, which may themselves cause hypotension due to decreased diastolic filling.

1. Atrial fibrillation with rapid ventricular response (Fig. 18–1)

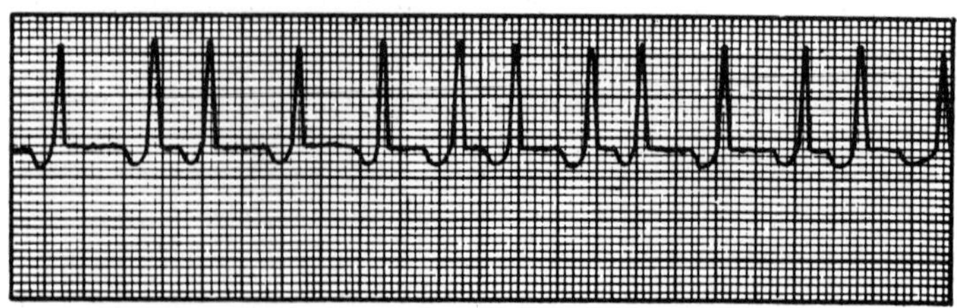

Figure 18–1 □ Atrial fibrillation with rapid ventricular response.

2. Supraventricular tachycardia (Fig. 18–2)
3. Ventricular tachycardia (Fig. 18–3)

If any one of these three rhythms is present in the hypotensive patient

- Ask the RN to notify your resident immediately.
- Ask the RN to bring the cardiac arrest cart into the room.
- Attach the patient to the ECG monitor.
- Ask the RN to draw up *diazepam* (Valium) 10 mg IV in a syringe.
- Ensure that an IV is in place. (Refer to Chapter 15, p. 116, for further treatment of rapid heart rates associated with hypotension.)

Selective Physical Examination

Determine the *cause* of hypotension or shock by *assessing the volume status.*

Only cardiogenic shock will result in a clinical picture of *volume overload.* Hypovolemic, septic, or anaphylactic shock will result in a clinical picture of *volume depletion.*

VITALS	Repeat now
HEENT	Elevated JVP (CHF), flat neck veins (volume depletion)
RESP	Stridor (anaphylaxis)
	Crackles ± pleural effusions (CHF)
	Wheezes (anaphylaxis, CHF)
CVS	Cardiac apex displaced laterally, S_3 (CHF)
ABD	Hepatomegaly with positive HJR (CHF)
EXT	Presacral or ankle edema (CHF)

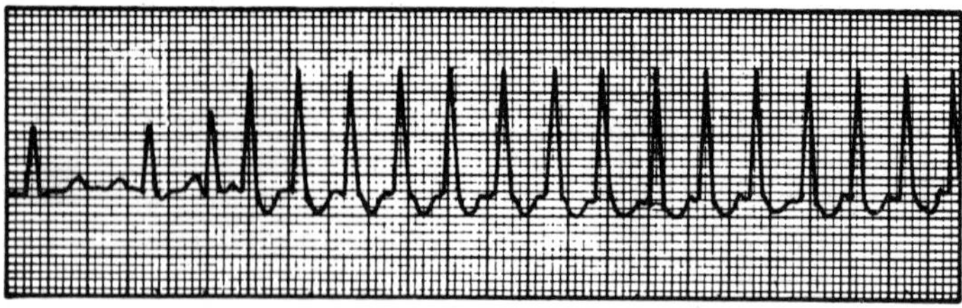

Figure 18–2 □ Supraventricular tachycardia.

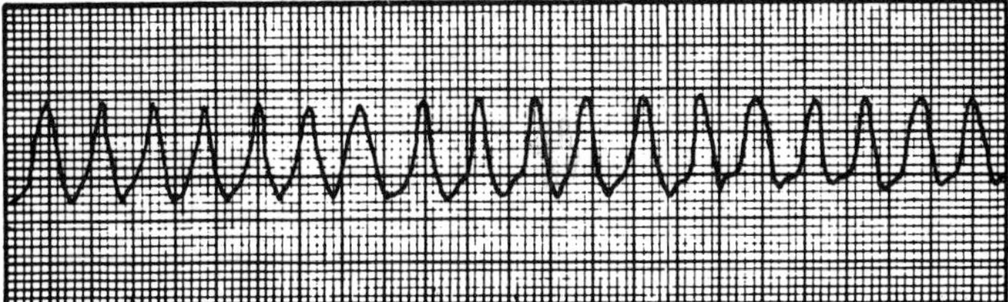

Figure 18–3 □ Ventricular tachycardia.

SKIN   Urticaria (anaphylaxis)
RECTAL   Melena or hematochezia (GI bleed)

Remember that *wheezing* may be seen in both CHF and anaphylaxis. Administration of epinephrine may save the life of someone with anaphylaxis but may kill someone with CHF. Anaphylactic shock comes on relatively suddenly and nearly always an inciting factor (e.g., IV contrast material, penicillin) can be identified. Usually, other clues, such as angioedema or urticaria, are present.

Management

What immediate measures need to be taken to correct or prevent shock from occurring?

Normalize the intravascular volume. In the case of *cardiogenic shock* (volume overload), stop the IV NS bolus (ordered over the phone) and replace with D5W TKVO. Proper management also will require preload reduction and further investigation, as outlined in Chapter 24.

All other forms of shock will require volume expansion. This can be achieved quickly by elevation of the legs (i.e., reverse Trendelenburg) and administration of repeated small volumes (200 to 300 ml over 15 to 30 minutes) of an IV fluid that will at least temporarily stay in the intravascular space, e.g., NS or Ringer's lactate. Reassess volume status after each bolus of IV fluid, aiming for a JVP of 2 to 3 cm H_2O above the sternal angle and concomitant normalization of HR, BP, and tissue perfusion.

If the patient is in *anaphylactic shock,* treat rapidly as follows.

1. IV NS wide open until normotensive.
2. *Epinephrine* 0.3 mg (3 ml of 1 : 10,000 solution) IV immediately or 0.3 mg (0.3 ml of a 1 : 1000 solution) SC immediately, with repeat doses q10–15min if indicated. Because the skin is usually hypoperfused during shock, it is better to administer epinephrine IV rather than SC.
3. *Salbutamol* (Ventolin) 2.5 mg/3 ml NS by nebulizer.
4. *Diphenhydramine* (Benadryl) 50 mg IV.
5. *Hydrocortisone* 250 mg IV bolus, followed by 100 mg IV q6h.

Correct hypoxia and acidemia. If the patient is in shock, obtain

ABGs and administer O_2. If the arterial pH is <7.2 in the absence of respiratory acidosis, order $NaHCO_3$ 0.5 to 1 amp (44.6 mmol) IV. Monitor the effects of your treatment by repeat ABGs every 30 minutes until the patient is stabilized.

While restoring the intravascular volume, determine the specific cause of hypotension or shock.

Cardiogenic Shock. This is commonly a result of acute MI. Order stat ECG, portable CXR, and cardiac enzyme tests. However, any of the CHF *etiological factors* listed on p. 239 may be operative.

Be certain that the patient is in CHF! Patients with four other conditions can experience hypotension and elevated JVP, as follows.
1. *Acute cardiac tamponade* may cause elevated JVP, arterial hypotension, and soft heart sounds (Beck's triad). Suspect this as the diagnosis if there is a pulsus paradoxus of >10 mm Hg during relaxed respirations (see p. 234).
2. A massive *pulmonary embolus* can cause hypotension, elevated JVP, and cyanosis and may be accompanied by additional evidence of acute right ventricular overload (e.g., positive HJR, RV heave, loud P_2, right-sided S_3, murmur of tricuspid insufficiency).
3. *Superior vena cava obstruction* may cause hypotension and elevated JVP that does not vary with respiration. Additional features may include headache, facial plethora, conjunctival injection, and dilatation of collateral veins on the upper thorax and neck.
4. *Tension pneumothorax* can also cause hypotension and elevated JVP due to positive intrathoracic pressure that decreases venous return to the heart. Look for severe dyspnea, unilateral hyperresonance, and decreased air entry, with tracheal shift *away* from the involved side. If a tension pneumothorax is suspected, do not wait for x-ray confirmation. Call for your resident and get a 14- to 16-gauge needle ready to aspirate the pleural space at the second intercostal space in the midclavicular line on the affected side. This is a medical emergency!

Hypovolemia. If there is suspicion that *GI bleed* or another *acute blood loss* is responsible for hypotension, refer to Chapter 13 for further investigation and management.

Excess fluid losses via sweating, vomiting, diarrhea, and polyuria and *third space losses* (e.g., pancreatitis, peritonitis) will respond to simple intravascular volume expansion with NS or Ringer's lactate and correction of the underlying problem.

Drugs are common causes of hypotension, resulting from relative hypovolemia due to their effects on the heart and peripheral circulation. Common offenders are morphine, meperidine, quinidine, nitroglycerin, beta blockers, calcium entry blockers, captopril, enalapril, and antihypertensives. In these instances, hypotension is seldom accompanied by evidence of inadequate tissue perfusion and usually can be avoided by reducing the dose or altering the schedule of administration of the drug.

Reverse Trendelenburg position or a small volume (300 to 500 ml) of NS or Ringer's lactate usually suffices to support the BP until the effect of most drugs wears off. The hypotension of narcotics (morphine, meperidine) can be reversed by *naloxone hydrochloride* (Narcan), 0.2 to 2.0 mg (maximum total dose 10 mg) IV, SC, or IM q5min until the desired degree of reversal is seen.

Sepsis. Occasionally, intravascular volume repletion and appropriate antibiotics are sufficient to resolve septic shock. Continuing hypotension despite intravascular volume repletion, however, requires ICU/CCU admission for inotropic or vasopressor support.

Anaphylactic Shock. This must be recognized and treated immediately to prevent fatal laryngeal edema. Treat as described on p. 155.

REMEMBER

1. Consider *toxic shock syndrome* in any hypotensive premenopausal female. Ask about tampon use, or if the patient is obtunded, perform a pelvic examination and remove the tampon, if present.
2. The skin is not a vital organ but gives valuable evidence of inadequate tissue perfusion. Remember that during the early stage of septic shock, the skin may be warm and dry owing to abnormal peripheral vasodilation.
3. Adequate BP is required to perfuse the three vital organs—the *brain, heart,* and *kidney.* After you have successfully rescued your patient from an episode of hypotension, look out for hypotensive sequelae during the next few days. Not surprisingly, the common sequelae involve these three vital organs.
   a. *Brain.* Thrombotic stroke in a patient with underlying cerebrovascular disease.
   b. *Heart.* MI in a patient with preexisting atherosclerosis.
   c. *Kidney.* Acute tubular necrosis. Monitor urine output and check urea and creatinine levels in a few days.

Centrilobular hepatic necrosis (manifested by jaundice and elevated liver enzymes) and bowel ischemia or infarction also may be seen as sequelae of hypotension in the critically ill patient.

19

LEG PAIN

The easiest approach to leg pain at night is to identify what part of the leg hurts. Most leg pain originates from the muscle, joints, bone, or the vascular supply to the legs. However, there are also several referred causes of leg pain.

PHONE CALL

Questions

1. **What part of the leg hurts? Is the leg swollen or discolored?**
2. **What are the vital signs?**
3. **Was the pain sudden in onset, or is it chronic?**
4. **What was the reason for admission?**
5. **Has there been a recent leg injury or fracture? Does the patient have a leg cast on?**
   Leg pain following a leg injury, fracture, or casting raises the possibility of a compartment syndrome.

Orders

None.

Inform RN

"Will arrive at the bedside in . . . minutes."

An acute pulseless limb, fever, or severe leg pain of any etiology requires you to see the patient immediately. Increasing leg pain 24 to 48 hours after casting also requires you to see the patient immediately.

ELEVATOR THOUGHTS (What causes leg pain?)

Bone and Joint Disease
- Lumbar disc disease (sciatica)
- Arthritis
  - Septic (*Staphylococcus aureus, Neisseria gonorrhoeae, Streptococcus pneumoniae, Haemophilus influenzae,* and gram-negative bacilli)
  - Inflammatory (gout, pseudogout, RA, SLE)
  - Degenerative (osteoarthritis)
- Osteomyelitis
- Ruptured Baker's cyst
- Skeletal tumors

Vascular Disease
- Arterial disease
  - Acute arterial insufficiency (e.g., thromboembolism, cholesterol embolism)
  - Arteriosclerosis obliterans (chronic arterial insufficiency)
  - Thromboangiitis obliterans (Buerger's disease)
- Venous disease
  - Deep venous thrombosis
  - Superficial thrombophlebitis

Muscle, Soft Tissue, or Nerve Pain
- Compartment syndrome
- Cellulitis
- Neuropathies (diabetes)
- Reflex sympathetic dystrophy syndrome
- Erythema nodosum
- Nodular liquefying panniculitis
- Benign nocturnal leg cramps

MAJOR THREAT TO LIFE
- Loss of limb from arterial insufficiency
- Pulmonary embolism from a DVT
- Septic arthritis
- Compartment syndrome

Acute arterial occlusion of the lower extremity, if left untreated, may result in gangrene in as little as 6 hours. A *deep venous thrombosis* may result in severe respiratory insufficiency or death if pulmonary embolism occurs. Although *septic arthritis* is not likely to result in loss of life overnight, its prompt recognition and management are essential to avoid permanent joint damage. Similarly, an unrecognized *compartment syndrome* can result in permanent ischemic muscle contractures within hours.

BEDSIDE

Although the list of possible diagnoses of leg pain is long, only the four Major Threats to Life require emergency treatment at night. You should perform a systematic inspection, looking for evidence of each of these in the patient with leg pain.

Quick Look Test

Does the patient look well (comfortable), sick (uncomfortable or distressed), or critical (about to die)?

Most patients with significant leg pain lie still, appear apprehensive, and are reluctant to move the affected extremity.

Airway and Vital Signs

Leg pain should not compromise the vital signs. However, abnormalities in the vital signs may provide clues to the cause of leg pain.

What is the HR? Is it regular or irregular?
Pain from any cause may result in tachycardia. However, an irregularly irregular rhythm suggests atrial fibrillation, raising the possibility of an embolic event.

What is the BP?
Pain or anxiety from any cause may raise the BP.

What is the temperature?
Fever suggests inflammation, as may be seen with DVT or septic arthritis.

■ ACUTE ARTERIAL INSUFFICIENCY

Selective History

Was the pain sudden in onset, suggesting an arterial embolism?

Is there a history of underlying cardiac disease (e.g., atrial fibrillation, mitral stenosis, ventricular aneurysm, prosthetic heart valve) that might predispose to arterial embolization?

Is there a history of intermittent claudication, which suggests long-standing chronic arterial insufficiency?

Selective Physical Examination

Look for the 4 Ps.
1. Pain
2. Pallor
3. Pulselessness
4. Paresthesias
These suggest a major arterial embolism.

SKIN	Pallor
	Focal areas of gangrene
	Bilateral brawny discoloration (arteriosclerosis obliterans)
	Diminished temperature, especially if unilateral
CVS	Check the femoral, popliteal, and pedal pulses.
	In an acute or chronic arterial occlusion, pulses will be absent distal to the site of occlusion.
NEURO	Paresthesias, diminished light touch in a stocking distribution

An *acute arterial embolism* tends to cause unilateral pain, pallor, paresthesias, and pulselessness (the 4 Ps), whereas *chronic arterial insufficiency* due to arteriosclerosis obliterans usually involves both lower limbs to a variable extent, with bilateral diminished pulses, trophic skin changes, loss of limb hair, and dependent rubor. Do not be fooled, however—although the presentation of arteriosclerosis obliterans is almost always chronic and progressive, fresh thrombosis on top of a fixed atherosclerotic plaque may completely obstruct arterial flow, resulting in an *acute on chronic* presentation.

Management

Acute arterial insufficiency is a surgical emergency. If you suspect that an arterial embolism has occluded a major artery

1. Notify your resident and a vascular surgeon immediately.
2. Draw a stat blood sample for CBC and aPTT.
3. If there are no contraindications, begin heparin 100 units/ kg IV bolus, followed by a maintenance infusion of 1000 to 1600 units/h, with the lower range selected for patients with a higher risk of bleeding. See page 242 for precautions in the use of heparin.
4. If limb viability is threatened, the patient may require emergency thrombectomy or bypass. If limb viability is not a concern, direct intraarterial streptokinase may achieve lysis of a thrombus, but this should only be initiated under the guidance of a vascular surgeon.

Chronic arterial insufficiency due to arteriosclerosis obliterans is not usually an emergency unless an acute thrombosis occurs on top of a longstanding fixed plaque. In this case, direct intraarterial streptokinase or urokinase may result in clot lysis, but this should be administered only under the guidance of a vascular surgeon. The more common scenario is the complaint of rest pain in a patient with chronic intermittent claudication. If there is no immediate concern regarding limb viability, rest pain can be treated with nonnarcotic analgesics, such as *acetaminophen* 325 to 650 mg PO q4h PRN, and placing the affected extremity in the dependent position. More definitive therapy, including lumbar sympathectomy or direct arterial surgery, is seldom required on an emergency basis.

■ DEEP VENOUS THROMBOSIS

Selective History

Look for predisposing causes.
- Stasis
  - Prolonged bedrest
  - Immobilized limb
  - Obesity
  - CHF
  - Pregnancy
- Vein injury
  - Trauma (especially hip fractures)
  - Surgery (especially abdominal, pelvic, and orthopedic procedures)

- Hypercoagulability
  - Malignancy
  - Inflammatory bowel disease
  - Nephrotic syndrome
  - Use of birth control pills
  - Deficiencies of antithrombin III, protein C or S

Selective Physical Examination

Look for the following signs involving the calf or thigh:
- Tenderness
- Erythema
- Edema
  Subtle degrees of swelling may be appreciated by measuring and comparing the circumferences of both calves or thighs at several different levels.
- Warmth
- Distention of the overlying superficial veins
- *Homan's sign:* With the patient supine, flex the knee and then sharply dorsiflex the ankle. Pain in the calf during ankle dorsiflexion is supportive evidence of a calf deep venous thrombosis; its absence in no way excludes the diagnosis.

Management

A *deep venous thrombosis* should be recognized and treated immediately to prevent embolization and pulmonary infarction. If your suspicion of a DVT is high, you are obligated to begin anticoagulation without further confirmation of the diagnosis at this point. Heparin will inhibit further growth and promote resolution of the thrombus. However, before ordering heparin, ensure that the patient has no history of bleeding disorders, peptic ulcer, and intracranial disease, e.g., recent stroke, subarachnoid hemorrhage, tumor, and recent surgery. All are contraindications to anticoagulation. These patients will require confirmation of DVT by an imaging modality and, if DVT is documented, consultation for consideration of interruption of the inferior vena cava by the insertion of a transvenous caval device or, occasionally, IVC ligation.

Draw a blood sample for CBC, aPTT, and platelet count immediately. If there are no contraindications, begin *heparin* 100 units/kg IV bolus (usual dose 5000 to 10,000 units IV) and follow with a maintenance infusion of 1000 to 1600 units/h, with the lower range selected for patients with a higher risk of bleeding.

Heparin should be delivered by infusion pump, with maintenance dosing ordered as in the following example: heparin 25,000 units/500 ml D5W to run at 20 ml/h = 1000 units/h. It is dangerous to put large doses of heparin in small volume IV bags, since runaway IVs filled with heparin can result in serious overdose.

Heparin and warfarin are dangerous drugs because of their potential for causing bleeding disorders. Write and double check your heparin orders carefully. Also, measure platelet counts once or twice a week to detect reversible heparin-induced thrombocytopenia, which may occur at any time while a patient is on heparin.

After starting heparin, the diagnosis should be confirmed in the morning by impedance plethysmography, lower limb Doppler studies, or a nuclear venogram (radiofibrinogen scanning).

Monitor the aPTT q4–6h and adjust the heparin maintenance dose until the aPTT is in the therapeutic range (1.8 to 2.8 × normal). After this, daily aPTTs are sufficient. Initial measurements of aPTT are made only to ensure adequate anticoagulation.

Continue IV heparin for 5 days. Add oral *warfarin* (Coumadin) on the first day, beginning at 10 mg PO and titrating the dose to achieve a PT with an international normalized ratio of 2.0 to 3.0 (this corresponds to a PT of 1.3 to 1.5 × control, using rabbit brain thromboplastin; if you are unsure of the method used by your laboratory, call them and ask). Measure aPTT and PT daily during this initial adjustment phase. Attainment of a therapeutic PT will usually take 5 days, at which time the heparin can be discontinued.

Numerous drugs interfere with warfarin metabolism to increase or decrease the PT. Before prescribing any drug to a patient on warfarin, look up its effect on warfarin metabolism and monitor PTs carefully if an interaction is anticipated.

Write an order that the patient should receive no aspirin-containing drugs, sulfinpyrazone, dipyridamole, or thrombolytic agents and no IM injections while on anticoagulation.

Ask your patient daily about signs of bleeding or bruising. Instruct your patient that prolonged pressure after venipuncture will be required to prevent local bruising while on anticoagulation.

■ SEPTIC ARTHRITIS
Selective History

In septic arthritis, the patient most often points to the painful joint involved. Your job is to determine whether the joint in question is infected or not. Two rules-of-thumb can be helpful. (1) If a single joint is swollen, red, and tender, it should be considered septic until proven otherwise. (2) In a patient with multiple joint involvement (as may be seen with rheumatoid arthritis or other inflammatory arthritides) if a single joint is inflamed out of proportion to the other joints involved, the joint in question should be considered possibly infected.

Look for predisposing factors.

Has there been a penetrating wound?

Has there been recent arthoscopy or intraarticular injection of steroids?

Does the patient have a joint prosthesis or other foreign body in the involved joint?

Has there been bacteremia (e.g., endocarditis)?

Selective Physical Examination

Fever may be present. The knee joint is most commonly affected. The joint is swollen, tender, restricted in range, and erythematous. These signs may be less marked, however, in the elderly patient or the patient on steroids.

Septic arthritis of the hip is often missed because of the deep location of the hip joint—swelling may not be detected easily. Conditions involving the hip joint are sometimes only manifested by referred pain to the groin, buttocks, lateral thigh, or anterior aspect of the knee. The affected extremity is usually held in adduction, flexion, and internal rotation.

Management

Septic arthritis is a medical emergency. Any suspected septic joint should be aspirated without delay. You will need your resident's help or the assistance of a rheumatologist to perform joint aspiration. The diagnosis of septic arthritis is made by demonstrating microorganisms on Gram's stain of synovial fluid. Prompt treatment with appropriate antibiotics is required, should not await confirmation by culture, and should be directed by the results of the Gram's stain. When microorganisms are not seen on the synovial fluid sample, empiric antibiotics should be administered. A good choice is a penicillinase-resistant penicillin and gentamicin until culture and sensitivity results are available.

Synovial fluid should be sent for
- WBC count and differential
- Glucose determination
- Gram's stain
- Aerobic and anaerobic cultures
- Gonococcal culture
- TB stain and culture

Blood samples should be sent for
- Simultaneous serum glucose determination
- Blood cultures for aerobes and anaerobes
- Gonococcal culture

In septic arthritis, the synovial fluid is usually cloudy or purulent, WBC $\geq$ 10,000/mm^3 with $\geq$90% neutrophils. Synovial glucose is $\leq$50% of a simultaneously drawn serum glucose.

■ COMPARTMENT SYNDROME

Some muscle groups in the leg are surrounded by well-fitted fascial sheaths, leaving no space for swelling should an injury occur. An increase in pressure within these sheaths may interfere with the circulation to the nerves and muscles within the compartment, resulting in a compartment syndrome.

Selective History

Look for predisposing causes.
- Recent fractures of the tibia and fibula
- Overly tight pressure bandages or casts
- Blunt leg trauma
- Prolonged, unaccustomed, vigorous exertion

Selective Physical Examination

The anterior compartment of the leg is affected most commonly. It contains the anterior tibial muscle, the extensor hallucis longus, and the extensor digitorum longus muscles.

Look for
- Pain and tenderness over the involved compartment
- Overlying skin possibly erythematous, glossy, and edematous
- Sensory loss on the dorsum of the foot between the first and second toes
- Increasing pain on passive stretching of the involved muscle groups
- Weakness of dorsiflexion of the ankles and toes (footdrop)

Caution: Do not be fooled by the pulses! The pedal pulses are rarely obliterated by the compartment swelling and may be easy to feel despite progressive muscle and nerve damage within the compartment.

If the patient has had a tibial fracture and has been casted, it may be difficult to examine the affected extremity properly. Any such patient who develops increasing pain 24 to 48 hours after casting should be suspected of having a compartment syndrome and should have the cast removed so that the leg can be properly examined.

Management

Once the diagnosis of compartment syndrome is confirmed, a *decompressing fasciotomy* must be performed immediately by a surgeon. A delay of greater than 12 hours may lead to irreversible muscle necrosis and contracture formation. Conservative measures are only temporizing and may involve ice packs and elevation. Pressure dressings should be removed.

If the four Major Threats to Life have been excluded, a more leisurely approach to the diagnosis can be taken, looking for other, less urgent conditions.

Selective Physical Examination II

SKIN
Localized skin and subcutaneous erythema, swelling, and warmth (cellulitis)
Painful subcutaneous red nodules (erythma nodosum, nodular liquefying panniculitis)
Tender superficial vein with surrounding erythema and edema (superficial thrombophlebitis)
"Blue toe syndrome" or levido reticularis (cholesterol emboli)
Focal areas of gangrene from cholesterol emboli (usually from the thoracic or abdominal aorta) may give one or more toes a bluish discoloration. Levido reticularis refers to cyanotic mottling of the skin in a fishnet-like pattern.
Erythema, swelling, dysesthesias, increased hair growth of one foot (reflex sympathetic dystrophy syndrome)

MSS
Posterior knee joint swelling (Baker's cyst)
Joint inflammation (RA, SLE, gout, pseudogout)
Hip palpation and ROM (hip joint pathology may cause leg pain with little or no evidence of inflammation)

NEURO
If no visible abnormality is found, a complete neurological examination is required to look for lumbar disc disease (sciatica) or peripheral neuropathy (e.g., diabetes). Benign nocturnal leg cramps often occur in the absence of physical findings.

Management of Selective Non-life-threatening Conditions

Acute Gout.   Acute gout results from the sudden release of monosodium urate crystals from the cartilage and synovial membranes into the joint space. The diagnosis is made by synovial fluid aspiration and demonstration of negatively birefringent monosodium urate crystals by polarizing microscopy.

At night, your main goal is to terminate the acute attack as quickly as possible. This can be done by administering *indomethacin* (Indocid) 100 mg PO, followed by 50 mg PO q6h until pain relief occurs. *Colchicine* is a good alternative choice and may be administered as 0.6 mg PO q2h until either the pain improves, intolerable GI side effects occur, or a total of 6 mg is given. Intraarticular *triamcinolone hexacetonide* (15 to 30 mg) or *depomedrol* (20 to 40 mg) is occasionally required.

Pseudogout.   Pseudogout is a result of release of calcium pyrophosphate dihydrate crystals from the joint cartilage into the joint space. Diagnosis is made by joint aspiration and demonstration of weakly positive birefringent rods when viewed under polarized light. Acute inflammation usually responds to *indo-*

methacin (Indocid) 25 to 50 mg PO TID × 10 to 14 days, aspiration of fluid, and steroid injection.

Lumbar Disc Disease. Lumbar disc disease initially can be treated conservatively with bedrest, analgesics, and muscle relaxants.

Thromboangiitis Obliterans (Buerger's Disease). The only known effective treatment for this condition is complete abstinence from tobacco.

Erythema nodosum. Erythema nodosum should be considered a symptom of some other underlying disorder, including drugs (oral contraceptives, penicillin, sulfonamides, bromides), inflammatory bowel disease, TB, fungal infections, and sarcoidosis. Treatment is that of the underlying condition.

Nodular Liquefying Panniculitis. The appearance of these nodules can be differentiated from erythema nodosum by their mobility with palpation. They are seen in association with acute pancreatitis or pancreatic neoplasms. Treatment is that of the underlying condition.

Reflex Sympathetic Dystrophy Syndrome. This disorder is often precipitated by an MI, stroke, or local trauma occurring weeks to months before characteristic redness, swelling (usually of the entire foot), and burning pain occur. Increased sweating and hair growth of the involved extremity also may occur. The condition may respond to analgesics and physiotherapy. Occasionally, surgical sympathectomy or a short course of steroids is required.

Baker's Cyst. A Baker's cyst is caused by extension of inflamed synovial tissue into the popliteal space, resulting in pain and swelling behind the knee. A well-known complication is rupture of the synovial sac into the adjacent tissues. This may mimic a calf DVT with tenderness, swelling, and a positive Homan's sign. The diagnosis can be confirmed by a popliteal ultrasonogram or arthrogram. Treatment involves drainage of the cyst or intra-articular steroid injection. Occasionally, surgical synovectomy is required.

Superficial Thrombophlebitis. This condition presents with a tender lower extremity vein with surrounding edema and erythema. Often fever is present. Superficial venous thrombosis seldom propagates into the deep venous system, and anticoagulation therapy is not recommended. Treatment involves local measures, such as leg elevation, heat, and NSAIDs, such as *indomethacin* (Indocid) 25 to 50 mg PO TID.

Cellulitis.   Cellulitis is most often caused by *Staphylococcus* or *Streptococcus*. Since it can be difficult to ascertain which culprit is responsible, treatment to cover both organisms is usual. Small, localized areas of cellulitis with intact skin may be treated with *cloxacillin, cephalexin,* or *erythromycin,* all at doses of 250 to 500 mg PO QID. If the patient is febrile, if the area of cellulitis is extensive, or if the patient is diabetic, IV antibiotics should be considered. A good choice is *cephalothin* 1 to 2 g IV q6h.

Cellulitis associated with skin ulcers in the diabetic patient should be swabbed for Gram's stain, culture, and sensitivity. In the diabetic, such infections are commonly caused by multiple organisms and often respond to *cefoxitin* 1 to 2 g IV q8h.

Benign Nocturnal Leg Cramps.   The cause of this condition is unknown. They frequently respond to *quinine sulfate* 300 mg PO QHS PRN.

20

LINES, TUBES, AND DRAINS

Almost every patient admitted to the hospital will have some form of IV line, tube, or drain inserted during their stay. These devices are useful in the care of patients but, on occasion, will clog, leak, or otherwise malfunction, requiring your expertise and common sense to remedy the problem.

Since the corrective measures that you may have to take when problems arise with lines, tubes, and drains carry the risk of contact with blood and body fluids, make sure you are familiar with and follow your institution's infection control guidelines.

This chapter describes some of the problems that can occur with commonly used lines, tubes, and drains.

Central Lines
1. Blocked central line (p. 170)
2. Bleeding at the central line entry site (p. 172)
3. SOB following central line insertion (p. 175)

Chest Tubes
1. Persistent bubbling in the drainage container (p. 178)
2. Bleeding around the chest tube entry site (p. 183)
3. Drainage of an excessive volume of blood (p. 184)
4. Loss of fluctuation of the underwater seal (p. 186)
5. SC emphysema (p. 189)
6. SOB (p. 191)

Urethral Catheters
1. Blocked urethral catheter (p. 194)
2. Gross hematuria (p. 196)
3. Inability to insert a urethral catheter (p. 198)

T-Tubes, J-Tubes, and Penrose Drains
1. Blocked T-tubes and J-tubes (p. 200)
2. Dislodged T-tubes, J-tubes, and Penrose drains (p. 203)

Nasogastric and Enteral Feeding Tubes
1. Blocked NG and enteral tubes (p. 204)
2. Dislodged NG and enteral feeding tubes (p. 205)

■ CENTRAL LINES
■ *Blocked Central Lines*
PHONE CALL
Questions

1 How long has the line been blocked?
2 What are the vital signs?
3 What was the reason for admission?

Orders

Ask the RN for a dressing set, two pairs of sterile gloves in your size, chlorhexidine (Hibitane) skin disinfectant, a 5-ml syringe, and a size 20- or 21-gauge needle to be at the bedside. You will probably have to remove the dressing that is securing the central line, and you must keep the site sterile. A second pair of sterile gloves is useful. It is easy to contaminate your gloves when on call at night.

Inform RN

"Will arrive at the bedside in . . . minutes."

A blocked central line requires you to see the patient immediately.

ELEVATOR THOUGHTS (What causes a central line to block [Fig. 20–1]?)

1. Kinked tubing
2. Thrombus at the catheter tip

MAJOR THREAT TO LIFE

- Failure of delivery of medications

Interruption of delivery of essential medications may temporarily deprive the patient of required treatment.

BEDSIDE
Quick Look Test

Does the patient look well (comfortable), sick (uncomfortable or distressed), or critical (about to die)?

A blocked central line, by itself, should not cause the patient to look sick or critical. If the patient looks unwell, search for another cause.

Airway and Vital Signs

A blocked central line should not compromise the airway or other vital signs.

Selective Physical Examination and Management

Inspect the central line. **Is the line kinked?**
If so, remove the dressing securing the line, straighten the line,

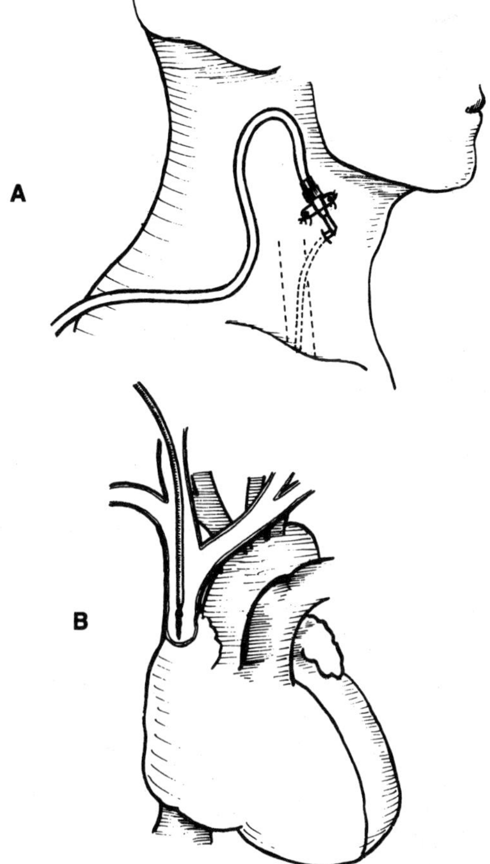

Figure 20–1 □ Causes of blocked central lines. **A.** Kinked tubing. **B.** Thrombosis at the catheter tip.

and see if there now is flow of IV fluid. If the problem is a kinked line, clean the area using sterile technique and secure the line with a plastic occlusive dressing without rekinking it.

If there is no flow of IV fluid with the line wide open, proceed as follows.

1. Turn the IV off.
2. Place the patient in the Trendelenburg position (head down). Take the 5-ml syringe and size 20- or 21-gauge capped needle and get ready to disconnect the central line from the IV tubing.

3. During the expiration phase of respiration, disconnect the central line from the IV tubing. Quickly attach the syringe to the central line and the capped needle to the IV tubing. The latter keeps the tubing sterile. The disconnection must be performed quickly to avoid an air embolus, which may result from air being sucked into the line owing to negative intrathoracic pressure generated during inspiration. The risk of an air embolus is diminished by clamping the IV tubing, placing the patient in Trendelenburg position, and disconnecting the line only during expiration.
4. Draw back gently on the syringe, as too much force will collapse the central line tubing. If the line is blocked with a small thrombus, this maneuver often is sufficient to dislodge the clot.
5. Draw back 3 ml of blood if possible. During the expiratory phase of respiration, remove the capped needle from the end of the IV tubing, remove the syringe from the central line, and reattach the IV tubing to the central line. Turn the IV on again. Blocked central lines should never be flushed. Flushing may dislodge a clot attached to the catheter tip, with subsequent pulmonary embolism.

If the previous maneuvers have been unsuccessful in unblocking the central line, ascertain whether indeed the central line is still necessary. Is the patient receiving medications that can be delivered only via a central line (e.g., amphotericin, dopamine, TPN)? Was the central line started because of lack of peripheral vein access? If so, reexamine the patient to see if there are now any peripheral veins suitable for IV access.

If central venous access is essential, the next step is to insert a new central line at a different site. A new central line should not be inserted over a guidewire placed through the blocked central line, since the insertion of the guidewire may also dislodge a clot.

In situations where central venous access is essential and no alternative sites are available, streptokinase or urokinase has been used to dissolve the obstructing clot. Significant risks are involved with the use of these agents, and routine use is not recommended.

■ *Bleeding at the Central Line Entry Site*
PHONE CALL
Questions

  1 **What are the vital signs?**
  2 **What was the reason for admission?**

Orders

Ask for a dressing set, two pairs of sterile gloves in your size, and chlorhexidine (Hibitane) skin disinfectant to be at the bedside.

You will probably have to remove the plastic occlusive dressing that is securing the central line, and you must keep the site sterile.

Inform RN

"Will arrive at the bedside in . . . minutes."

Bleeding at the central line site requires you to see the patient immediately.

ELEVATOR THOUGHTS (What causes bleeding at the line insertion site?)

1. Oozing of subcutaneous and cutaneous blood vessels (capillaries)
2. Coagulation disorders
   a. Drugs (warfarin, heparin, aspirin, NSAIDs, streptokinase, tPA)
   b. Thrombocytopenia, platelet dysfunction
   c. Clotting factor deficiency

MAJOR THREAT TO LIFE

- Upper airway obstruction

Bleeding into the soft tissues of the neck may cause tracheal compression, resulting in life-threatening upper airway obstruction. The patient may look sick or critical if excessive blood loss has occurred.

BEDSIDE
Quick Look Test

Does the patient look well (comfortable), sick (uncomfortable or distressed), or critical (about to die)?

These patients look well unless there is an upper airway obstruction.

Airway and Vital Signs

Check the airway. **What is the RR?**

If there is any evidence of an upper airway obstruction (inspiratory stridor or significant soft tissue swelling of the neck), call your resident for help immediately.

Selective Physical Examination and Management

1. Remove the dressing and try to identify a specific area of bleeding.
2. If you are unable to identify a specific site of bleeding, clean the site using sterile technique and reinspect the area. Usually, generalized oozing of blood is seen at the entry site, with no one specific skin vessel identified as the culprit.
3. Apply continuous pressure to the entry site for the next 20 minutes. This is performed by applying, with a gloved hand,

a folded, sterile 2 cm × 2 cm gauze dressing to the site with firm, continuous pressure. Do not release this pressure during the 20 minutes, since the platelet plug you are allowing to form may be broken (Fig. 20–2).

4. Reinspect the entry site. If the bleeding has stopped, clean the area using sterile technique and secure the line with plastic occlusive dressing. If there is still bleeding at the site, repeat the previous maneuver for another 20 minutes. Provided *continuous* pressure has been applied, any bleeding should have stopped. In the unusual circumstance where bleeding has not stopped, a coagulation disorder should be suspected. Refer to Chapter 31 for management of coagulation problems. Alternatively, a single suture may be placed at the site of bleeding in an attempt to provide hemostasis.

5. Removal of the central line should be considered if bleeding

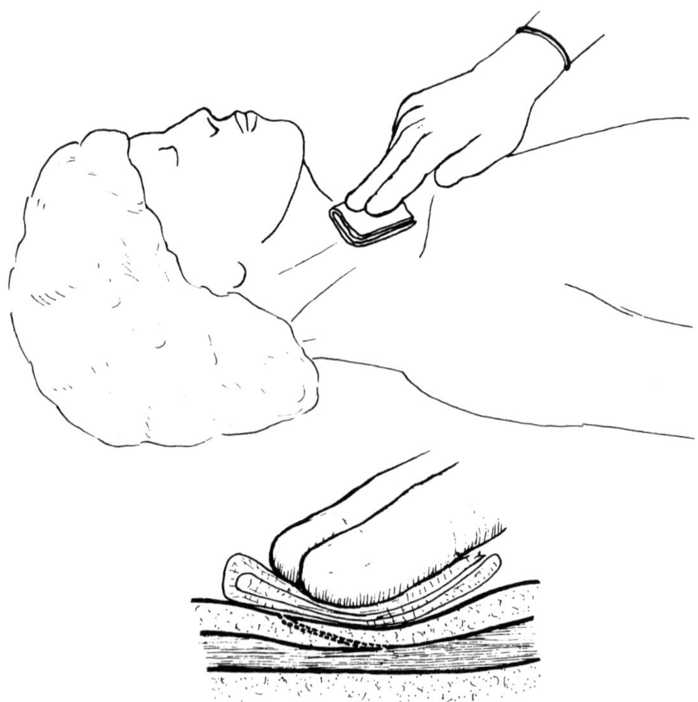

Figure 20–2 □ Continuous firm local pressure is required for 20 minutes to stop the oozing of blood from the central line entry site. Make sure the pressure is applied over the puncture site in the vein and not at the skin entry site.

at the insertion site is excessive and resistant to the previous measures.

■ *Shortness of Breath Following Central Line Insertion*
PHONE CALL
Questions

1 **How long has the patient been SOB?**
2 **What are the vital signs?**
3 **What was the reason for admission?**

Orders

1. Ask the RN for a dressing set, two pairs of sterile gloves in your size, chlorhexidine (Hibitane) skin disinfectant, and a size 16 IV catheter to be at the bedside. If the patient has a tension pneumothorax, you will need to insert a size 16 IV catheter into the second intercostal space on the hyperresonant side, with your resident's guidance.
2. If you suspect a pneumothorax, order a stat portable CXR in the upright position in expiration. Hypotension, tachypnea, and pleuritic chest pain after central line insertion are suggestive of a pneumothorax.
3. Order O_2 mask at 10 L/min.

Inform RN

"Will arrive at bedside in . . . minutes."

SOB after central line insertion requires you to see the patient immediately.

ELEVATOR THOUGHTS (What causes shortness of breath following central line insertion [Fig. 20–3]?)

1. Pneumothorax or tension pneumothorax
2. Massive soft tissue hematoma from inadvertent carotid artery puncture, resulting in upper airway obstruction
3. Cardiac tamponade
4. Air embolus
5. Pleural effusion

MAJOR THREAT TO LIFE

- Upper airway obstruction
- Tension pneumothorax
- Cardiac tamponade
- Air embolus

Upper airway obstruction may result from a massive soft tissue hematoma (e.g., from inadvertent carotid artery puncture). A *tension pneumothorax* may develop minutes to days after the insertion of a central line, if pleural perforation occurred during insertion. Rarely, *cardiac tamponade* results from perforation by the

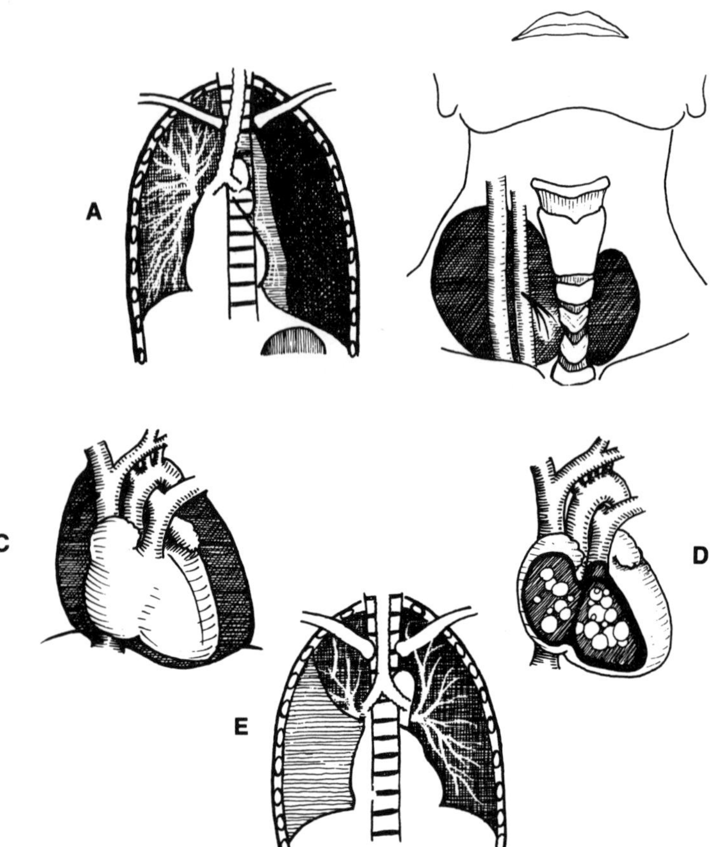

Figure 20–3 □ Causes of SOB following central line insertion. **A.** Pneumothorax. **B.** Massive soft tissue hematoma from inadvertent carotid artery puncture, resulting in upper airway obstruction. **C.** Cardiac tamponade. **D.** Air embolus. **E.** Pleural effusion.

catheter of the right atrium or right ventricle. Air may be inadvertently introduced if the line is disconnected incorrectly, resulting in an *air embolus*.

BEDSIDE
Quick Look Test

Does the patient look well (comfortable), sick (uncomfortable or distressed), or critical (about to die)?

A patient with a tension pneumothorax or upper airway obstruction looks sick or critical.

Airway and Vital Signs

Check the airway. If there is any evidence of an *upper airway obstruction* (i.e., inspiratory stridor or significant soft tissue swelling of the neck), call the ICU/CCU team immediately for possible intubation.

What are the BP and RR?

Hypotension and tachypnea in a patient with a recently inserted central line may indicate a tension pneumothorax or cardiac tamponade, inadvertently caused at the time of line insertion. See page 156 for the assessment and pages 177–178 for the management of tension pneumothorax and cardiac tamponade.

Selective Physical Examination

RESP	Tracheal deviation (tension pneumothorax or massive pleural effusion)
	Unilateral hyperresonance to percussion with decreased breath sounds (pneumothorax)
	Stony dullness to percussion, decreased breath sounds, decreased tactile fremitus (pleural effusion)
CVS	Pulsus paradoxus (cardiac tamponade or tension pneumothorax)
	Pulsus paradoxus is present when the decrease in systolic BP with inspiration is >10 mm Hg (the normal variation in systolic BP with quiet respiration is 0 to 10 mm Hg). A pulsus paradoxus is definitely present if the radial pulse disappears during inspiration.
	Elevated JVP (cardiac tamponade or tension pneumothorax)
	Distant heart sounds (pericardial effusion or cardiac tamponade)
	Mill wheel murmur, hypotension, elevated JVP (major air embolism)
CENTRAL LINE	Check all IV connections to ensure that they are not loose (air embolus)

Management

Tension pneumothorax is a medical emergency requiring urgent treatment. You will need supervision by your resident or attending physician.

1. Identify the second intercostal space in the midclavicular line on the affected (hyperresonant) side.
2. Mark this point with the pressure from a capped needle or ballpoint pen.
3. Open the dressing set and pour the chlorhexidine (Hibitane) into the appropriate space.
4. Put on the sterile gloves, and clean the identified area.
5. Insert the size 16 IV catheter into the designated site. Re-

move the inner needle, leaving the plastic cannula in the chest. If a tension pneumothorax is present, there will be a loud sound of air rushing out through the catheter. You will not need to connect the catheter to suction, since the lung will decompress itself.

6. Order a chest tube sent to the room immediately. The definitive treatment is the insertion of a chest tube.

Small pneumothoraces usually undergo spontaneous reabsorption over a few days.

Large or symptomatic pneumothoraces require chest tube drainage.

Cardiac tamponade is a medical emergency.

1. Clamp the IV tubing and turn off the IV.
2. Call the ICU/CCU team immediately for possible urgent pericardiocentesis. An emergency echocardiogram, if available, will confirm the diagnosis before pericardiocentesis.
3. Volume expansion with NS through a large-bore IV may be a useful temporizing measure to help maintain adequate CO.

Massive unilateral pleural effusion should be managed as follows.

1. Clamp the IV tubing and stop the IV fluid.
2. Thoracentesis will be required if the patient is markedly SOB.

Air embolism may be helped by placing the patient on the right side in Trendelenburg position (head down) in order to trap the air bubbles in the right ventricle and prevent them from entering the pulmonary artery. The patient should be kept in this position until the air bubbles have been reabsorbed. (Aspiration of air bubbles from the right ventricle is advocated by some experts.) Reinspect all the IV connections and make certain they are secure. If necessary, a new central line may have to be inserted.

■ CHEST TUBES

Chest tubes are inserted to drain air (pneumothoraces), blood (hemothoraces), fluid (pleural effusions), or pus (empyemas) (Fig. 20–4). They should always be connected to an underwater seal. They may be left to straight drainage (no suction) or, more commonly, to suction. Figure 20–5 illustrates the various chest tube drainage apparatuses. Common chest tube problems are illustrated in Figure 20–6.

■ *Persistent Bubbling in the Drainage Container (Air Leak)*
PHONE CALL
Questions

1 Why was the chest tube inserted?
2 What are the vital signs?

3 Is the patient SOB?

4 What was the reason for admission?

Orders

None.

Inform RN

"Will arrive at the bedside in . . . minutes."

Persistent bubbling in the drainage container is a potential emergency, requiring you to see the patient as soon as possible. Any malfunctioning of the chest tube, if associated with SOB, requires you to see the patient immediately.

ELEVATOR THOUGHTS (What causes persistent bubbling in the drainage compartment?)

1. Loose tubing connection.
2. Air leaking into the chest around the chest tube at the insertion site.
3. Traumatic tracheobronchial injury. A large, persistent air leak in traumatic pneumothorax suggests a concomitant tracheobronchial injury.

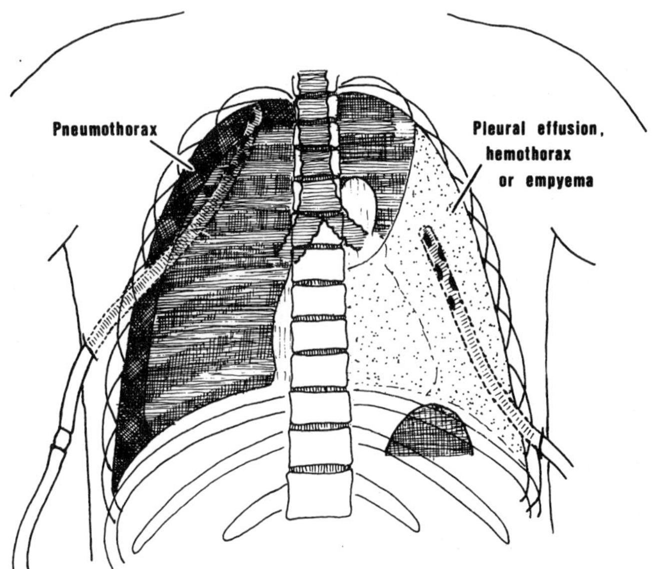

Figure 20–4 □ Chest tubes are inserted to drain air (pneumothoraces), blood (hemothoraces), fluid (pleural effusions), and pus (empyemas).

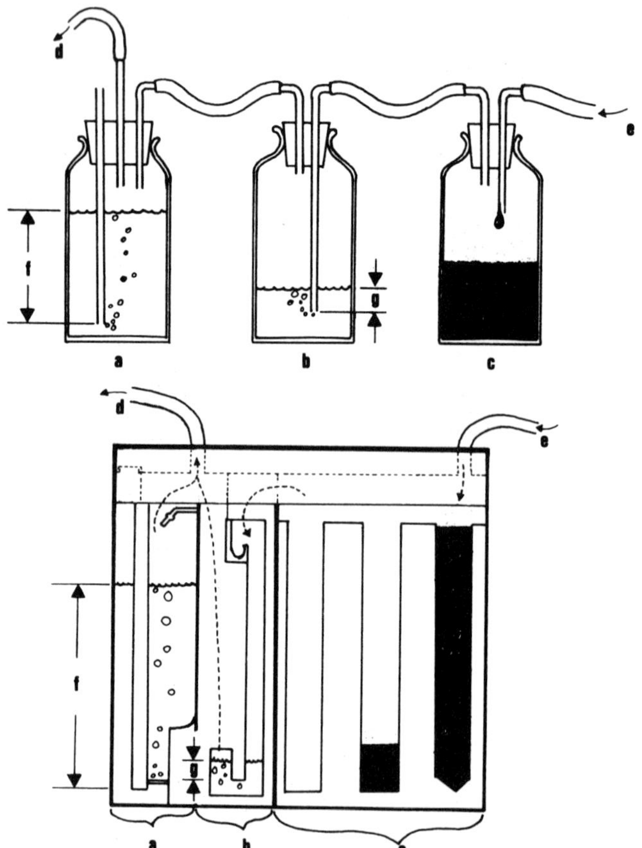

Figure 20–5 □ Chest tube apparatuses. *a.* Suction control chamber. *b.* Underwater seal. *c.* Collection chamber. *d.* To suction. *e.* From patient. *f.* Height equals amount of suction in cm H₂O. *g.* Height equals underwater seal in cm H₂O.

4. Persistent bronchopleural air leak
    a. Postlobectomy
    b. Ruptured bleb or bulla (e.g., asthma, ephysema)
    c. Following intrathoracic procedures (e.g., needle biopsy,
       thoracentesis)

MAJOR THREAT TO LIFE

A persistent air leak suggests either a pneumothorax from in-trathoracic injury or a loose connection of the drainage apparatus.

Hence, the major threat to life is the underlying intrathoracic disease process responsible for the persistent air leak. As long as air continues to bubble through the collection chamber, one can be reasonably certain that excessive intrapleural air will not accumulate.

BEDSIDE
Quick Look Test

Does the patient look well (comfortable), sick (uncomfortable or distressed), or critical (about to die)?

If a small air leak is the problem, the patient may look well. A patient who looks sick may be developing a larger pneumothorax or may look sick for unrelated reasons.

Airway and Vital Signs

Providing all tubing connections are snug and the chest tube dressing is airtight, a persistent air leak means that the patient

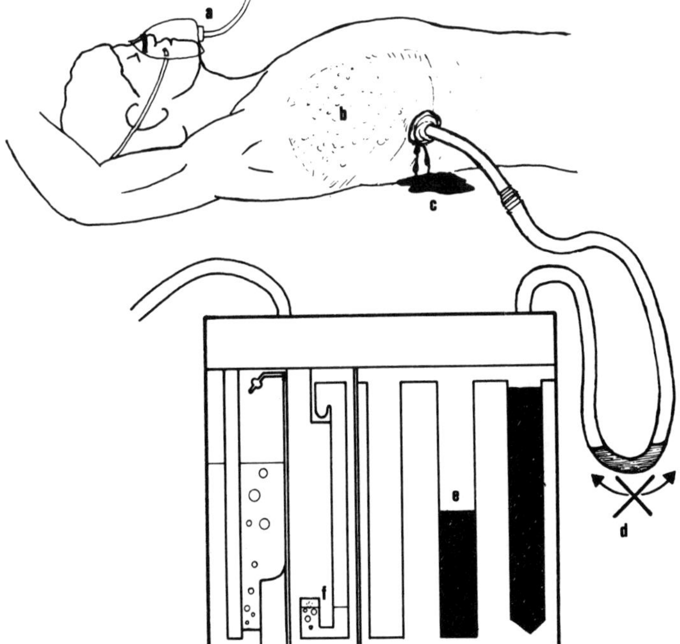

Figure 20–6 □ Common chest tube problems. *a.* SOB. *b.* Subcutaneous emphysema. *c.* Bleeding at the entry site. *d.* Loss of fluctuation. *e.* Excessive drainage. *f.* Persistent bubbling.

has a pneumothorax. As long as air continues to bubble through the collection chamber, the pneumothorax should drain and thus not result in alteration of vital signs.

Selective History and Chart Review

Why was the chest tube inserted?
If the chest tube was inserted to drain a pneumothorax, the tube should be bubbling unless the lung is fully expanded and the leak has sealed.

If the chest tube was inserted to drain a hemothorax, a pleural effusion, or an empyema with straight drainage (no suction), new onset of bubbling in the collection chamber represents either loose tubing connections, air leaking into the chest from around the chest tube insertion site, or the development of a pneumothorax.

Selective Physical Examination and Management

Provided a pneumothorax is not present, a persistent air leak is indicated by air bubbles in the underwater seal section of the Pleur-evac while the suction is turned off. If the air leak is small, it may be seen only with measures that increase intrapleural pressure (e.g., coughing) (Fig. 20–6).

Clamping of chest tubes before obtaining an x-ray may be dangerous, especially if there is a persistent pneumothorax. *Never leave a patient with a clamped chest tube unattended.* A tension pneumothorax may develop rapidly if a ball-valve mechanism is present. The following procedure is recommended when there is persistent bubbling in the drainage compartment.

1. Inspect the tubing connections to ensure that all seals are airtight.
2. Remove the dressing at the entry site of the chest tube, listen for sucking sounds, and observe the incision area. If the incision is too large and inadequately closed, insert one or two sterile 2-0 sutures to seal the opening. If the incision is adequately closed with sutures, reapply a pressure dressing, ensuring that the petrolatum (Vaseline) gauze occlusive dressing seals the incision.
3. Disconnect the suction from the Pleur-evac. Persistent air leak (spontaneous or with coughing) usually means an air leak from the lung (persistent pneumothorax).
4. Obtain a CXR to ensure correct tube placement. The chest tube holes should be inside the thorax, and the tip of the tube should be away from mediastinal and subclavicular structures.
5. If on CXR the lung is not reexpanded, call surgery for consideration of placing a second chest tube and for management of the persistent air leak from the lung.

■ *Bleeding Around the Chest Tube Entry Site*
PHONE CALL
Questions

1 Why was the chest tube inserted?
2 What are the vital signs?
3 Is the patient SOB?
4 What was the reason for admission?

Orders

Ask the RN for a dressing set, two pairs of sterile gloves in your size, and chlorhexidine (Hibitane) skin cleanser to be at the bedside. You will have to remove the dressing around the chest tube, and you must keep the site sterile.

Inform RN

"Will arrive at the bedside in . . . minutes."

Bleeding around the chest tube entry site is a potential emergency, requiring you to see the patient as soon as possible. Any malfunctioning chest tube in association with SOB requires you to see the patient immediately.

ELEVATOR THOUGHTS (What causes bleeding around the chest tube entry site?)

1. Inadequate pressure bandage
2. Inadequate closure of the incision with suture
3. Coagulation disorders
4. Trauma to intercostal vessels or lung during insertion of the chest tube
5. Blockage of chest tube or inadequate sized chest tube with drainage of the hemothorax around the entry site

Major Threat to Life

- Hemorrhagic shock

Continuous oozing, if allowed to progress, may eventually lead to intravascular volume depletion and, in the extreme case, hemorrhagic shock.

BEDSIDE
Quick Look Test

Does the patient look well (comfortable), sick (uncomfortable or distressed), or critical (about to die)?

If there is only a small amount of bleeding from the chest tube entry site, the patient will probably look entirely well. A patient who has lost more blood may look sick or critical.

Airway and Vital Signs

What are the BP and RR?
Hypotension and tachycardia may indicate major loss of blood. Tachypnea may indicate a large hemothorax.

Selective History and Chart Review

1. Why was the chest tube inserted?
2. Check the following recent laboratory results: Hb, PT, aPTT, and platelet count.

Selective Physical Examination and Management

Remove the dressing at the chest tube entry site and inspect the incision. If the incision is too large and inadequately closed, insert one or two sutures to seal the opening. If the incision is adequately closed with sutures, reapply a pressure dressing over the site, taking care to ensure that the pressure is maintained. Such maneuvers, when performed adequately, will stop the bleeding in the majority of situations.

Is the chest tube obstructed, resulting in blood draining around the entry site? Try milking the chest tube. Reinspect to see if this maneuver reestablished fluctuation in the underwater seal. The connecting tube is made of rubber and may be carefully stripped using the chest tube strippers. These two maneuvers help dislodge blood clots and debris that may be blocking the tube.

Is the chest tube too small, thus unable to drain a large hemothorax adequately? A larger size chest tube may be required.

■ *Drainage of an Excessive Volume of Blood*
PHONE CALL

Questions

1 Why was the chest tube inserted?
2 What are the vital signs?
3 Is the patient SOB?
4 What was the reason for admission?

Orders

None.

Inform RN

"Will arrive at the bedside in . . . minutes."

Drainage of an excessive volume of blood via the chest tube is a potential emergency and requires you to see the patient immediately. Any malfunctioning chest tube, if associated with SOB, requires you to see the patient immediately.

ELEVATOR THOUGHTS (What causes excessive blood to drain via the chest tube?)

Intrathoracic bleeding.

MAJOR THREAT TO LIFE

- Hemorrhagic shock

Hemorrhagic shock may result from excessive intrathoracic blood loss.

BEDSIDE

Quick Look Test

Does the patient look well (comfortable), sick (uncomfortable or distressed), or critical (about to die)?

A patient with hemorrhagic shock will look pale, sweaty, and restless.

Airway and Vital Signs

What are the BP and HR?

Hypotension and tachycardia may indicate hemorrhagic shock.

What is the RR?

Tachypnea and hypotension may indicate a tension pneumo-thorax.

Management I

1. Give supplemental oxygen, e.g., 4 L/min by nasal prongs.
2. If the patient is hypotensive, draw 20 ml of blood and start a large-bore IV (size 16 if possible). Give 500 ml of NS or Ringer's lactate IV as fast as possible.
3. Send blood for an immediate crossmatch for 4 to 6 units of packed RBCs on hold, Hb,PT, aPTT, and platelet count.
4. Order a stat CXR.

Selective Chart Review and Management

Is the patient receiving anticoagulant medication (heparin, warfarin)?

If so, review the initial indication for anticoagulation. Can the anticoagulant be safely discontinued or reversed? Consult the hematology department for assistance in the management of this difficult and potentially life-threatening situation.

Estimate how much blood the patient has lost over the past 48 hours by reviewing the intake/output chart.

If the patient has lost more the 500 ml over 8 hours, consultation with a thoracic surgeon is recommended. The patient may need immediate transfer to the operating room for an emergency thoracotomy to localize the site of hemorrhage and achieve hemostasis.

If the patient has lost less than 500 ml over 8 hours, order hourly monitoring of the blood lost via the chest tube, noting that a physician needs to be informed if the blood loss is greater than 50 ml/h.

■ *Loss of Fluctuation of the Underwater Seal*
PHONE CALL
Questions

   1 **Why was the chest tube inserted?**
   2 **What are the vital signs?**
   3 **Is the patient SOB?**
   4 **What was the reason for admission?**

Orders

None.

Inform RN

"Will arrive at the bedside in . . . minutes."

Loss of fluctuation of the underwater seal is a potential emergency and requires you to see the patient as soon as possible. Any malfunctioning chest tube, if associated with SOB, requires you to see the patient immediately.

ELEVATOR THOUGHTS (What causes loss of fluctuation of the underwater seal?)

   1. Kinked chest tube
   2. Plugged chest tube
   3. Improper chest tube positioning

The underwater seal is essentially a one-way, low-resistance valve. During expiration, the intrapleural pressure increases, becoming higher than atmospheric pressure, forcing air or fluid that is in the pleural space through the chest tube and underwater seal (Fig. 20–7).

MAJOR THREAT TO LIFE

   ■ Tension pneumothorax

Inadequate drainage of a pneumothorax because of a blocked chest tube may lead to a tension pneumothorax (Figs. 20–8 and 20–9).

BEDSIDE
Quick Look Test

Does the patient look well (comfortable), sick (uncomfortable or distressed), or critical (about to die)?

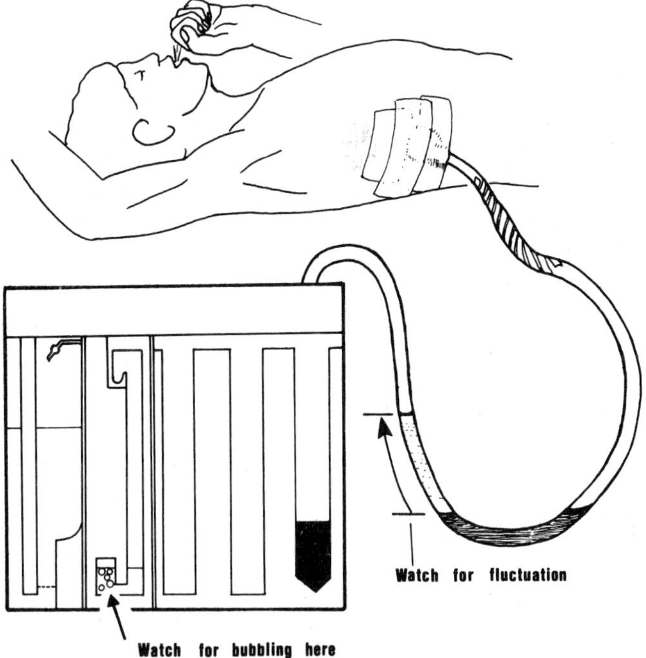

Figure 20-7 □ Loss of fluctuation of the underwater seal. Ask the patient to cough, and observe for any fluctuation or bubbling.

A patient who looks sick may be developing a tension pneumothorax or may look sick for unrelated reasons.

Airway and Vital Signs

What are the BP and RR?

Hypotension and tachypnea may indicate a tension pneumothorax.

Selective History and Chart Review

1. Why was the chest tube inserted?
2. How long ago did the chest tube stop fluctuating?
3. What has been draining from the chest tube? What volume has drained over the past 24 hours?

Selective Physical Examination and Management

1. Inspect the underwater seal. Is there any fluctuation? Ask the patient to cough, and observe the tube for any fluctua-

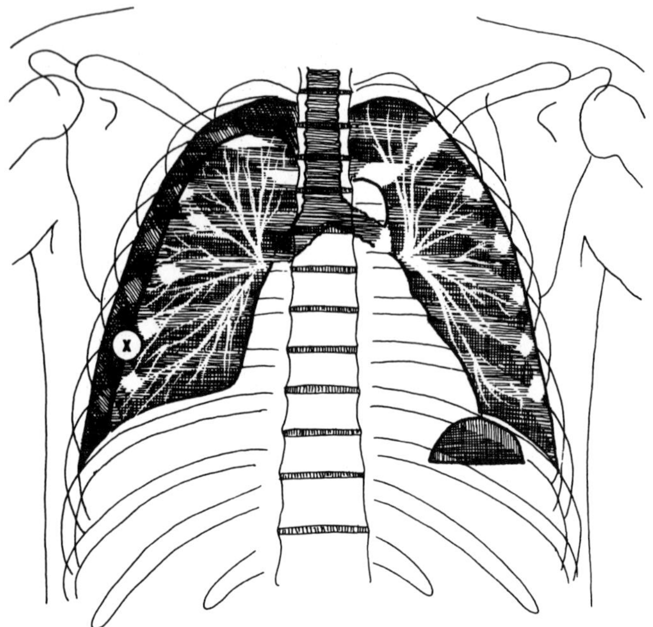

Figure 20-8 □ Pneumothorax. *x.* Edge of visceral pleura or lung.

tion. A chest tube with its distal aperture located within the pleural space fluctuates with respiration.

2. Inspect the chest tube for kinking. You may need to remove the dressing at the chest tube site. If the chest tube is kinked, reposition and reinspect it for fluctuation of the underwater seal.
3. Try milking the chest tube. Reinspect to see if this maneuver reestablishes fluctuation in the underwater seal. The connecting tubing is rubber and may be carefully stripped using chest tube strippers. These two maneuvers help dislodge blood clots and debris that may be blocking the tube.
4. Order a portable CXR. Improper positioning of the chest tube may result in loss of fluctuation of the underwater seal.
5. If the tube is not fluctuating after all the aforementioned maneuvers are attempted, a new chest tube may have to be inserted.

■ *Subcutaneous Emphysema*
PHONE CALL
Questions

1 Why was the chest tube inserted?
2 What are the vital signs?
3 Is the patient SOB?
4 What was the reason for admission?

Orders

Ask the RN for a dressing set, two pairs of sterile gloves in your size, and chlorhexidine (Hibitane) skin cleanser to be at the bedside. You will have to remove the dressing around the chest tube, and you must keep the site sterile.

Inform RN

"Will arrive at the bedside in . . . minutes."

Subcutaneous emphysema is a potential emergency requiring you to see the patient immediately. Any malfunctioning chest tube, if associated with SOB, requires you to see the patient immediately.

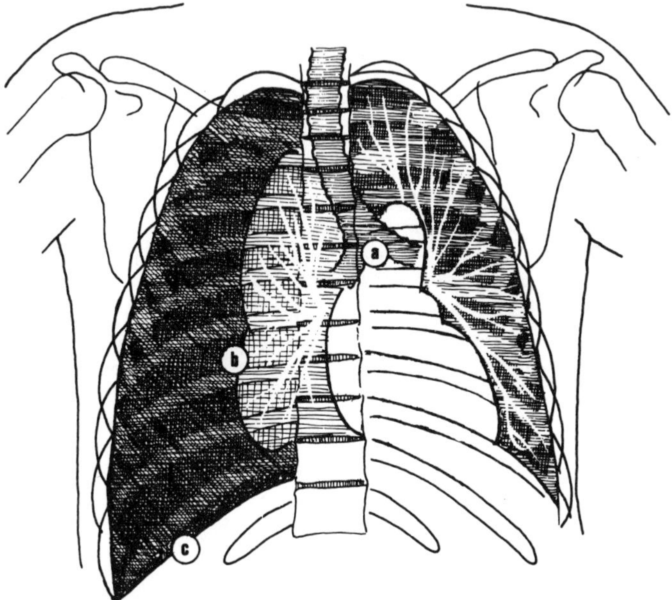

Figure 20–9 □ Tension pneumothorax. *a.* Shifted mediastinum. *b.* Edge of collapsed lung. *c.* Low flattened diaphragm.

ELEVATOR THOUGHTS (What causes subcutaneous emphysema?)

1. Chest tube may be too small for the size of the leak.
2. Inadequate suction.
3. One of the chest tube apertures may be in the chest wall.
4. Chest tube may be in the chest wall or abdominal cavity.
5. Insignificant localized subcutaneous emphysema around the entry site is not uncommon after chest tube insertion.

MAJOR THREAT TO LIFE

- Upper airway obstruction

Subcutaneous emphysema extending up into the neck rarely may result in tracheal compression.

BEDSIDE

Quick Look Test

Does the patient look well (comfortable), sick (uncomfortable or distressed), or critical (about to die)?

The patient with upper airway obstruction will look sick or critical, and there may be audible inspiratory stridor.

Airway and Vital Signs

1. Inspect and palpate the neck for SC emphysema.
2. **What is the RR?** The patient with upper airway obstruction will be tachypneic.
3. **What are the BP and HR?** SC emphysema may be accompanied by a tension pneumothorax. If so, the patient will be tachycardic.

Selective History and Chart Review

Why was the chest tube inserted?

Selective Physical Examination and Management

1. If there is significant upper airway obstruction (palpable SC emphysema over the trachea, inspiratory stridor, tachypnea), call the ICU/CCU team immediately for probable intubation and transfer to the ICU/CCU. Cardiothoracic surgery may be required if mediastinal decompression is indicated.
2. **What size chest tube has been inserted? Is the chest tube too small in diameter?** Multifenestrated vinyl chest tubes are available in two sizes: 20F and 36F. The 20F may not be large enough, and air may escape from the pleural cavity into the chest wall, resulting in SC emphysema. If the chest tube is too small, a larger one will need to be inserted. Sometimes, two large chest tubes may be required for adequate drainage.

3. **Is the chest tube connected to suction?** A large pneumothorax may not be drained adequately if it is connected only to an underwater seal, as opposed to suction.
4. Remove the dressing at the chest tube site and inspect the chest tube. **Are any of the drainage holes in the distal end of the chest tube visible?** None of the drainage lines should be visible. They should all be inside the pleural cavity. SC emphysema may be caused by misplacement of the chest tube, with one of the drainage holes inadvertently in the soft tissues of the chest wall. A new chest tube should be inserted. Do not reintroduce the partially extruded chest tube, since you may introduce infection into the pleural space.

■ *Shortness of Breath*
PHONE CALL
Questions

1 **Why was the chest tube inserted?**
2 **What are the vital signs?**
3 **What was the reason for admission?**

Orders

Ask the RN for a dressing set, two pairs of sterile gloves in your size, chlorhexidine (Hibitane) skin cleanser, and a size 16 IV catheter. A tension pneumothorax, if present, is most effectively treated with insertion of a size 16 IV catheter into the pleural space on the affected side.

Inform RN

"Will arrive at the bedside in . . . minutes."

SOB in a patient with a chest tube in place is a potential emergency and requires you to see the patient immediately.

ELEVATOR THOUGHTS (What causes shortness of breath in a patient with a chest tube?)
Causes Related to the Chest Tube

1. Tension pneumothorax
2. Increasing pneumothorax. Both 1 and 2 may occur because of
   a. Inadequate suction
   b. Misplaced tube (i.e., chest tube not in the pleural cavity)
   c. Blocked or kinked tube
   d. Bronchopulmonary fistula
3. Subcutaneous emphysema
4. Increasing pleural effusion or hemothorax
5. Reexpansion pulmonary edema (sometimes this occurs after

rapid expansion of a pneumothorax, drainage of pleural fluid, or both)

Causes Unrelated to the Chest Tube

See Chapter 24, page 232.

MAJOR THREAT TO LIFE

- Tension pneumothorax
- Upper airway obstruction

Inadequate drainage of a pneumothorax produced through a ball-valve mechanism may result in a life-threatening *tension pneumothorax*. Tracheal compression from interstitial emphysema rarely causes *upper airway obstruction*.

BEDSIDE

Quick Look Test

Does the patient look well (comfortable), sick (uncomfortable or distressed), or critical (about to die)?

A sick or critical looking patient may have a tension pneumothorax or may have an unrelated reason for SOB (Chapter 24).

Airway and Vital Signs

1. Inspect and palpate the neck for SC emphysema.
2. **What is the RR?** Rates >20/min suggest hypoxia, pain, or anxiety. Look for thoracoabdominal dissociation, which may indicate impending respiratory failure. Remember that the rib cage and abdominal wall normally move in the same direction during inspiration and expiration.
3. **What are the BP and HR?** Hypotension and tachycardia may indicate a tension pneumothorax or another unrelated cause of SOB (Chapter 24).

Selective Physical Examination

Does the patient have a tension penumothorax?

VITALS	Tachypnea
	Hypotension
HEENT	Tracheal deviation away from the hyperresonant side
RESP	Unilateral hyperresonance
	Decreased air entry on hyperresonant side
CVS	Elevated JVP
CHEST TUBE	Is there bubbling in the collection chamber? Absence of bubbling suggests malposition or malfunction of the chest tube.

Selective Chart Review

Why was the chest tube inserted?

Management

1. If there is *significant upper airway obstruction* (palpable subcutaneous emphysema over the trachea, inspiratory stridor, tachypnea), call the ICU/CCU team immediately for probable intubation and transfer to the ICU/CCU.
2. *Tension pneumothorax* is a medical emergency requiring urgent treatment. You will need supervision by your resident or attending physician.
   a. Identify the second intercostal space in the midclavicular line on the affected (hyperresonant) side.
   b. Mark this point using pressure from the cap of a needle or ballpoint pen.
   c. Open the dressing set and pour the chlorhexidine (Hibitane) into the appropriate container.
   d. Put on sterile gloves.
   e. Clean the area previously identified.
   f. Insert the size 16 IV catheter into the designated area. If a tension pneumothorax is present, there will be a loud sound of air rushing out through the catheter. You will not need to connect the catheter to suction, since the pleural space will decompress itself.
   g. Order a chest tube sent to the room immediately. The definitive treatment is insertion of a chest tube.
3. If there is an *increasing pneumothorax* but no evidence of a tension pneumothorax, order a stat upright CXR in expiration. Meanwhile, look for any correctable causes, e.g., kinked or blocked tubing, inadequate suction, and dislodged chest tube.
4. For the management of other causes of SOB, i.e., causes unrelated to chest tubes, see Chapter 24.

■ URETHRAL CATHETERS

There are five types of urethral catheters (Fig. 20–10). The *Foley (balloon retention) catheter* is the most commonly used of these. It consists of a double-lumen tube. The larger lumen drains urine, and the smaller lumen admits 5 to 30 ml of water to inflate the balloon tip. *Straight (Robinson) catheters* are used to obtain in–out collections of urine, to obtain sterile specimens in patients who are unable to void voluntarily, and to obtain postvoiding residual urine volume measurements. A *coudé catheter* has a curved tip that facilitates insertion when a urethral obstruction (e.g., benign prostatic hypertrophy) makes passage of a Foley catheter difficult. *Three-way irrigation catheters* have, in addition to lumens for urine drainage and balloon inflation, a third lumen for bladder irrigation. These catheters are used commonly after transurethral prostate resection to facilitate bladder irrigation and drainage of blood

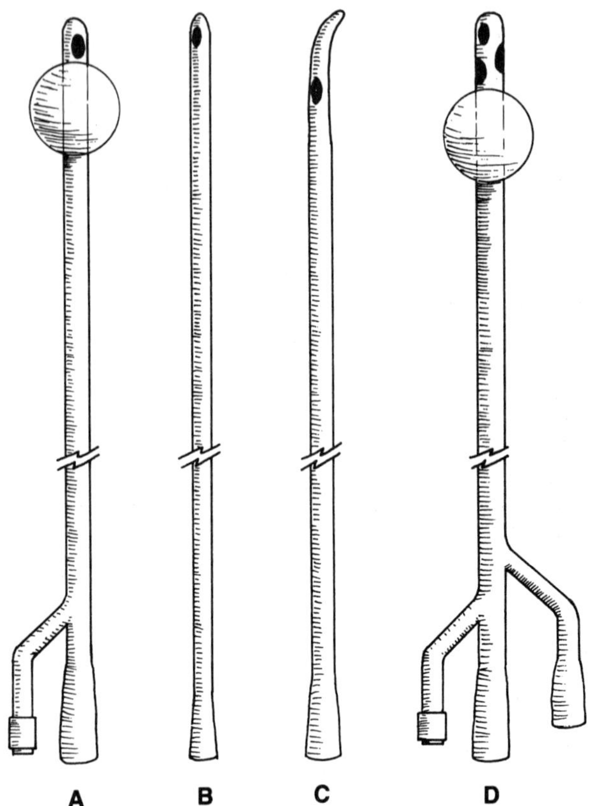

Figure 20–10 □ Urethral catheters. **A.** Foley catheter. **B.** Straight (Robinson) catheter. **C.** Coudé catheter. **D.** Three-way irrigation catheter.

clots. A *Silastic catheter* is similar to a Foley catheter but is constructed of softer, less reactive plastic. It is used when a urethral catheter is required on a long-term basis.

■ *Blocked Urethral Catheter*
PHONE CALL
Questions

1 How long has the catheter been blocked?
2 What are the vital signs?
3 Does the patient have suprapubic pain?
   Urinary retention secondary to a blocked catheter can result in suprapubic pain due to bladder distention.
4 What was the reason for admission?

Orders

Ask the RN to try flushing the catheter with 30 to 40 ml of sterile NS if this has not been done.

Inform RN

"Will arrive at the bedside in . . . minutes."

Provided the patient does not have suprapubic pain (bladder distention), assessment of a blocked urinary catheter can wait an hour or two if other problems of higher priority exist.

ELEVATOR THOUGHTS (What causes blocked urethral catheters?)

1. Urinary sediment
2. Blood clots
3. Kinked catheter (look under the bedsheets!)
4. Improperly placed or dislodged catheter

MAJOR THREAT TO LIFE

- Bladder rupture
- Progressive renal insufficiency

Bladder rupture may occur if bladder distention progresses without decompression. Since bladder distention is painful, bladder rupture from this cause usually is seen only in the unconscious or paraplegic patient. Persistent lower urinary tract obstruction may lead to hydronephrosis and *renal failure*.

BEDSIDE
Quick Look Test

Does the patient look well (comfortable), sick (uncomfortable or distressed), or critical (about to die)?

Most patients with blocked urethral catheters look well. However, patients with acute bladder distention may look distressed because of abdominal pain.

Airway and Vital Signs

A blocked urethral catheter is not usually responsible for alterations in vital signs unless pain due to bladder distention causes tachypnea or tachycardia.

Selective Physical Examination and Management

1. Percuss and palpate the abdomen to determine whether the bladder is distended. Suprapubic dullness and tenderness suggest a distended bladder.
2. Examine the tubing for kinking of the catheter, blood clots, or sediment.
3. Order a sterile dressing tray, a 50-ml bulb syringe (or a 50-ml syringe and an adapter), and two pairs of sterile gloves

in your size. Aspirate and irrigate the catheter with 30 to 40 ml of sterile NS as follows.

   a. Ask an assistant to hold the distal part of the catheter close to the connection between the tubing and urinary drainage bag.

   b. Wear sterile gloves and clean the distal catheter and the proximal connecting tubing with chlorhexidine.

   c. Disconnect the drainage tubing from the catheter. Ask an assistant to hold the connecting tubing in the air to maintain a sterile tip.

   d. Using a 50-ml syringe, aspirate the catheter vigorously to dislodge and extract any blood clots or sediment that may have blocked the catheter. If the maneuver is unsuccessful, flush the catheter with 30 to 40 ml of sterile NS. Several attempts at aspiration should be made before abandoning this technique.

   e. Reconnect the catheter to the connecting tubing, using sterile technique. The majority of blocked Foley catheters will become unplugged with this maneuver.

4. If flushing of the catheter fails to relieve obstruction, a new catheter should be inserted if one is still required.

■ *Gross Hematuria*

PHONE CALL

Questions

   1 **Why was the urethral catheter inserted?**
   2 **What are the vital signs?**
   3 **Is the patient receiving anticoagulant drugs or cyclophosphamide?**
   4 **What was the reason for admission?**

Orders

None.

Inform RN

"Will arrive at the bedside in . . . minutes."

Gross hematuria in the anticoagulated patient requires you to see the patient immediately.

ELEVATOR THOUGHTS (What causes gross hematuria in the catheterized patient?)

1. Urethral trauma
   a. Inadvertent or partial removal of the catheter with the balloon still inflated
   b. During catheter insertion (false passage)

2. Drugs
   a. Anticoagulants (heparin, warfarin)
   b. Thrombolytic agents (streptokinase, tPA, urokinase)
   c. Cyclophosphamide
3. Coagulation abnormalities
   a. DIC
   b. Specific factor deficiencies
   c. Thrombocytopenia
4. Unrelated problems
   a. Renal stones
   b. Carcinoma of the kidney, bladder, or prostate
   c. Glomerulonephritis
   d. Prostatitis
   e. Rupture of a bladder vein

MAJOR THREAT TO LIFE

- Hemorrhagic shock

Although gross hematuria is dramatic and most distressing to the patient, it is quite rare for bleeding to be significant enough to result in hemorrhagic shock. It only requires 1 ml of blood in 1 L of urine to change the color from yellow to red.

BEDSIDE

Quick Look Test

Does the patient look well (comfortable), sick (uncomfortable or distressed), or critical (about to die)?

It is unusual for these patients to look other than well. If they look sick or critical, search for a separate unrecognized problem.

Airway and Vital Signs

What is the BP?

Hypotension in the patient with gross hematuria may be a sign of hemorrhagic shock.

What is the HR?

A resting tachycardia, though a nonspecific finding, may indicate hypovolemia if significant blood loss has occurred.

Selective History and Chart Review

Is the patient receiving any of the following medications?
- Heparin, warfarin
- Streptokinase, tPA, urokinase
- Cyclophosphamide

Is there any abnormality in the coagulation profile?
- PT, aPTT, platelet count

Is there a history of urethral trauma?
- Recent inadvertent removal of Foley catheter with the balloon still inflated (especially in the elderly, confused patient)
- Recent GU surgery
- Recent difficulty with insertion of a urethral catheter

Has there been a recent decrease in the Hb value? How much blood has the patient lost?
- Bleeding via the urinary tract is unlikely to cause significant hemodynamic changes unless there has been recent GU surgery.

Management

1. If the patient is anticoagulated, review the initial indication for the anticoagulation. Decide, in consultation with your resident and a hematologist, whether the risk of anticoagulation is still warranted.
2. If a coagulation abnormality is identified, refer to Chapter 31 for discussion of investigation and management.
3. If there is a history of recent urethral trauma, continued significant blood loss is unlikely. Have the vital signs taken every 4 to 6 hours for the next 24 hours. Significant bleeding may be manifested by tachycardia and orthostatic hypotension.

■ *Inability to Insert a Urethral Catheter*
PHONE CALL
Questions

1 Why was the urethral catheter ordered?
2 What are the vital signs?
3 Does the patient have suprapubic pain?
4 How many attempts have been made to catheterize the patient?
5 What was the reason for admission?

Orders

Ask the RN for a catheter insertion set, two pairs of sterile gloves in your size, and chlorhexidine (Hibitane) skin disinfectant to be at the bedside.

Inform RN

"Will arrive at the bedside in . . . minutes."

Provided the patient does not have suprapubic pain (bladder distention), insertion of a urethral catheter can wait an hour or two if other problems of higher priority exist.

ELEVATOR THOUGHTS (What causes difficulty in urethral catheterization?)

1. Urethral edema
   a. Multiple insertion attempts
   b. Inadvertent removal of a Foley catheter with the balloon still inflated
2. Urethral obstruction
   a. Benign prostatic hypertrophy
   b. Carcinoma of the prostate
   c. Urethral stricture
   d. Anatomic anomaly (diverticulum, false passage)

MAJOR THREAT TO LIFE

- Bladder rupture
- Progressive renal insufficiency

Bladder rupture may occur if bladder distention is not relieved by placement of a urinary catheter. A suprapubic catheter may be required if urethral catheterization is impossible. Persistent bladder obstruction may lead to hydronephrosis and *renal failure.*

BEDSIDE

Quick Look Test

Does the patient look well (comfortable), sick (uncomfortable or distressed), or critical (about to die)?

Patients with acute bladder distention may look distressed because of abdominal pain.

Airway and Vital Signs

Inability to insert a urethral catheter should not compromise the vital signs.

Selective History and Chart Review

1. Is there a history of recent, multiple attempts at catheterization or removal of a catheter with the balloon still inflated (urethral edema)?
2. Is there a history of benign prostatic hypertrophy, carcinoma of the prostate, urethral stricture, or an anatomic abnormality of the urethra?
3. What was the original indication for urethral catheter placement? Does the indication still exist?

Selective Physical Examination and Management

1. Percuss and palpate the abdomen to determine whether the bladder is distended. Suprapubic tenderness and dullness are suggestive of a distended bladder.
2. If urethral edema is suspected, try inserting a smaller sized catheter.

3. If there is a history of urethral obstruction, try inserting a coudé catheter.
4. If you are unable to catheterize the patient, consult the urology department for assistance.

■ T-TUBES, J-TUBES, AND PENROSE DRAINS

T-tubes are usually used for postoperative drainage of the common bile duct following common bile duct exploration or choledochotomy (Fig. 20–11). A T-tube cholangiogram is commonly performed on the seventh to tenth postoperative day. If the cholangiogram is normal, the T-tube is removed. If a blockage (strictures, tumors, retained common duct stones) exists, the T-tube is left in place.

J-tubes are *jejunostomy tubes*, surgically inserted to provide enteral nutrition on a long-term basis. They are particularly useful when gastroesophageal reflux and aspiration are a problem. *Gastrostomy tubes* may be inserted percutaneously under direct vision (e.g., gastroscopy or fluoroscopy) and are used for long-term feeding when there is no gastroesophageal reflux.

Penrose drains are flat rubber drains inserted into wounds or operative sites with potential dead spaces to prevent the accumulation of pus, intestinal contents, blood, bile, or pancreatic juice.

Closed suction (Davon or Jackson-Pratt) *drains* are used with operative, large potential dead spaces where bacterial ingress may contaminate sterile cavities.

Sump drains have filters incorporated into them to prevent airborne bacteria from entering. They are usually used to drain peripancreatic fluid collections. Interventional radiologists sometimes insert various percutaneous drains into the biliary tree and intraabdominal abscesses. Problems with these drains should be referred to the radiologist or surgeon.

■ *Blocked T-Tubes and J-Tubes*
PHONE CALL
Questions

1 How long has the tube been blocked?
2 What type of tube is in place?
3 Has the tube been dislodged?
4 What operation was performed and how many days ago?
5 What are the vital signs?
6 What was the reason for admission?

Orders

Ask the RN for a dressing set, two pairs of gloves in your size, and chlorhexidine (Hibitane) skin disinfectant to be at the bedside.

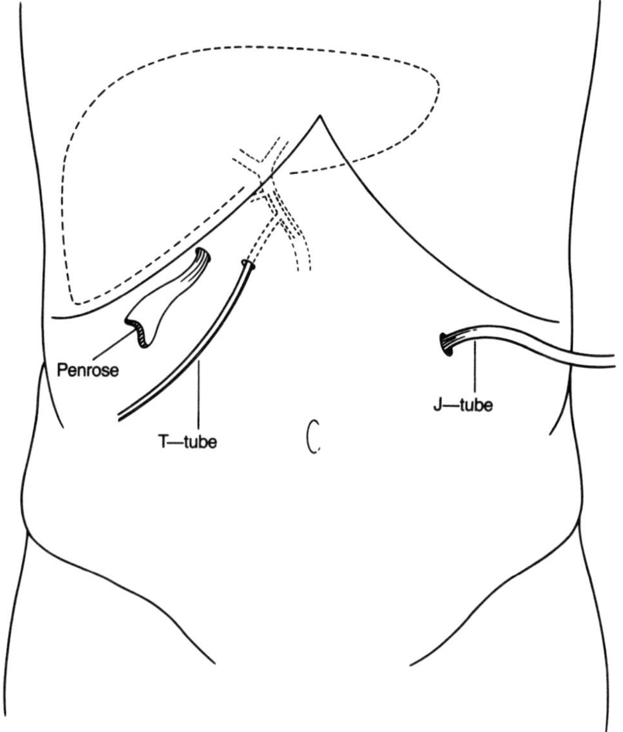

Figure 20–11 □ T-tube, J-tube, and Penrose drain.

You will have to remove the dressing around the drainage tube, and you must keep the site sterile.

Inform RN

"Will arrive at the bedside in . . . minutes."

Provided you are certain the tube has not been dislodged, assessment of blocked T-tubes and J-tubes can wait an hour or two if other problems of higher priority exist.

ELEVATOR THOUGHTS (What causes blocked T-tubes or J-tubes?)

1. Blood clots within the tube
2. Debris within the tube
3. Failure to irrigate the tube regularly

MAJOR THREAT TO LIFE

- Sepsis with blocked T-tubes

Blocked T-tubes may lead to postoperative infection with resultant abscess formation or systemic *sepsis*. Blocked J-tubes, provided they are not dislodged, present no immediate threat to life. The risk of further surgery exists if replacement of the tube is required.

BEDSIDE

Quick Look Test

Does the patient look well (comfortable), sick (uncomfortable or distressed), or critical (about to die)?

The patient with a blocked T-tube or J-tube will look well unless the underlying problem causes the patient to look sick or critical.

Airway and Vital Signs

A blocked T-tube or J-tube should not compromise the airway or vital signs.

Selective Physical Examination and Management

Aspirate and irrigate the tube as follows.

1. Ask an assistant to hold the distal part of the T-tube or J-tube close to the connection between the tube and the drainage bag.
2. Wear sterile gloves and clean the distal end of the T-tube or J-tube and the proximal connecting tubing with chlorhexidine (Hibitane).
3. Disconnect the tube from the connecting tubing and give the connecting tubing to the assistant to maintain a sterile field.
4. Using a 5-ml syringe, aspirate *very gently* (i.e., withdraw the syringe plunger) to dislodge and extract the obstruction.
5. If this maneuver is unsuccessful, fill a second 5-ml syringe with 3 ml of sterile NS and *very gently* flush the T-tube or J-tube by applying slow, careful pressure to the syringe plunger. Only gentle pressure should be used. After flushing with saline, attempt to aspirate gently. If this maneuver fails, *do not try again.*
6. Reconnect the T-tube or J-tube and the drainage bag, maintaining sterile technique.

If the aspiration and irrigation are unsuccessful, the surgeon should be informed immediately. The decision between a T-tube cholangiogram to visualize the problem and a closed exploration of the obstructed tube with a Fogarty catheter will have to be made. Closed exploration should be performed only by someone experienced in the procedure. It can be done only when a large, intact T-tube has been used or when the back wall of the T-limb has been cut away. An adequately functioning T-tube usually drains 100 to 250 ml/8 h.

■ *Dislodged T-Tubes, J-Tubes, and Penrose Drains*
PHONE CALLS
Questions

1 How long ago was the tube or drain dislodged?
2 What type of tube is in place?
3 What operation was performed and how many days ago?
4 What are the vital signs?
5 What was the reason for admission?

Orders

Ask the RN for a dressing set, two pairs of gloves in your size, and chlorhexidine (Hibitane) skin cleanser to be at the bedside. You will have to remove the dressing around the drainage tube, and you must keep the site sterile.

Inform RN

"Will arrive at the bedside in . . . minutes."

Assessment of dislodged T-tubes and J-tubes requires you to see the patient immediately, since urgent replacement of the tube is mandatory if it was inserted recently. A delay in this replacement may result in the patient's requiring emergency surgery to replace the tube.

ELEVATOR THOUGHTS (What causes dislodgement of tubes and drains?)

1. Failure to secure the tube or drain adequately
2. Confused, uncooperative patient

MAJOR THREAT TO LIFE

■ Sepsis

Dislodged T-tubes and Penrose drains may lead to postoperative sepsis with resultant abscess formation or systemic *sepsis*. Dislodged J-tubes and T-tubes that cannot be replaced early may require surgical replacement, thus increasing the risk of morbidity and mortality from a second anesthetic.

BEDSIDE
Quick Look Test

Does the patient look well (comfortable), sick (uncomfortable or distressed), or critical (about to die)?

The patient with a recently dislodged T-tube, J-tube, or Penrose drain will look well unless the underlying problem causes the patient to look sick or critical.

Airway and Vital Signs

A dislodged T-tube, J-tube, or Penrose drain should not compromise the vital signs acutely.

Selective Physical Examination and Management

A dislodged *T-tube* draining the common bile duct is a potentially life-threatening situation, since septic shock can follow rapidly. If dislodgement is suspected, order an immediate T-tube cholangiogram and inform the surgeon. The patient will need surgery to reestablish drainage if dislodgement is confirmed by the cholangiogram.

A dislodged *J-tube* (enterostomy tube) must be reinserted immediately as follows.

1. Wear sterile gloves and clean and drape the tube exit site.
2. If the tube is only partially dislodged, carefully clean the exposed tubing and gently advance the tube to the appropriate (previous) depth.
3. If the tube has been completely dislodged, select a similar sterile tube and introduce it gently through the track left by the previous tube. *Do not force the tube.*
4. If this maneuver is successful, secure the tube well by suturing it in place with a 3-0 suture.
5. Order a water-soluble radiocontrast x-ray to confirm the correct positioning of the replaced or repositioned tube.

If replacement of the J-tube (enterostomy tube) is unsuccessful, notify the surgeon, who will decide if an urgent reoperation is indicated.

Dislodged *Penrose drains* should not be reinserted into the wound, since bacteria will be introduced into the site. Secure the Penrose drain into the position you find it and examine the area for abscess formation (heat, tenderness, swelling) daily for the next few days. Inform the surgeon that the Penrose drain has become dislodged.

■ NASOGASTRIC AND ENTERAL FEEDING TUBES
■ *Blocked Nasogastric and Enteral Tubes*
PHONE CALL
Questions

1 How long has the tube been blocked?
2 What type of tube is in place?
3 Has the tube been dislodged?
4 What are the vital signs?
5 What was the reason for admission?

Orders

Ask the RN for a 50-ml syringe, sterile NS, and a bowl to be at the bedside.

Inform RN

"Will arrive at the bedside in . . . minutes."

A blocked NG or enteral tube is not an emergency. Assessment can wait an hour or two if other problems of higher priority exist.

ELEVATOR THOUGHTS (What causes blocked NG or enteral feeding tubes?)

1. Debris within the tube
2. Blood clots within the tube
3. Failure to irrigate the tube regularly

MAJOR THREAT TO LIFE

- Aspiration pneumonia

If the NG tube is blocked and thus fails to drain the stomach, gastric contents can be aspirated into the lungs.

BEDSIDE

Quick Look Test

Does the patient look well (comfortable), sick (uncomfortable or distressed), or critical (about to die)?

Failure to drain the gastric contents by a blocked NG tube may result in the patient's developing nausea and vomiting, thus looking sick.

Airways and Vital Signs

What is the RR?

A blocked NG tube should not compromise the airway unless gastric contents accumulate and are aspirated into the lungs.

Selective Physical Examination and Management

1. Irrigate the tube with 25 to 50 ml of NS. As the tube is being irrigated, listen over the stomach region for the gurgling of fluid that indicates that the tube is in the stomach.
2. If the previous maneuver is unsuccessful, remove the tube, and replace with a new tube if there is ongoing gastric stasis with the potential for aspiration.
3. Ensure that the usual nursing protocols are being followed for regular irrigation of the tube.

■ *Dislodged Nasogastric and Enteral Feeding Tubes*

PHONE CALL

Questions

1 How long has the tube been dislodged?
2 What type of tube is in place?
3 What are the vital signs?
4 What was the reason for admission?

Orders

None.

Inform RN

"Will arrive at the bedside in . . . minutes."

Assessment of a dislodged NG or enteral feeding tube may wait an hour or two if other problems of higher priority exist. Be careful, however, not to leave the diabetic patient who has received insulin without caloric intake for too long.

ELEVATOR THOUGHTS (What causes an NG or enteral feeding tube to become dislodged?)

1. Failure to secure the tube adequately
2. Confused, uncooperative patient

MAJOR THREAT TO LIFE

- Aspiration pneumonia

If the NG tube is dislodged and thus fails to drain the stomach, gastric contents may accumulate and can be aspirated into the lung. The danger of a dislodged or misplaced enteral feeding tube is the risk of infusing the enteral feeding solution into the lung.

BEDSIDE

Quick Look Test

Does the patient look well (comfortable), sick (uncomfortable or distressed), or critical (about to die)?

Patients who have aspirated because of a dislodged NG tube or a malpositioned feeding tube may appear tachypneic and unwell.

Airway and Vital Signs

A dislodged NG or enteral feeding tube should not compromise the vital signs unless aspiration of gastric contents or enteral feeding solutions has occurred.

Selective Physical Examination and Management

1. Inspect the tube. **Are there any markings on the tube that indicate how far the tube is situated?** If you are not familiar with these markings, ask the RN to bring a similar tube so you will be able to estimate how far in the tube is.
2. Aspirate the tube to see if gastric contents can be obtained. Instill 25 to 50 ml of air using the 50-ml syringe while listening over the stomach region with your stethoscope. If the tube is properly positioned, you should be able to hear a gurgling swoosh as air is introduced into the stomach.
3. A small-bore enteral feeding tube should not be pushed farther down if it has been dislodged. Do *not* insert the

guidewire down the tube blindly, as laceration or perforation of the esophagus, stomach, or duodenum may occur if the tip of the guidewire exits from one of the distal apertures in the tube. Dislodged enteral feeding tubes must be removed and replaced. The same tube may be reused, with the guidewire being inserted into the tube under direct vision ex vivo. The tube, stiffened by the guidewire, may then be reinserted.

4. Ensure that the usual nursing protocols are being followed for regular irrigation of the tube.

21

POLYURIA—FREQUENCY—INCONTINENCE

You will receive many calls at night regarding patients' urinary volumes. The patients are voiding either too much or too little. It is often difficult for a patient to differentiate between problems of *polyuria* and *frequency,* and for many elderly patients, either one of these problems may present as *incontinence.* Once you clarify which one of the three problems is present, you will find the rest easy.

PHONE CALL
Questions

1 **Clarify the symptom.**
   Polyuria refers to a urine output of greater than 3 L/day. This usually comes to the attention of the nurse when reviewing the fluid balance record or when the urinary drainage bag needs frequent emptying. *Frequency* of urination refers to the frequent passage of urine, whether of large or small volume, and may occur in concert with polyuria or urinary incontinence. *Urinary incontinence* refers to the involuntary loss of urine.
2 **What are the vital signs?**
3 **What was the admitting diagnosis?**

Orders

Polyuria, frequency, and incontinence are seldom urgent problems. Urinary incontinence is a common problem in hospitalized elderly patients and is a frequent source of frustration for nurses. Avoid ordering a Foley catheter as the first line of treatment.

Inform RN

"Will arrive at the bedside in . . . minutes."

If the patient's vital signs are stable and other sick patients require assessment, a patient with polyuria, frequency, or incontinence need not be seen immediately.

ELEVATOR THOUGHTS

What causes **polyuria?**
- Diabetes mellitus
- Diabetes insipidus (central, nephrogenic)
- Psychogenic polydipsia
- Large volumes of oral or IV fluids
- Diuretics

- Diuretic phase of acute tubular necrosis
- Postobstructive diuresis
- Salt-losing nephritis
- Hypercalcemia

What causes **frequency?**
- Urinary tract infection
- Partial bladder outlet obstruction (e.g., prostatism)
- Bladder irritation (tumors, stones, infections)

What causes **incontinence?**
- Urinary tract infection
- Detrusor instability (stroke, Alzheimer's disease, normal pressure hydrocephalus, prostatic hypertrophy, pelvic tumor)
- Stress incontinence (in multiparous women, lax pelvic bladder support; in men, after prostatic surgery)
- Overflow incontinence (bladder outlet obstruction as in BPH, urethral stricture; spinal cord disease, autonomic neuropathy)
- Environmental factors (inaccessibility to call bell, obstacle course to the bathroom)
- Iatrogenic factors (diuretics, sedatives)

MAJOR THREAT TO LIFE

- *Polyuria:* Intravascular volume depletion. If polyuria is not due to fluid excess and continues without adequate fluid replacement, the intravascular volume will drop, and the patient may become hypotensive.
- *Frequency or incontinence:* Sepsis. Frequency or incontinence does not pose a major threat to life unless an underlying urinary tract infection goes unchecked and progresses to pyelonephritis or sepsis.

BEDSIDE
Quick Look Test

Does the patient look well (comfortable), sick (uncomfortable or distressed), or critical (about to die)?

Most often, patients with polyuria, frequency, or incontinence look well. If sick or critical, search for a previously unrecognized problem. For example, if *polyuria* is due to previously undetected diabetes mellitus, the patient may be ketoacidotic and appear sick. Similarly, *frequency* or *incontinence* may prove to be the presenting manifestation of urinary tract infection in a patient who appears sick.

Airway and Vital Signs

Check for postural changes. A rise in HR > 15 beats/min or a fall in systolic BP > 15 mm Hg or any fall in diastolic BP indicates significant hypovolemia. *Caution:* A resting tachycardia alone may indicate decreased intravascular volume.

Fever suggests possible urinary tract infection.

Selective Physical Examination I

Is the patient volume depleted?

CVS	Pulse volume, JVP
	Skin temperature and color
NEURO	Level of consciousness

Management

What immediate measure needs to be taken to correct or prevent intravascular volume depletion?

Replace intravascular volume. If volume depleted, give IV NS or Ringer's lactate, aiming for a JVP of 2 to 3 cm H_2O above the sternal angle and normalization of the vital signs. Remember that aggressive fluid repletion in a patient with a history of CHF may compromise cardiac function. Do not overshoot the mark!

Selective History and Chart Review

Identify the specific problem.

Polyuria. The assessment of polyuria can be estimated by history but accurately confirmed only by scrutiny of meticulously kept fluid balance sheets. If these are not available, order strict intake/output monitoring. It is worthwhile to document polyuria (>3 L/day) before embarking on an exhaustive workup of a possibly nonexistent problem.

1. Ask about associated symptoms. "Polyuria + polydipsia" suggests diabetes mellitus, diabetes insipidus, or compulsive water drinking (psychogenic polydipsia). Of these, diabetes mellitus is the most common.
2. Check the chart for recent laboratory results.
   a. Blood glucose (diabetes mellitus)
   b. Potassium
   c. Calcium

   Hypokalemia and hypercalcemia are important reversible causes of nephrogenic diabetes insipidus. Refer to Chapter 33 for management of hypokalemia and Chapter 30 for management of hypercalcemia.
3. Make sure the patient is not on any drugs that may cause either nephrogenic diabetes insipidus (lithium carbonate, demeclocycline) or diuresis (diuretics, mannitol).

Frequency. Frequency can be assessed by questioning the patient. Estimate from the nursing notes or fluid balance sheets if the patient is an unreliable historian. Ask about associated symptoms. Fever, dysuria, hematuria, and foul-smelling urine suggest urinary tract infection. Poor stream, hesitancy, dribbling, or nocturia suggests prostatism.

Incontinence.   Incontinence is obvious when it occurs and is often embarrassing to the patient. You need an honest history from the patient to make a proper diagnosis. Address the subject nonjudgmentally.

Selective Physical Examination II

Look for specific causes and complications of polyuria, frequency, or incontinence.

VITALS	Fever (UTI)
HEENT	Visual fields (pituitary neoplasm)
RESP	Kussmaul's respiration (diabetic ketoacidosis)
	Kussmaul's respirations are characterized by deep, pauseless breathing at a rate of 25 to 30/min.
ABD	Enlarged bladder (neurogenic bladder, bladder outlet obstruction with overflow incontinence)
	Suprapubic tenderness (cystitis)
NEURO	Level of consciousness
	Localizing findings
	An alert, conscious person with polyuria and with free access to fluids and salt will not become volume depleted. If volume depletion is present, suspect metabolic or structural neurological abnormalities impairing the normal response to thirst. Perform a complete neurological examination, looking for evidence of stroke, subdural hemorrhage, or metabolic abnormalities.
SKIN	Perineal skin breakdown (a complication of repeated incontinence and a source of infection)
RECTAL	Enlarged prostate (bladder outlet obstruction)
	Perineal sensation, resting tone of anal sphincter, anal wink
	An anal wink is elicited by gently stroking the perineal mucosa with a tongue depressor. A normal response is manifested by contraction of the external sphincter.
	If abnormalities in perineal sensation, anal sphincter tone, or anal wink are discovered, the bulbocavernosus reflex should also be tested. To elicit this reflex, the index finger of the examining hand is introduced into the rectum, and the patient is asked to relax the sphincter as much as possible. The glans penis is then squeezed with the opposite hand, which normally results in involuntary contraction of the anal sphincter.
	Innervation of the anus is similar to that of the lower

urinary tract. Therefore, abnormalities in perineal sensation or in the sacral reflexes may provide a clue that a spinal cord lesion is responsible for the incontinence.

Management

What more needs to be done tonight?

Polyuria

1. Once intravascular volume is restored, ensure adequate continuing replacement (usually IV) fluid as estimated by urinary, insensible (400 to 800 ml/day), and other (nasogastric suction, vomiting, diarrhea) losses. Recheck the volume status periodically to ensure that your mathematic estimates for replacement correlate with an appropriate clinical response.

2. Order strict intake/output records to be kept.

3. Serum glucose, Chemstrip, or Glucometer testing. This will identify diabetes mellitus before it progresses to ketoacidosis (IDDM) or hyperosmolar coma (NIDDM). The presence of glycosuria on urinalysis will provide more rapid evidence of hyperglycemia as a possible cause of polyuria. Random blood glucose levels of <10 mmol/L are seldom accompanied by osmotic diuresis. If hyperglycemia of more than 10 mmol/L exists, refer to Chapter 32, page 303, for further management.

4. Serum calcium level is often not available as a stat test at night. If there is strong suspicion of hypercalcemia (polyuria or lethargy in a patient with malignancy, hyperparathyroidism, or sarcoidosis), contact the laboratory for permission to measure the serum calcium level on an urgent basis.

5. Maximal urine concentrating ability measured by the water deprivation test can help differentiate among central diabetes insipidus, nephrogenic diabetes insipidus, and psychogenic polydipsia. This test can be arranged on an elective basis in the morning.

Frequency

1. If other symptoms (urgency, dysuria, low-grade fever, suprapubic tenderness) of urinary tract infection (cystitis) are present, empiric treatment with antibiotics may be warranted, pending urine culture and sensitivity results, which will usually take 48 hours to complete. Scrutiny of the patient's chart may reveal a previous urine culture or previous antibacterial therapy that may affect the selection of empiric treatment. *Amoxicillin* 500 mg PO q8h for 7 to 10 days or *trimethoprim-sulfamethoxazole* (Septra D.S.) (160 mg–800 mg) 1 tablet PO BID for 7 to 10 days may be used. In young outpatient females, single-dose therapy has been successful, e.g., *amoxicillin* 3 g PO × 1 dose or *trimethoprim-sulfamethoxazole* (160 mg–800 mg) PO × 1 dose. Although they may be tried, these single-dose regimens have not been definitely proved efficacious in the hospitalized population.

Allergies to penicillin and its derivatives and to sulfonamides are common. Ensure the absence of allergies to these drugs before initiating treatment. If the patient is allergic to penicillin and to sulfonamides, *cephalexin* (Keflex) 500 mg PO QID for 7 days can be given, recognizing a 10% to 15% cross-reactivity in penicillin-allergic patients. Inform these patients of this risk.

Phenazopyridine (Pyridium) 200 mg PO TID after meals may help alleviate dysuria in cases of urethritis during the first day or two of treatment. Warn the patient that this drug may turn the urine orange. Also, encourage high fluid intake to promote washout of the urinary tract.

2. If history and physical examination suggest partial bladder outlet obstruction, examine the abdomen carefully for an enlarged bladder. If in urinary retention, a Foley catheter should be placed. (Refer to Chapter 9, p. 66, for further investigation and management of urinary retention.)

Always check for heart murmurs before catheterizing a patient. Patients with cardiac valvular abnormalities are at risk for development of infective endocarditis following GU procedures, including catheterization with a Foley catheter. Any patient with a documented valvular abnormality, including mitral valve prolapse with a persistent systolic murmur, should receive antibiotic prophylaxis directed primarily against enterococci before catheterization. Current recommendations are as follows: *ampicillin* 2 g IM or IV plus *gentamicin* 1.5 mg/kg IM or IV. Both antibiotics should be given 30 minutes before the procedure and once again 8 hours later. Patients who are allergic to penicillin may be treated with *vancomycin* 1 g IV over 1 hour plus *gentamicin* 1.5 mg/kg IM or IV. Both of these antibiotics should be given 1 hour before the procedure and once again 8 to 12 hours later.

A brief in-and-out catheterization, in the presence of sterile urine, may not require antibiotic prophylaxis. If, however, the patient has a prosthetic cardiac valve, you may want to err on the safe side and administer prophylactic antibiotics. Ask your resident or the patient's cardiologist for advice in this situation.

3. Other causes of frequency, such as bladder irritation by stones or tumors, can be addressed by urological consultation in the morning. You may be able to expedite the diagnosis of bladder tumor by ordering a collection of urine for cytologic study.

Incontinence

1. Even if incontinence is the only symptom, order a urinalysis and urine culture to ensure that a urinary tract infection is not contributing to the patient's symptoms.

2. Check for hyperglycemia, hypokalemia, and hypercalcemia if there is a question of polyuria. These conditions may present as incontinence in the elderly or bedridden patient, and specific treatment may alleviate the incontinence.

3. If neurological examination (e.g., abnormal sacral reflexes, diminished perineal sensation, lower limb weakness or spasticity) suggests the presence of a *spinal cord lesion*, consultation should be arranged with a neurologist.

4. In the case of *overflow incontinence*, one must differentiate between overflow due to bladder outlet obstruction (e.g., BPH, uterine prolapse) and impaired ability of detrusor contraction (e.g., lower motor neuron bladder). This is best done in the morning by assessment of urinary bladder dynamics under the direction of a urologist. If the bladder is palpably enlarged and the patient is distressed, bladder catheterization may be attempted. Forceful attempts at catheterization should be avoided, and a urologist should be called for assistance if the catheter does not pass easily (see Chapter 20, p. 198). If no correctable obstruction is found, long-term treatment may involve intermittent straight catheterization q4–6h, which is less likely to cause infection than a chronic indwelling Foley catheter. Aim for a urine volume of less than 400 ml q4–6h. Greater volumes result in ureterovesical reflux, which promotes ascending urinary tract infection. A young motivated patient with a neurogenic bladder can be taught to self-catheterize. In these cases, a silicone elastomer (Silastic) Foley catheter should be used. This type has the advantage of less predisposition to calcification and encrustation and may be kept in place up to 6 weeks at a time.

5. *Detrusor instability* is a condition in which the bladder escapes central inhibition, resulting in reflex contractions. It is the most common cause of incontinence in the elderly population and is often manifested by *urge incontinence* (involuntary micturition preceded by a warning of a few seconds or minute). Ensure that there are no physical barriers preventing the patient from reaching the bathroom or commode in time. Is there easy access to the call bell? Are the nurses responding promptly? Are the bedrails kept up or down? Does the patient have a medical condition (e.g., Parkinson's disease, stroke, arthritis) that prevents easy mobilization when the urge to void occurs? If there is no evidence of perineal skin breakdown, *urinary incontinence pads* with frequent checks and changes by the nursing staff are entirely adequate. (Babies exist for years in such a state!) If perineal skin breakdown or ulceration is present, a Foley or condom catheter is justified to allow skin healing. Long-term treatment involves regular toileting q2–3h while awake and limiting the evening fluid intake.

6. Urinary spillage with coughing or straining suggests *stress incontinence*. Again, if there is no evidence of perineal skin breakdown, urinary incontinence pads are perfectly adequate until urological consultation can assess the need for surgery.

REMEMBER

Urinary incontinence is an understandable source of frustration for nurses caring for these patients. Listen to the concerns of the nurses looking after your patients and discuss with them the reasons for your actions.

22

PRONOUNCING DEATH

One of the required duties of medical students and interns on call at night is the pronouncement of death in patients who have recently died. This is a situation that is seldom addressed in medical school, and you will certainly wonder what needs to be done to pronounce a patient dead. Unfortunately, there has long been uncertainty surrounding what constitutes the medical and legal definition of death.

Traditionally, the determination of death has been solely a medical decision. In the United States, legislative action on the criteria of death falls within state jurisdiction. Many states have opted to follow the recommendations set forth by the Harvard Medical School Ad Hoc Committee,[1] Capron and Kass,[2] or the Kansas legislation of 1971.[3] It is best to be familiar with the medical and legal criteria accepted for the determination of death in the state in which you work.

The recommended criteria of death to be used for all purposes within the jurisdiction of the Parliament of Canada, issued by the Law Reform Commission of Canada[4] in 1981, were as follows.

1. A person is dead when an irreversible cessation of all that person's brain function has occurred.
2. The irreversible cessation of brain function can be determined by the prolonged absence of spontaneous circulatory and respiratory functions.
3. When the determination of the prolonged absence of spontaneous circulatory and respiratory functions is made impossible by the use of artificial means of support, the irreversible cessation of the brain function can be determined by any means recognized by the ordinary standards of current medical practice.

Although criterion 1 alone may imply that a complete neurological examination is required for pronouncement of death, we know that this is neither practical nor necessary. Criterion 2 accounts for this by assuming that when "prolonged absence of spontaneous circulatory and respiratory functions" exists, irreversible cessation of the patient's brain function has occurred. Hence, there will be no question in the majority of cases that most of the patients you will be asked to pronounce dead will indeed be medically and legally dead, as they will fulfill the criterion set out in 2 alone. Thus, legally, in most cases all that is required of you to pronounce a patient dead is to verify that there has been a prolonged absence of spontaneous circulatory and respiratory functions. A slightly more detailed assessment is recommended, however, and will take only a few minutes to complete.

The RN will page you and inform you of the death of the patient, requesting that you come to the unit and pronounce the patient dead.

1. Identify the patient by the hospital identification tag worn on the wrist.
2. Ascertain that the patient does not rouse to verbal or tactile stimuli.
3. Listen for heart sounds and feel for the carotid pulse. The deceased patient is pulseless and without heart sounds.
4. Look and listen to the patient's chest for evidence of spontaneous respirations. The deceased patient shows no evidence of breathing movements or of air entry on examination.
5. Record the position of the pupils and their reactions to light. The deceased patient shows no evidence of pupillary reaction to light. Though the pupils are usually dilated, this position is not invariable.
6. Record the time at which your assessment was completed. Although other emergencies take precedence over pronouncing a patient dead, one should try not to postpone this task too long, since the time of death is legally the time at which you pronounce the patient dead.
7. Document your findings on the chart. A typical chart entry may read as follows: Called to pronounce Mr. Doe dead. Patient unresponsive to verbal or tactile stimuli. No heart sounds heard, no pulse felt. Not breathing, no air entry heard. Pupils fixed and dilated. Patient pronounced dead at 2030 hours, December 7, 1993.
8. Notify the family physician, attending physician, or both if the nurses have not already done so. Decide together with the attending physician whether an autopsy would be useful and appropriate in this patient's case.
9. Notification of relatives. Next of kin should be notified as soon as possible after you have pronounced the patient dead and notified the family physician, attending physician, or both. Normally, it is the responsibility of the family physician to notify the relatives once he or she has been told of the patient's death. Occasionally, you may experience the situation where the family physician has signed over his or her nighttime call to a partner or another physician who does not know the patient or family. In this situation, it is best to inform the physician on call, and if he or she is uncomfortable with speaking to the family, a member of the house staff who knows the patient or family best should then notify the next of kin. The family will appreciate hearing the news from a familiar voice.

    If neither the family physician on call nor the house staff

knows the patient, spend a few minutes familiarizing yourself with the patient's medical history and mode of death. If you are appointed to deliver the news to the family, the following guidelines may be helpful.

a. Identify yourself, e.g., "This is Dr. Jones calling from St. Paul's Hospital."

b. Ask for the next of kin, e.g., "May I speak with Mrs. Doe, please?"

c. Deliver the message, e.g., "Mrs. Doe, I am sorry to inform you that your husband died at 8:30 this evening."

d. You may be surprised to find that in many instances this news is not unexpected. It is, however, always comforting to a family to know that a relative has died peacefully—e.g., "As you know, your husband was suffering from a terminal illness. Although I was not with your husband at the time of his death, the nurses looking after him assure me that he was very comfortable at the time of his death and that he passed away peacefully."

e. If an autopsy is desired by one of the medical staff, this question should be broached now—e.g., "Your husband had an unusual illness, and if you are agreeable, it would be very useful to us to perform an autopsy. Although it obviously won't change the course of events in terms of your husband's illness, it may provide some valuable information for other patients suffering from similar problems to your husband's." If there is any hesitation on the part of the next of kin, emphasize that they are under no obligation to grant permission for an autopsy to be performed if it is against the perceived wishes of the patient or family. If the next of kin refuses, do not argue, no matter how interested you may be in the outcome of the case. Accept the family's decision graciously—e.g., "We understand completely, and, of course, we will respect your wishes."

f. Ask the next of kin if he or she would like to come to the hospital to see the patient one last time. Inform the nurses of this decision. Questions pertaining to funeral homes and the patient's personal belongings are best referred to the nurse in charge.

SPECIAL SITUATIONS

Medical technology has introduced two other scenarios in the pronouncement of a patient's death.

The Mechanically Ventilated Patient Without Circulatory Function

There is general understanding that those patients whose hearts have stopped beating despite being mechanically ventilated will all meet the criteria for legal death through a lack of spontaneous ventilation once the ventilator is turned off. Thus, it is reasonable practice to

1. Ensure that connections are intact and properly attached if the patient is on the ECG monitor. (This assures that the absence of cardiac electrical activity is not an artifact due to faulty electrical connections.)
2. Follow the usual procedure for pronouncing death.
3. Discuss your findings with the attending physician *before* disconnecting the ventilator.
4. After agreement with the attending physician, disconnect the ventilator. Observe the patient for 3 minutes for evidence of spontaneous respiration.
5. Document your findings in the chart—e.g., "Called to pronounce Mr. Doe dead. Patient unresponsive to verbal or tactile stimuli. No heart sounds heard, no pulse felt. Pupils fixed and dilated. Patient being mechanically ventilated. Ventilator disconnected at 2030 hours after discussion with attending physician, Dr. Smith. No spontaneous respirations noted for 3 minutes. Patient pronounced dead at 2033 hours, December 7, 1993."

The Mechanically Ventilated Patient With Circulatory Function Intact

This type of patient is usually being cared for in the ICU. A variety of controversial criteria exists for the determination of brain death, and criteria may differ between geographic locations. The task of pronouncing a mechanically ventilated patient dead and the discussion of organ procurement are best left to the ICU staff and associated subspecialists in consultation with the patient's family.

REFERENCES

1. Report of the Ad Hoc Committee of the Harvard Medical School to Examine the Definition of Brain Death. JAMA 205, 337 (1968).
2. Capron and Kass. A Statutory Definition of the Standards for Determining Human Death, 121 U. Pa. L. Rev. 87 (1972a).
3. Kan. Stat. Ann. 77-202 (Supp. 1974).
4. Report on the Criteria for the Determination of Death. Law Reform Commission of Canada, 1981.

23

SEIZURES

A seizure is one of the more dramatic events you may witness while on call. Usually, everyone around you will be in a panic. The key to controlling the situation is to remain calm.

PHONE CALL

Questions

1 Is the patient still seizing?
2 What type of seizure was witnessed? Was the seizure generalized tonic-clonic, or was it focal?
3 What is the patient's level of consciousness?
4 Has there been any obvious injury?
5 What was the reason for admission?
6 Does the patient have diabetes mellitus?

Orders

1. Ask the RN to make sure the patient is positioned on his or her side. During both the seizure and the postictal state, the patient should be kept in the lateral decubitus position to prevent aspiration of gastric contents.
2. Ask the RN to have the following available *at the bedside.*
    a. Oral airway
    b. IV setup with NS (flushed through and ready for immediate use)
    c. Two blood tubes (one for chemistry and one for hematology)
    d. *Diazepam* (Valium) 20 mg
    e. *Thiamine* 100 mg
    f. D50W 50 ml (1 ampule)
    g. Chart
3. If the patient is postictal, ask the RN to remove any dentures, suction the oropharynx, and insert an oral airway.
4. Order a stat blood glucose, Chemstrip, or Glucometer reading if the patient is in the postictal state (unconscious).

Inform RN

"Will arrive at bedside in . . . minutes."

A seizure requires you to see the patient immediately.

ELEVATOR THOUGHTS (What causes seizures?)

Drugs

1. Antiepileptic medication inadvertently discontinued or nontherapeutic level
2. Alcohol withdrawal. *Caution:* **Does the patient have delirium tremens in addition to the seizures?**
3. Meperidine (Demerol) overdose (an easily missed diagnosis in the elderly postoperative patient)
4. Benzodiazepine or barbiturate withdrawal
5. Penicillin at high doses
6. Theophylline toxicity
7. Lidocaine HCl infusion
8. Isoniazid
9. Lithium carbonate
10. Neuroleptics (e.g., chlorpromazine)

CNS

1. Tumor
2. Previous stroke
3. Previous head injury
4. Meningitis/encephalitis
5. Idiopathic epilepsy

ENDO

1. Hypoglycemia
2. Hyponatremia
3. Hypocalcemia
4. Hypomagnesemia

} The four hypos

MISC

1. Uremia
2. CNS vasculitis
3. Hypertensive encephalopathy
4. Hypoxia/hypercapnia
5. Pseudoseizure

Common Causes of Seizures in Patients With AIDS

1. Mass lesions (toxoplasmosis, CNS lymphoma)
2. HIV encephalopathy
3. Meningitis (cryptococcal, herpes zoster, toxoplasmosis, aseptic)
4. Any of the usual causes of seizures seen in immunocompetent hosts

MAJOR THREAT TO LIFE

- Aspiration
- Hypoxia

The patient should be lying in the lateral decubitus position to prevent the tongue from falling posteriorly, blocking the airway, and to minimize the risk of aspiration of gastric contents while in the postictal state. Patients usually keep breathing throughout seizure activity. Most patients can be in status epilepticus for 30 minutes with no subsequent neurological damage.

The majority of seizures will have stopped by the time you arrive at the bedside. The procedures and protocols to follow if the seizure has stopped are discussed subsequently. The procedures and protocols to follow if the seizure persists begin on page 222.

■ IF THE SEIZURE HAS STOPPED
BEDSIDE
Quick Look Test

Does the patient look well (comfortable), sick (uncomfortable or distressed), or critical (about to die)?

Most patients after a generalized tonic-clonic seizure are unconscious (the postictal state).

Airway, Vital Signs, and Blood Glucose Results

In what position is the patient lying?

The patient should be positioned in the lateral decubitus position to prevent aspiration of gastric contents (Fig. 23–1).

Remove any dentures and suction the airway. Insert an oral airway if one is not already in place (Fig. 23–2). You are not out of the woods yet! The patient might begin to experience another seizure, so make sure the airway is protected.

Give oxygen by face mask or nasal prongs.

What is the Chemstrip result?

Hypoglycemia needs to be treated immediately to prevent further seizures.

Management I

Draw blood (20 ml) and establish IV access. Send the blood for the following tests.

Chemistry tube: Electrolytes, urea, creatinine, random blood glucose, Ca, Mg, albumin, and antiepileptic drug levels (if the patient is receiving these medications). If the patient is undergoing a 3-day fast for investigation of possible hypoglycemia, order an insulin level as well.

Hematology tube: CBC and manual differential.

Once the IV is established keep the line open with NS. NS is the IV fluid of choice, as phenytoin is not compatible with dextrose-containing solutions.

If the *Chemstrip* result or *Glucometer* reading reveals hypogly-

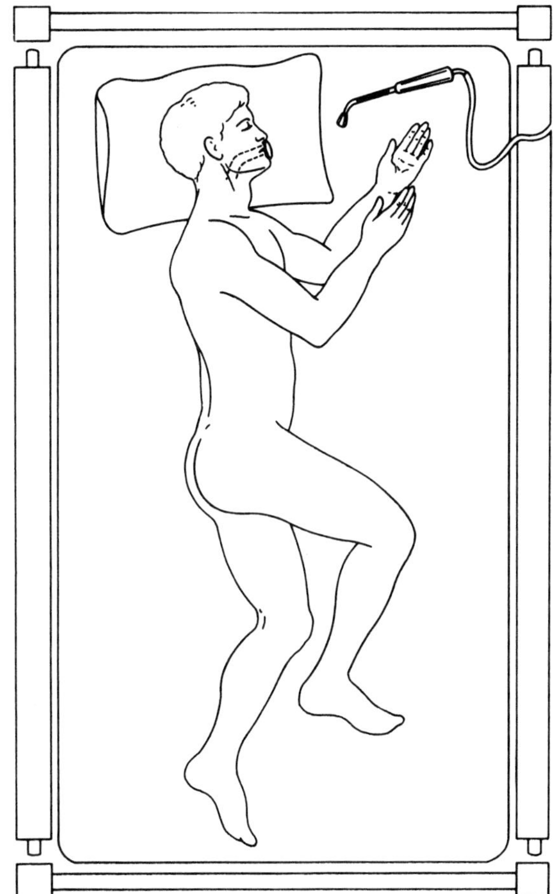

Figure 23–1 □ Positioning of the patient to prevent aspiration of gastric contents.

cemia, give *thiamine* 100 mg IV by slow, direct injection over 3 to 5 minutes, followed by D50W 50 ml IV by slow, direct injection. Thiamine is given before administration of glucose to protect against an exacerbation of Wernicke's encephalopathy.

Draw *ABGs* if the patient appears cyanotic.

Selective Physical Examination I

Assess LOC. **Does the patient respond to verbal or painful stimuli? Is the patient in a postictal state** (i.e., decreased level of consciousness)? Remember, if the patient does not regain con-

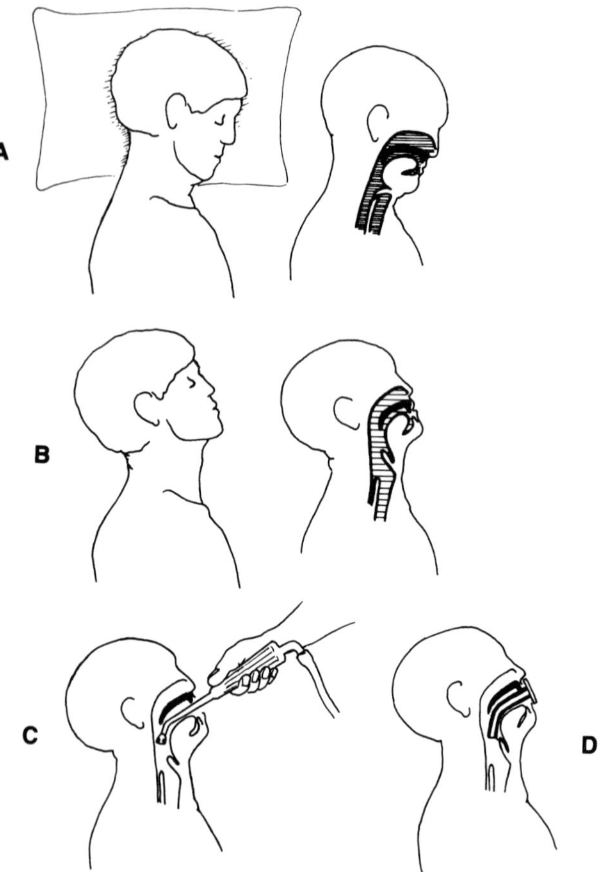

Figure 23–2 □ Airway management. Correct positioning of the head, correct suctioning, and correct inserting of an oral airway. **A.** Neck flexion closes the airway. **B.** Neck extension to sniffing position opens the airway. **C.** Suctioning. **D.** Placement of the airway.

sciousness between seizures, after 30 minutes the diagnosis becomes *status epilepticus*.

Selective History and Chart Review

1. Ask any witnesses the following details about the seizure.
   a. **Length of time?**
   b. **Generalized tonic-clonic or focal?**

    c. **Onset generalized or focal?** A focal onset of a generalized tonic-clonic seizure suggests structural brain disease, which may be old or new.

    d. **Any injury observed during the seizure?**

2. Is there a **history of epilepsy, alcohol or sedative withdrawal, head injury** (e.g., recent fall while in hospital), **stroke, CNS tumor** (primary or secondary), or **diabetes mellitus?**

3. **Is the patient receiving any of the following medications, which may induce seizures?**
   a. Penicillin
   b. Meperidine (Demerol)
   c. Insulin
   d. Oral hypoglycemics
   e. Antidepressants, lithium carbonate
   f. Isoniazid
   g. Lidocaine
   h. Neuroleptics (e.g., chlorpromazine)
   i. Theophylline

4. **Is the patient HIV positive or otherwise immunosuppressed?** Seizures are a common manifestation of CNS disease in the HIV-positive patient.

5. **What are the most recent laboratory results?**
   a. Glucose
   b. Na
   c. Ca
   d. Albumin
   e. Mg
   f. Antiepileptic drug levels
   g. Urea
   h. Creatinine

The chart is reviewed before the physical examination because an immediate, treatable cause (e.g., insulin or meperidine overdose, hyponatremia) is more likely to be found in the chart.

Selective Physical Examination II

VITALS	Repeat now
HEENT	Tongue or cheek lacerations, nuchal rigidity
RESP	Signs of aspiration
NEURO	Complete CNS examination within the limits of LOC Can the patient speak, follow commands? Is there any asymmetry of pupils, visual fields, reflexes, or plantar responses? Asymmetry suggests structural brain disease.
MSS	Palpate skull and face, spine and ribs Passive ROM of all four limbs Are there any lacerations, hematomas, or fractures?

Management II

Establish the *provisional and differential diagnoses* of the seizure—this must be a *causally defined* diagnosis (e.g., "Generalized tonic-clonic seizure secondary to hypoglycemia").

Are there any *complications* of the seizure giving rise to a second diagnosis? For example, if a head injury has been sustained, the provisional diagnosis might be "forehead hematoma" and the differential diagnosis would include subdural hematoma, frontal bone fracture,

Treat the underlying cause! Seizure is a symptom, not a diagnosis.

Maintain IV access for 24 hours with NS. If there is a concern regarding volume overloading, use a heparin lock instead of maintaining the IV open with NS.

In most patients with a single seizure, it is not necessary to administer antiepileptic medications, particularly if a rapidly correctable metabolic cause is found. Exceptions include the patient already on antiepileptic medication but with inadequate serum concentrations, the patient with suspected structural CNS abnormality, and the HIV-positive patient (in whom seizures tend to be recurrent). If further seizures are anticipated, a long-acting antiepileptic drug (e.g., phenytoin rather than diazepam) is recommended (see p. 229 for dosage). Although diazepam is useful as an anticonvulsant to halt seizures, it is not useful as a prophylactic. The antiepileptic medication of choice is *phenytoin*.

The *elderly* and other patients suspected of having *structural CNS disease* as a cause of their seizure should have a CT head scan performed. The *HIV-positive patient* should have a CT head scan (because of the high incidence of CNS mass lesions), and if there is no risk of herniation, an LP also should be performed. Occasionally, cryptococcal meningitis may coexist in an HIV-positive patient who also has a mass lesion on CT head scan.

Seizure precautions should be instituted for the next 48 hours and then reviewed (Table 23–1).

■ IF THE PATIENT IS STILL SEIZING

Don't panic (almost everybody else will)! Most seizures will resolve without treatment within 2 minutes.

BEDSIDE
Quick Look Test

Does the patient look well (comfortable), sick (uncomfortable or distressed), or critical (about to die)?

A patient having a generalized tonic-clonic seizure often engenders anxiety in the observer. Remember, if the patient is seizing, you can be assured that he or she has both a BP and a pulse.

Table 23–1 □ SEIZURE PRECAUTIONS

1 Bed placed in lowest position
2 Oral airway at head of bed
3 Side rails up when patient in bed. In case of generalized tonic-clonic seizure, side rails should be padded
4 Provide patient with a firm pillow
5 Suction at bedside
6 Oxygen at bedside
7 Bathroom privileges with supervision only
8 Baths or showers only with a nurse in attendance
9 Axilla temperature only
10 Direct supervision when using sharp objects, e.g., straight razor, nail scissors

Ask the RN to notify your resident of the situation—a seizure is a medical emergency.

Airway, Vital Signs, and Blood Glucose Result

In what position is the patient lying?
The patient should be positioned and maintained in the lateral decubitus position to prevent aspiration of gastric contents. One or two assistants may be required to hold the patient in this position if the seizure is violent.

Suction the airway. Do not insert an oral airway or attempt to remove dentures if force is required. You will break the patient's teeth.

Give oxygen by face mask or nasal prongs.

What is the patient's BP?
It is virtually impossible to take a BP during a generalized tonic-clonic seizure, so palpate the femoral pulse. (You may need an assistant to hold the patient's knee against the bed.) A palpable femoral pulse indicates a systolic BP of >60 mm Hg.

What is the Chemstrip result?
Hypoglycemia needs to be treated immediately, if present.

Management I

How long has the patient been seizing?
If the seizure has stopped, refer to page 222.

If the seizure has lasted < 3 minutes
Do not give diazepam yet.
- Recheck the airway.
- Observe the seizure activity.

- Do *not* attempt to start an IV yet; it will be much easier in 1 or 2 minutes, after the seizure has stopped.
- Ensure that IV tubing is flushed through with NS and that thiamine, D50W, diazepam, and two blood tubes are all available at the bedside.

If the seizure has lasted > 3 minutes
Draw blood (20 ml) and establish IV access.

Tips on Starting the IV.   When the patient is seizing, it is very difficult to start an IV. This is an emergency and not the time for a novice to try his or her hand at starting an IV. Appoint the most experienced person present to obtain IV access. The patient's arm should be held firmly by one or two assistants (Fig. 23–3) while maintaining the patient on the side. Sit down—it is much easier to start an IV when sitting rather than standing. Try for the largest vein available but not the antecubital vein unless forced, since the elbow will then have to be splinted to avoid losing the IV access.

Medications.   Order the following medications to be given immediately.
- *Thiamine* 100 mg IV by slow, direct injection over 3 to 5 minutes.
- *D50W* 50 ml IV by slow, direct injection. If hypoglycemic, the patient will become conscious abruptly while receiving the first 30 ml of D50W. Do not proceed with any further medication; change the IV to D5W. Thiamine is given before ad-

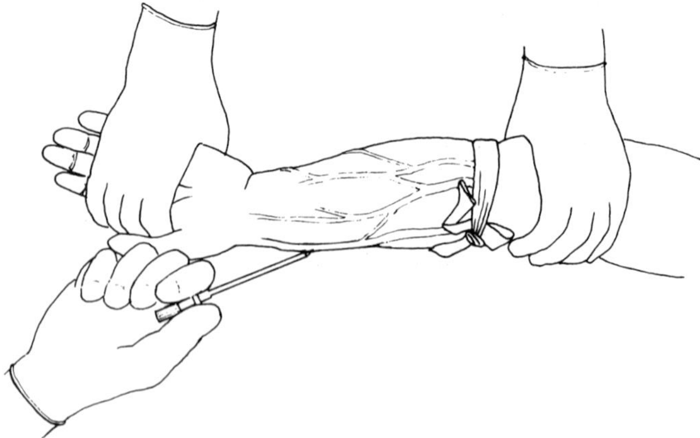

Figure 23–3 □ Positioning required when starting an IV during a generalized tonic-clonic seizure.

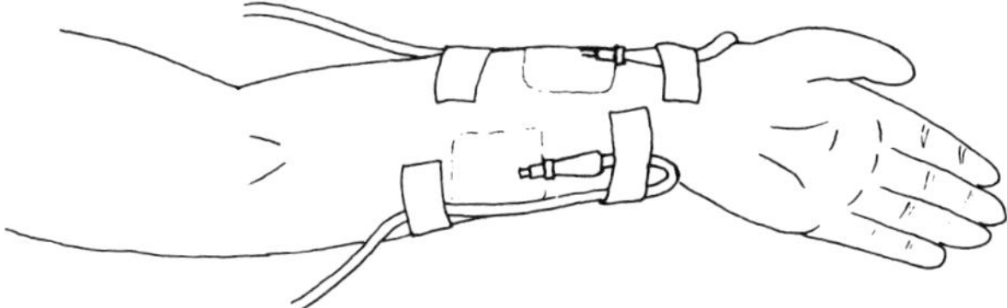

Figure 23–4 □ Two IVs are needed if both diazepam (Valium) and phenytoin (Dilantin) are to be administered.

ministration of glucose to protect against an exacerbation of Wernicke's encephalopathy.

- *Diazepam* (Valium) at a rate of 2 mg/min IV until the seizure stops or to a maximum dose of 20 mg. It will take 10 minutes to deliver 20 mg of diazepam at this rate. (An Ambu bag should be available at the bedside whenever diazepam is being given IV, since diazepam may cause respiratory depression.) If diazepam is not available a good alternative is *lorazepam* (Ativan) 2 to 4 mg IV over 3 to 5 minutes.
- *Phenytoin.* Ask an assistant to obtain the following.
  - A second IV setup with NS (Fig. 23–4). Diazepam and phenytoin are not compatible, so they cannot be given via the same IV.
  - Phenytoin, loading dose 18 mg/kg (1250 mg for a 70 kg patient), to be available at the bedside. The phenytoin loading dose may be injected directly via an NS IV at a rate no faster than 25 to 50 mg/min or as an infusion (add the loading dose to 100 ml of NS) given at a rate not greater than 25 to 50 mg/min. Following phenytoin administration, the IV should be flushed through with NS to avoid local venous irritation from the drug's alkalinity.

Phenytoin may cause hypotension and cardiac dysrhythmias. Monitor the femoral pulse for decrease of volume (hypotension) and for irregularities of rhythm (Fig. 23–5). If either of these problems occurs, slow the phenytoin infusion rate.

If seizing continues despite administering half the maximum dose of diazepam (10 mg), begin administering the loading dose of phenytoin (Dilantin) (no faster than 25 to 50 mg/min) but continue with the diazepam until the maximum dose has been given.

If the patient has *already received phenytoin* or has an inadequate level, give *half* the phenytoin loading dose IV. The most frequent side effects of overshooting with an extra loading dose are dizziness, nausea, and blurred vision for a few days. These are not major risks.

If the seizure now stops, stop giving the diazepam but give

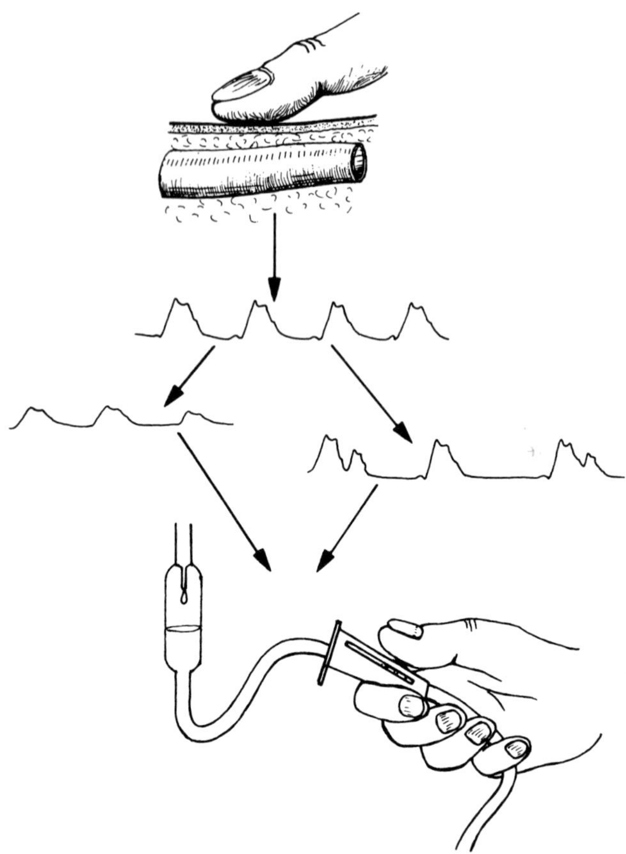

Figure 23–5 □ Phenytoin (Dilantin) may cause hypotension or cardiac dysrhythmias, detectable by palpating the femoral pulse. If either one is present, the phenytoin infusion rate should be slowed.

the full loading dose of phenytoin. See page 222 for further instructions. Most seizures can be controlled with diazepam and phenytoin. If not, CNS infection or structural brain disease should be considered.

If the seizure has persisted for 30 minutes, the patient is now in *status epilepticus*. This is an emergency! A neurologist, intensivist, or anesthesiologist should be consulted immediately. The patient should be transferred to the ICU/CCU for management of the airway and probable intubation.

Status epilepticus is rare. It is defined as a single seizure lasting 30 minutes or repetitive seizures without intervening periods of normal consciousness, lasting more than 30 minutes.

Additional treatment in the ICU/CCU may include an intravenous phenobarbital infusion or, rarely, general anesthesia with halothane and neuromuscular blockade.

24

SHORTNESS OF BREATH

Calls at night to assess a patient's breathing are common. Do not become overwhelmed by the myriad causes of SOB that you learned about in medical school. In hospitalized patients, as you will see, there are only four common causes of SOB.

PHONE CALL

Questions

1 **How long has the patient been SOB?**
2 **Did the SOB begin gradually or suddenly?**
  Sudden onset of SOB suggests pulmonary embolus or pneumothorax.
3 **Is the patient cyanosed?**
4 **What are the vital signs?**
5 **What was the reason for admission?**
6 **Does the patient have COPD?**
  What you really need to know is whether or not the patient is a CO_2 retainer. In most cases, this will apply to patients with COPD or with a history of heavy smoking.
7 **Does the patient have O_2 ordered?**

Orders

1. Oxygen. If you are certain that the patient is not a CO_2 retainer, you may safely order any concentration of O_2 in the short-term situation. If you are not certain, order O_2 28% by Venturi mask and reassess on arrival at the bedside.
2. If the admitting diagnosis is asthma and the patient has not received a nebulized bronchodilator within the last 2 hours, order nebulized *salbutamol* (Ventolin) 2.5 to 5 mg in 3 ml NS immediately.
3. ABG set at bedside. Not all patients with SOB will require ABG determination, but it is best to have the equipment ready on arrival if needed. Alternatively, ask for an urgent measurement of pulse oximetry, if available.

Inform RN

"Will arrive at bedside in . . . minutes."

SOB requires you to see the patient immediately.

ELEVATOR THOUGHTS (What causes SOB?)

Cardiovascular Causes
- CHF
- Pulmonary embolism

Pulmonary Causes
- Pneumonia
- Bronchospasm (asthma and COPD)

Miscellaneous Causes
- Anxiety, upper airway obstruction, pneumothorax, massive pleural effusions, massive ascites, postoperative atelectasis, cardiac tamponade, aspiration of gastric contents.

MAJOR THREAT TO LIFE

- Hypoxia

Inadequate tissue oxygenation is the most worrisome end result of any process causing SOB. Hence, you must direct your initial assessment toward ascertaining whether or not hypoxia is present.

BEDSIDE
Quick Look Test

Does the patient look well (comfortable), sick (uncomfortable or distressed), or critical (about to die)?

This simple observation will help determine the necessity of immediate intervention. If the patient looks sick, order ABGs, O_2, IV D5W TKVO. Ask the nurse to bring the cardaic arrest cart to the bedside, attach the patient to the ECG monitor, and prepare for possible intubation. Consult ICU immediately.

Airway and Vital Signs

Check that the upper airway is clear.

What is the RR?

Rates <12/min suggest a central depression of ventilation, which is usually due to a stroke, narcotic overdose, or some other drug overdose. Rates >20/min suggest hypoxia, pain, or anxiety. Look also for thoracoabdominal dissociation that may indicate impending respiratory failure. Remember that the chest cage and abdominal wall normally move in the same direction.

What is the HR?

Sinus tachycardia is an expected accompaniment of hypoxia.

What is the temperature?

An elevated temperature suggests *infection* (pneumonia, pyothorax, or bronchitis) but is consistent with *pulmonary embolism.*

What is the BP?

Hypotension may indicate CHF, septic shock, massive pulmonary embolism, or tension pneumothorax (Chapter 18). Also, measure the amount of *pulsus paradoxus*, which, in asthmatics, roughly correlates with the degree of airflow obstruction. Pulsus paradoxus is an inspiratory fall in systolic BP>10 mm Hg. To determine whether a pulsus paradoxus is present, inflate the BP cuff 20 to 30 mm Hg above the palpable systolic BP. Deflate the cuff slowly. Initially, Korotkoff's sounds will be heard only in expiration. At some point during cuff deflation, Korotkoff's sounds will appear in inspiration as well, giving an impression of a doubling of the HR. The number of millimeters of mercury (mm Hg) between the initial appearance of Korotkoff's sounds and their appearance throughout the respiratory cycle represents the degree of pulsus paradoxus (Fig. 24–1).

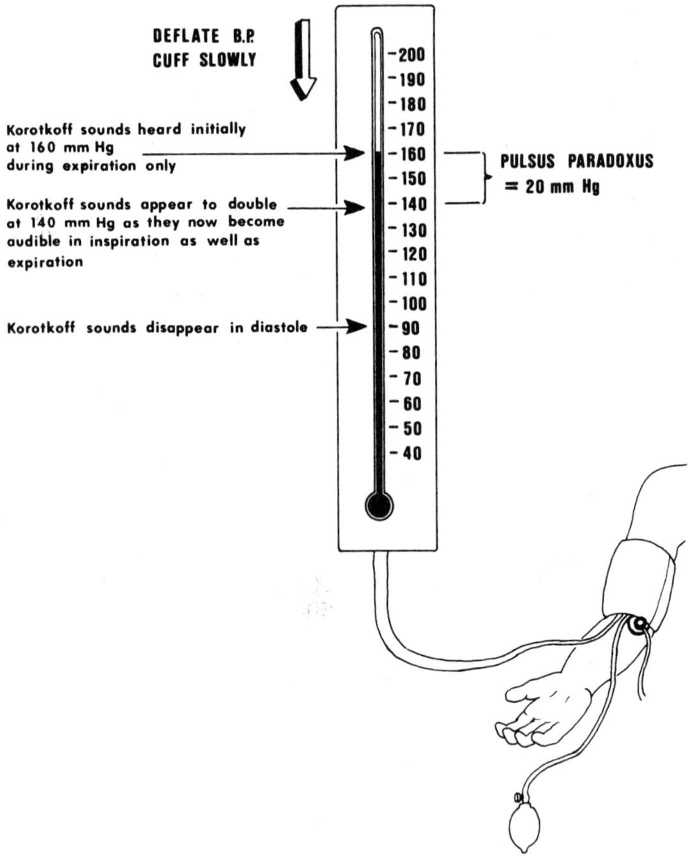

Figure 24–1 □ Determination of pulsus paradoxus.

Selective Physical Examination

Is the patient hypoxic?

VITALS	Repeat now. Again, ensure airway patency.
HEENT	Check for central cyanosis (blue tongue and mucous membranes). Check that the trachea is midline.
RESP	Are breath sounds present and of normal intensity? Check for crackles, wheezing, consolidation, or pleural effusion.
NEURO	Check level of sensorium. Is the patient alert, confused, drowsy, or unresponsive?

Cyanosis often does not occur until there is severe hemoglobin desaturation and may not occur at all in the anemic patient. If hypoxia is suspected, confirm by ABG measurement. *Remember:* Cyanosis is only helpful if it is present—its absence does not mean that the Po_2 is adequate.

Management

What immediate measure needs to be taken to correct hypoxia?

Supply adequate O_2. The initial concentration of O_2 ordered depends on your judgment of how sick the patient is. An accurate assessment can be made by drawing ABG samples, beginning empiric O_2 treatment, and adjusting Fio_2, depending on the results of subsequent ABGs or pulse oximetry. If pulse oximetry is available, gradually increase the Fio_2 until the O_2 saturation is >90%, then recheck with ABGs. [Remember that pulse oximetry tells you nothing about Pco_2, pH, or $(A\text{-}a)O_2$ gradient.] In most cases, a Po_2 >60 mm Hg or an O_2 saturation of 90% is adequate.

What harm can your treatment cause?

Some patients with COPD are CO_2 retainers and are dependent on mild hypoxia to stimulate the respiratory center. An Fio_2>0.28 may remove this hypoxia drive to breath. Unless there is or has been hypercarbia (check the old chart), it is difficult to predict which patients with COPD will be CO_2 retainers, and it is, therefore, prudent to assume that all patients with COPD and heavy smoking histories are CO_2 retainers.

Administering 100% O_2 can cause atelectasis or O_2 toxicity if given over a period of days. This is of more concern in the mechanically ventilated patient, since these Fio_2 levels are impossible to attain unless the patient is intubated.

Why is the patient SOB or hypoxic?

There are four common causes of SOB in hospitalized patients, as follows:

Cardiovascular causes	**CHF**
	Pulmonary embolism

Pulmonary causes	**Pneumonia**
	Bronchospasm (asthma and COPD)

In most cases, you will find it easy to distinguish among these four conditions. Look for specific associated signs and symptoms, as outlined in Table 24–1, that will help you identify which one of the four major causes of SOB your patient is most likely to have and treat him or her accordingly. Once you have established which pattern of SOB your patient most likely

Table 24–1 □ DISCRIMINATING FEATURES IN THE HISTORY AND PHYSICAL EXAMINATION OF A PATIENT WITH SOB

	CHF	Pulmonary Embolism and Infarction	Pneumonia	Asthma/ COPD
History				
Onset	Gradual	Sudden	Gradual	Gradual
Other	Orthopnea PND	Risk factors (see p. 240)	Cough Fever Sputum production	Previous history
Physical Examination				
Temperature	Normal	Normal or slightly elevated	High	Normal
Pulsus paradoxus	No	No	No	Yes
JVP	Elevated	Elevated or normal	Normal	Normal
S_3	Present	Occasional RVS_3 present	Absent	Absent
Respiratory				
Crackles	Bibasal	Unilateral	Unilateral	No
Wheezes	±	±	±	Present
Friction rub	No	±	±	No
Other	Pleural effusions		Consolidation Bronchial breath sounds Whispering pectoriloquy	

has, take a more thorough selective history and physical examination.

■ CARDIOVASCULAR CAUSES
■ *Congestive Heart Failure (CHF)*
Selective History

- Is there a history of CHF or cardiac disorder?
- Is there orthopnea?
- Is there PND?
- Are there trends in daily weight or fluid balance records that may heighten your suspicion of fluid retention and hence CHF?

Selective Physical Examination

Assess the *volume status.* **Is the patient volume overloaded?**

VITALS	Tachycardia, tachypnea
HEENT	Elevated JVP
RESP	Inspiratory crackles ± pleural effusions (more often on the right side)
CVS	Cardiac apex displaced laterally S_3 Systolic murmurs (aortic stenosis, mitral regurgitation, VSD, tricuspid regurgitation)
ABD	Hepatomegaly with positive HJR
EXT	Presacral or ankle edema

Crackles and S_3 are the most reliable indication of left-sided heart failure, whereas elevated JVP, enlarged liver, positive HJR, and peripheral edema indicate right-sided heart failure.

CXR (Fig. 24–2)
- Cardiomegaly
- Perihilar congestion
- Bilateral interstitial (early) or alveolar (more advanced) infiltrates
- Redistribution of pulmonary vascular markings
- Kerley's B lines
- Pleural effusions

Treatment
General Measures
- IV D5W TKVO. IV access is required to deliver medications. Switch to heparin lock when the acute episode has resolved.
- O_2
- Restricted sodium diet
- Bedrest
- SC heparin (5000 U SC q12h)
- Fluid balance charting
- Daily weight

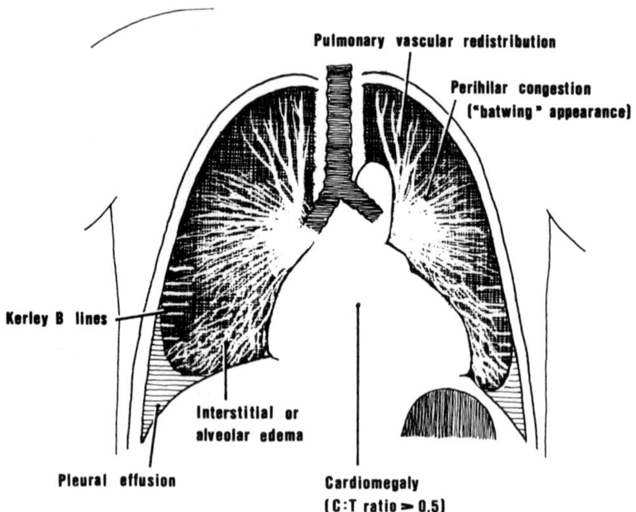

Figure 24–2 □ Chest x-ray features of congestive heart failure.

Specific Measures.   Cardiac function can be improved by altering preload, afterload, or contractility. In the acute situation, all of your intervention will involve decreasing the preload.

- Sit the patient up; this position pools blood in the legs.
- *Morphine sulfate* 2 to 4 mg IV q5–10 min up to 10 to 12 mg pools blood in the splanchnic circulation. Morphine sulfate may cause hypotension or respiratory depression. Take the BP and RR before and after each dose is given. If necessary, *naloxone hydrochloride* 0.2 to 2.0 mg IV, IM, or SC may be used to reverse the hypotension or respiratory depression of morphine, up to a total of 10 mg. Nausea or vomiting also may occur and usually can be controlled with *dimenhydrinate* (Dramamine, Gravol) 25 mg IV/IM or 50 mg PO q4h PRN.
- *Nitroglycerin ointment* (Nitrol) 2.5 to 5.0 cm (1–2 inches) topically q4h. If nitroglycerin ointment is not readily available, you may instead give *nitroglycerin tablets* 0.3 to 0.6 mg SL or *nitroglycerin spray* one puff SL q15 min until the patient feels less SOB, as long as the systolic BP remains above 90 mm Hg. All nitroglycerin preparations pool blood in the peripheral circulation. Nitroglycerin preparations commonly cause headaches, which can be treated with *acetaminophen* (Tylenol) 325 to 650 mg PO q4h PRN.

These three measures are temporary, shifting the excessive intravascular volume from the central veins. Only the diuretics actually reduce extracellular volume.

- *Furosemide* (Lasix) 40 mg IV given over 2 to 5 minutes. If there is no response (e.g., a lessening of the symptoms and signs of CHF, a diuresis), double the dose q1h (i.e., 40–80–160 mg) to a total dose of about 400 mg. Larger initial doses (e.g., 80–120 mg) may be required if the patient has renal insufficiency, is in severe CHF, or is already on maintenance furosemide. Doses of furosemide greater than 100 mg should be infused at a rate not exceeding 4 mg/min to avoid ototoxicity. Smaller initial doses (e.g., 10 mg) may suffice for frail, elderly (80- to 90-year-old) patients.
- A more effective diuresis may be achieved by the concomitant use of furosemide (which acts on the ascending loop of Henle) and a thiazide diuretic (which inhibits reabsorption of sodium in the distal nephron). *Hydrochlorothiazide* 25 to 50 mg may be given once or twice a day in conjunction with furosemide or other loop diuretics. *Metolazone* (Zaroloxyn) 5 to 10 mg PO may be more effective in patients with renal insufficiency.
- If furosemide is ineffective, try *ethacrynic acid* (Edecrin) 50 mg IV q60 min × 2 doses or *bumetanide* (Bumex) 1 to 10 mg IV over 1 to 2 minutes. (Bumetanide is a loop diuretic with a potency 40 times that of furosemide.)

  All the diuretics mentioned may cause hypokalemia, which is of particular concern in the digitalized patient. Monitor the serum potassium level once or twice daily in the acute situation. High doses of these diuretics also may lead to serious sensorineural hearing loss, especially if the patient is also receiving other ototoxic agents, such as aminoglycoside antibiotics.

If diuretics are ineffective, it is unlikely that the patient is going to produce urine. Other methods of removing intravascular volume, such as *phlebotomy* (200–300 ml) and *rotating tourniquets*, are seldom required in the hospital setting. If there is a persistent component of bronchospasm (cardiac asthma), an inhaled beta agonist or IV theophylline preparation may improve oxygenation.

Digoxin is not of benefit acutely unless the CHF was precipitated by a bout of supraventricular tachycardia (e.g., rapid atrial fibrillation or flutter), which can be slowed by digoxin. (Refer to Chapter 15 for the management of tachydysrhythmias.)

Causes of CHF. *CHF is a symptom* and a very serious one! After you have treated the symptom, sit down and ascertain *why* the patient developed CHF. This requires you to identify the *etiological factor*, of which there are six possibilities.

1. Myocardial infarction
2. Hypertension
3. Valvular heart disease

   4. Congenital heart disease
   5. Pericardial disease
   6. Cardiomyopathy (dilated, restrictive, hypertrophic)

If the patient has a *history* of CHF, the *etiological factor* may already be identified for you in the patient's chart. However, the job does not end there, for now you must also identify a *precipitating factor*, of which the following 10 are most common.

   1. Pulmonary embolism
   2. Noncompliance with diet or medication
   3. Cardiac depressant drugs (e.g., beta blockers, disopyramide, calcium entry blockers)
   4. Sodium-retaining agents (e.g., NSAIDs)
   5. Increased sodium load (dietary, medicinal, parenteral)
   6. Dysrhythmias
   7. Renal disease
   8. Anemia
   9. Fever, infection
  10. Pregnancy

Remember, that any *new etiological factor* may also act as a *precipitating factor* in a patient with a history of CHF. Document the suspected *etiological* and *precipitating* factors in the chart.

■ *Pulmonary Embolism*

The classic triad of SOB, hemoptysis, and chest pain actually occurs in only a minority of cases. The best way to avoid missing this diagnosis is to consider it in each case of SOB you see.

Selective History

Look for predisposing causes.

Stasis
- Prolonged bedrest
- Immobilized limb
- Obesity
- CHF
- Pregnancy

Vein Injury
- Trauma (especially hip fractures)
- Surgery (especially abdominal, pelvic, and orthopedic procedures)

Hypercoagulability
- Malignancy
- Inflammatory bowel disease
- Nephrotic syndrome

- Use of birth control pills
- Deficiencies of antithrombin III, protein C or S

Selective Physical Examination

Features suggestive of pulmonary embolism include the following.

- Pleural friction rub
- Pulmonáry consolidation
- Unilateral or bilateral pleural effusion
- Sudden onset cor pulmonale
- New onset tachydysrhythmia
- Simultaneous deep venous thrombosis (DVT)

CXR (Fig. 24–3)

- Atelectasis (loss of volume)
- Unilateral wedge-shaped pulmonary infiltrate
- Unilateral pleural effusion
- Raised hemidiaphragm
- Areas of oligemia
- Entirely normal

ECG.   Only a massive pulmonary embolism will give you the classic right ventricular strain pattern of S_1, Q_3, right axis deviation, and RBBB. The most common ECG finding is a *sinus tachycardia*, but other supraventricular tachycardias also may occur.

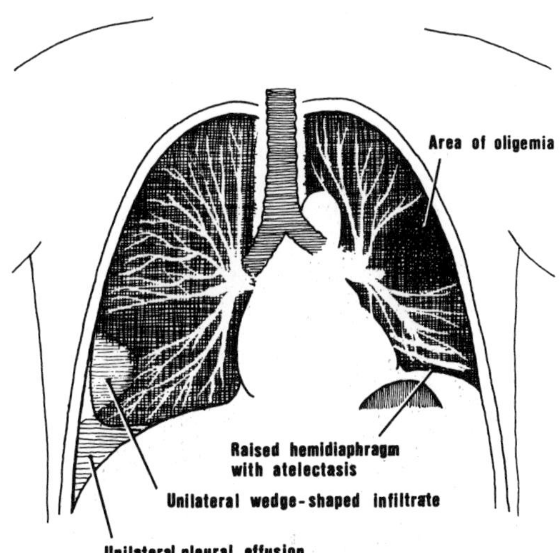

Figure 24–3 □ Variable chest x-ray features of pulmonary embolism.

ABGs.   The most common finding on ABG determination is acute respiratory alkalosis. Of patients with pulmonary embolism, 85% have $Po_2 < 80$ mm Hg on room air. If the Po_2 is > 80 mm Hg and pulmonary embolism is still suspected, look for an elevated $P(A\text{-}a)o_2$. (See Appendix, p. 340, for calculation.)

Management

If your suspicion for pulmonary embolism is high, you are obligated to begin anticoagulation therapy without further confirmation of the diagnosis at this point. *However, before ordering heparin, ensure that the patient has no history of bleeding disorders, peptic ulcers, and intracranial disease, e.g., recent stroke, subarachnoid hemorrhage (SAH), tumor, and recent surgery.* All are contraindications to anticoagulation. These patients will require confirmation of pulmonary embolism with V/Q scan or pulmonary angiography and, if embolism is documented, consultation for consideration of interruption of the inferior vena cava by the insertion of a transvenous intracaval device or, occasionally, IVC ligation.

Draw a blood sample for CBC, aPTT, and platelet count immediately. If there are *no contraindications*, begin *heparin* 100 units/ kg IV bolus (usual dose 5000 to 10,000 units IV) and follow with maintenance infusion of 1000 to 1600 units/h, with the lower range selected for patients with a higher risk of bleeding.

Heparin should be delivered by infusion pump, with maintenance dosing ordered as in the following example: heparin 25,000 units/500 ml D5W to run at 20 ml/h = 1000 units/h. It is dangerous to put large doses of heparin in small-volume IV bags, since runaway IVs filled with heparin can result in serious overdose.

Heparin and warfarin are dangerous drugs because of their potential for causing bleeding disorders. Write and double check your heparin orders carefully. Also, measure platelet counts once or twice a week to detect reversible heparin-induced thrombocytopenia, which may occur at any time while a patient is on heparin.

After starting heparin, obtain a V/Q scan as soon as possible to confirm the diagnosis of pulmonary embolism. A *high probability* V/Q scan is sufficient evidence to continue anticoagulation. A *normal* V/Q scan rules out pulmonary embolism. A *low* or *intermediate* probability V/Q scan in the presence of high clinical suspicion should be confirmed by pulmonary angiography before committing the patient to long-term anticoagulation. Alternatively, demonstration of simultaneous DVT by nuclear or contrast venography or impedance plethysmography is sufficient evidence to continue anticoagulation.

Monitor aPTT q4–6h and adjust the heparin maintenance dose until aPTT is in the therapeutic range (1.8–2.8 times normal).

After this, daily aPTTs are sufficient. Initial measurements of aPTT are made only to ensure adequate anticoagulation.

Continue IV heparin for 5 days. Add oral *warfarin* (Coumadin) on the first day, beginning at 10 mg PO and titrating the dose to achieve a PT with an international normalized ratio of 2.0 to 3.0. (This corresponds to a PT of 1.3 to 1.5 times control, using rabbit brain thromboplastin. If you are unsure of the method used by your laboratory, call them and ask.) Measure aPTT *and* PT daily during this initial adjustment phase. Attainment of a therapeutic PT will usually take 5 days, at which time the heparin can be discontinued.

Numerous drugs interfere with warfarin metabolism to increase or decrease the PT. Before prescribing *any* drug to a patient on warfarin, look up its effect on warfarin metabolism and monitor PTs carefully if an interaction is anticipated.

Write an order that the patient should receive no aspirin-containing drugs, sulfinpyrazone, dipyridamole, or thrombolytic agents and no IM injections while on anticoagulation.

Ask your patient daily about signs of bleeding or bruising. Instruct your patient that prolonged pressure after venipuncture will be required to prevent local bruising while on anticoagulation.

■ PULMONARY CAUSES
■ *Pneumonia*

Selective History and Physical Examination

- Cough: A cough productive of purulent sputum is typical. However, the cough may be dry in the early stages of pneumonia.
- Fever, chills
- Pleuritic chest pain
- Is the patient immunocompromised?
- Pulmonary consolidation ± pleural effusion

CXR.   There are variable findings, from patchy diffuse infiltrates to consolidation ± pleural effusion. Remember that a volume depleted patient may not manifest the typical CXR findings of pneumonia until the intravascular volume is restored to normal. Trust your clinical examination.

Identify the Organism
- Sputum Gram stain and culture. If the patient is not able to spontaneously cough up sputum, you may induce it with ultrasonic nebulization or chest physiotherapy. Take a sputum sample to the laboratory yourself and examine the Gram stain. (See Appendix, p. 332 for interpretation of the Gram stain.)

- Blood culture ($\times 2$)
- Thoracentesis. Moderate to large pleural effusions should be tapped to exclude empyema. Pleural biopsy also will be necessary if TB is a consideration. Send pleural fluid to the laboratory for
    - Gram stain and aerobic and anaerobic cultures
    - ZN stain and TB cultures
    - Cell count and differential
    - LDH
    - Protein
    - Glucose

If appropriate, send for
    - Fungal cultures
    - pH
    - Cytology
    - Amylase
    - Triglycerides

A simultaneous serum glucose, protein, and LDH should be drawn immediately after the pleural tap has been completed. These serum determinations are necessary to compare with pleural fluid values in assessing whether the fluid is a transudate or exudate.

Always consider TB in your differential diagnosis. Order ZN stains and sputum for culture if TB is suspected.

Pneumocystis carinii is the commonest cause of pneumonia in the patient who is HIV positive. Although this organism occasionally may be demonstrated by immunofluorescent staining of sputum, bronchoscopy is the best method for confirming the diagnosis.

Management

General Measures

- O_2
- Chest physiotherapy

Specific Measures

- Antimicrobials

Your choice will depend on the Gram stain results. If no sputum is available, several rules-of-thumb will help you out.

Outpatient-acquired pneumonia in the nonimmunocompromised host—*Streptococcus pneumoniae, Mycoplasma pneumoniae, Legionella pneumophila* (in some geographic locations). *Penicillin G* 1 to 2 million units IV q4–6h should be used in the patient suspected of having a pneumococcal pneumonia. Otherwise, a good antibacterial choice is *erythromycin* 500 mg PO or IV q6h.

Administration of erythromycin is painful and can cause thrombophlebitis when given IV. This can be minimized by diluting each 500 mg dose in 500 ml IV fluid and administering slowly over 6 hours. If volume overload is a concern, each 500 mg dose can be added to 250 ml IV fluid and given over 6 hours.

Chronic obstructive pulmonary disease (COPD)—*S. pneumoniae, Haemophilus influenzae. Ampicillin* 1 g PO or IV q6h is a good choice.

Aspiration pneumonias should be considered in any situation in which a decreased level of consciousness or an interference with the cough reflex has occurred (e.g., alcoholism, stroke, seizure, postsurgery). Episodes of aspiration do not require antibiotic treatment unless there are clinical signs of bacterial infection (fever, sputum production, leukocytosis). Aspiration pneumonias acquired before hospital admission involve mouth anaerobes and can be treated with *penicillin G* 2 million units IV q4h or *clindamycin* 300 to 600 mg PO or IV q6h. Hospital-acquired aspirations should also be treated using gram-negative coverage (e.g., gentamicin).

Elderly (>65 years of age) or *institutionalized* patients have an increased frequency of gram-negative pneumonias. A good choice for therapy is *cefuroxime* 750 mg IV q8h.

Hospital-acquired pneumonias also require gram-negative coverage with a cephalosporin or an aminoglycoside until culture and sensitivity results are available. *Pseudomonas* and *Acinetobacter* are common ICU/CCU pathogens and can be treated by using the known local antimicrobial sensitivities of these organisms in your hospital.

Alcoholics, in addition to aspiration pneumonias, have a high frequency of *Klebsiella pneumoniae*. This should be treated with two drugs—usually a cephalosporin and aminoglycoside, e.g., *cefazolin* (Ancef) 1 to 2 g IV q8h and *gentamicin* 1.5 to 2 mg/kg IV loading dose, followed by 1 to 1.5 mg/kg IV q8h of gentamicin if renal function is normal. Aminoglycosides can cause nephrotoxicity and ototoxicity. Avoid these side effects by following serum aminoglycoside levels, usually after the third or fourth maintenance dose, and serum creatinine levels. If the patient already has renal insufficiency, *give the same loading dose* but adjust the maintenance dose interval according to the creatinine clearance (see Appendix, p. 339).

The most common infecting pulmonary pathogen in *HIV-positive* patients is *Pneumocystis carinii*. Urgent diagnostic bronchoscopy is advisable when this organism is suspected. If the patient looks sick and bronchoscopy is not immediately available, the attending physician may want to give one dose of *trimethoprim-sulfamethoxasole* or *pentamidine isethionate* and arrange for bronchoscopy as soon as possible. Steroids also may be helpful in patients who are particularly ill with *P. carinii* pneumonia.

Pentamidine has numerous side effects, including hypotension, tachycardia, nausea, vomiting, unpleasant taste, and flushing. Some of these side effects can be minimized by administering the dose in 500 ml D5W over 2 to 4 hours. In addition, biochemical abnormalities may include hyperkalemia, hypocalcemia, megaloblastic anemia, leukopenia, thrombocytopenia, hyperglycemia or hypoglycemia, elevated liver enzyme levels, and dose-related, reversible nephrotoxicity.

■ *Bronchospasm (Asthma and COPD)*

Asthma is a condition characterized by airflow obstruction that varies significantly over time.

Chronic obstructive pulmonary disease (COPD) may take the form of *chronic bronchitis*, which is a clinical diagnosis (production of mucoid sputum on most days for 3 months of the year in 2 consecutive years), or *emphysema*, which is a pathological diagnosis (enlargement of airways distal to the terminal bronchioles). Most patients with COPD have features of both.

Selective History

- Does the patient smoke cigarettes?
- Is the patient on theophylline or steroids?
- Has the patient ever required intubation?
- Can precipitating factors (e.g., specific allergies, nonspecific irritants, URTI, pneumonia, beta blocker administration) be identified?
- Is the patient having an anaphylactic reaction? Look for evidence of systemic autocoid (e.g., histamine) release, i.e., wheezing, itch (urticaria), and hypotension. Anaphylactic reactions in hospitalized patients are most commonly seen after administration of IV dye, penicillin, or aspirin. If there is suspicion of anaphylaxis, refer immediately to Chapter 18, page 155, for appropriate management. This is an emergency!

Selective Physical Examination

Is there evidence of obstructive airways disease?

VITALS	Pulsus paradoxus
HEENT	Cyanosis
	Elevated JVP (cor pulmonale): Cor pulmonale is defined as right-sided heart failure secondary to pulmonary disease.
	Position of trachea: A pneumothorax may be a complication of asthma/COPD and results in a shift of the trachea away from the affected side.
RESP	Intercostal indrawing
	Use of accessory muscles of respiration
	Increased A/P diameter
	Hyperinflated lungs with depressed hemidiaphragms
	Wheezing: Diffuse wheezing is most often a manifestation of asthma or COPD but may also be seen in CHF (cardiac asthma), pulmonary embolism, pneumonia, or anaphylactic reactions. Ensure that the patient has not undergone

IV dye studies within the last 12 hours.
Prolonged expiratory phase
CVS   Loud P_2
RV heave, RVS_3 (pulmonary hypertension, cor pulmonale)

CXR

- Hyperinflation of lung fields
- Flattened diaphragms
- Increased A/P diameter
- Look also for infiltrates (suggesting concomitant pneumonia), atelectasis (suggesting mucous plugging), pneumothorax, or pneumomediastinum.

Management

General Measures

- O_2
- Hydration

Special Measures

STEP 1.   Inhaled beta agonists, such as *salbutamol* (Ventolin) 2.5 to 5.0 mg in 3 ml NS by nebulizer q4h or *fenoterol* (Berotec) 0.5 to 1.0 mg in 3 ml NS by nebulizer q4–6h. An anticholinergic agent, such as *ipratropium bromide* 0.5 ml in 3 ml NS by nebulizer, may also improve oxygenation but should always be preceded or followed by an inhaled beta agonist because it occasionally can worsen bronchoconstriction.

Although standard dosing intervals for beta agonists are q4–6h, they may be given almost continuously in severe bronchospasm, as long as you watch closely for potential side effects (supraventricular tachycardias, PVCs, muscle tremors).

STEP 2A.   Theophylline preparation in patients not receiving theophylline in the last 24 hours *(most useful in patients with COPD)*. *Aminophylline* 6 mg/kg IV loading dose over 20 minutes, followed by maintenance dosage of 0.6 mg/kg/h IV infusion. Give 0.3 mg/kg/h in patients with CHF or liver disease and elderly patients and 0.9 mg/kg/h in smokers. If the patient has received a theophylline-containing preparation in the past 24 hours, administer half the recommended loading dose, then follow with a full maintenance dose as previously recommended.

The therapeutic serum range for theophylline is 30 to 100 mmol/L. Higher levels cause cardiac stimulation (tachycardia, PVCs), GI upset (nausea, vomiting), and CNS irritability (headache, seizures). Remember that theophylline clearance is decreased by the addition of erythromycin, cimetidine (but usually not ranitidine), propranolol, allopurinol, and a number of other drugs.

STEP 2B.   Steroids, e.g., *hydrocortisone* 250 mg IV bolus, followed by maintenance dose of 100 mg IV q6h *(most useful in patients with pure asthma)*. The optimal steroid preparation and dosage are controversial. However, since pure asthma is predominantly a response to airway inflammation, steroids should be used early in the management of exacerbations. In addition, steroids take 6 hours to work, so they must be given now if persistent wheezing is anticipated in the next 6 to 24 hours. Beclomethasone dipropionate (Beclovent) is not useful in acute bronchospasm.

Steroids have few side effects in the short-term situation. Sodium retention is of concern in the patient with CHF or hypertension; hyperglycemia may occur in diabetics.

There has been a great deal of concern about tapering steroids too rapidly. A person on IV steroids for less than 2 weeks can have the steroids discontinued abruptly without fear of steroid withdrawal. Of more concern is exacerbation of wheezing as steroids are tapered. This may limit the rate at which steroids can be withdrawn.

When a patient develops an exacerbation of bronchospasm, a general rule-of-thumb is to administer medications *one step beyond* what is usually required as an outpatient. For example, an asthmatic patient normally controlled on a salbutamol inhaler at home will probably require both nebulized beta agonist and IV steroids during an exacerbation. If a COPD patient is wheezing despite outpatient treatment with a beta agonist and a theophylline preparation or if the patient is already on a small dose of prednisone, he or she should be given IV steroids during the acute attack. In the severe asthmatic, nebulized ipratropium may also be helpful.

Look for evidence of bronchitis or pneumonia as the precipitant of bronchospasm. In patients so affected, bronchospasm may persist until appropriate *antibiotics* are given.

Five Warning Signs in Asthma
1. Sudden acute deterioration in an asthmatic patient may represent a *pneumothorax*.
2. *Rising* $P\text{CO}_2$. Patients with an acute attack of asthma hyperventilate. A normal $P\text{CO}_2$ of 40 mm Hg in the acute situation may signify impending respiratory failure.
3. *Disappearance of wheezing*. In the acute situation, this is an ominous sign, indicating that the patient is not moving enough air in and out to generate a wheeze.
4. *Sedatives are contraindicated in asthma and COPD*. The RN may not be aware of this and may unknowingly request a sleeping pill from your colleague while you are off duty. To avoid this pitfall, write clearly in your orders "No sedatives or sleeping pills."
5. Some asthmatic patients have a triad of asthma, nasal polyps, and aspirin sensitivity. When prescribing analgesics in asthmatics, it is best to *avoid NSAIDs*, including aspirin, since fatal anaphylactoid reactions have occurred in some patients given these medications.

■ RESPIRATORY FAILURE

Any of the four conditions causing SOB and a variety of others may lead to respiratory failure. Suspect that this is occurring if the RR is less than 12/min or if there is thoracoabdominal dissociation. Confirm the diagnosis of acute respiratory failure by ABG determination. A Po_2 of <60 mm Hg or Pco_2 >50 mm Hg with a pH < 7.30 while breathing room air indicates *acute respiratory failure.*

1. Ensure that the patient has not received narcotic analgesics in the last 24 hours, which may depress the RR. Pupillary constriction may give you a hint that a narcotic is the culprit. If a narcotic has been given or if you are uncertain, order *naloxone hydrochloride* (Narcan) 0.2 to 2.0 mg IV immediately.
2. If no response to naloxone occurs, arrange for transfer of the patient to the ICU/CCU. Acute respiratory acidosis with pH < 7.30 *may* respond to aggressive treatment of the underlying respiratory or neuromuscular disorder, but make arrangements for possible endotracheal intubation if there is not rapid improvement. Acute respiratory acidosis with pH < 7.20 usually requires mechanical ventilation until the precipitating cause of respiratory deterioration can be reversed.

REMEMBER

1. Abdominal problems can masquerade as SOB. [One of us (SM) was once called to see a patient whose SOB resolved as soon as urinary retention was relieved by placement of a Foley catheter and 1300 ml of urine was drained.] Massive ascites and obesity may also compromise respiratory function.
2. Do not be worried about your inexperience with endotracheal intubation. A patient in respiratory failure can be bagged and masked effectively for hours until someone with intubation experience is available to assist you.
3. Notice that *epinephrine* does not appear in the protocol for treatment of asthma. There is no need to use epinephrine in the adult with an attack of asthma or COPD unless bronchospasm as a component of an anaphylactic reaction is present. Epinephrine given inadvertently in cases of cardiac asthma has resulted in fatal MI.
4. An occasional patient has SOB as a manifestation of anxiety. In this instance, SOB is often qualitatively unique, in that the patient describes "shortness of the *deep* breath," with the sensation that he or she cannot get a satisfactory deep breath. Sighing and yawning are common accompaniments.

25

SKIN RASHES AND URTICARIA

This chapter will not transform you into a dermatologist, able to diagnose any rash with one quick glance. It will, however, help you to describe accurately rashes for which you are called at night. This ability will facilitate confirmation of the diagnosis in the morning by more experienced physicians. Urticarial rashes are rare in hospitalized patients. However, they are important to recognize, since they may be the prodrome of anaphylactic shock.

PHONE CALL

Questions

1 **How long has the patient had the rash?**
2 **Is there any urticaria (hives)?**
3 **Is there any audible wheezing or SOB?**
4 **What are the vital signs?**
5 **What drugs has the patient received within the past 12 hours?**
6 **Has the patient received IV contrast material within the past 12 hours?**
   Remember that patients undergoing CT scans are often given IV contrast material.
7 **Does the patient have any known allergies?**
8 **What was the reason for admission?**

Orders

If the patient has evidence of anaphylaxis (urticaria, wheezing, SOB, or hypotension), order the following to be available at the bedside immediately.

1. IV to be started immediately with NS.
2. *Epinephrine* 5 ml (0.5 mg) of 1:10,000 for IV administration (this is available in a predrawn syringe from the emergency cart) or *epinephrine* 0.5 ml (0.5 mg) of 1:1000 for SC administration. Epinephrine may be required *either* IV *or* SC depending on the severity of the reaction. Do not confuse these doses and routes of administration.
3. Diphenhydramine (Benadryl) 50 mg IV.
4. Hydrocortisone (Solu-Cortef) 250 mg IV.

Inform RN

"Will arrive at bedside in . . . minutes."

Evidence of anaphylaxis (urticaria, wheezing, SOB, or hypotension) requires you to see the patient immediately. Assessment of a skin rash, with no associated symptoms of anaphylaxis, can wait an hour or two if other problems of higher priority exist.

ELEVATOR THOUGHTS (What causes skin rashes?)

The majority of calls at night regarding skin rashes are due to drug eruptions. The lesions may be urticarial, which is rare but potentially life-threatening, erythematous, vesicular, bullous, or purpuric. The distribution of the rash is usually generalized except for fixed drug eruptions (see following section).

Urticaria (Rare but Life Threatening)
- Drugs causing release of histamine
  - IV contrast material
  - Opiates (codeine, morphine, meperidine)
  - Antibiotics (penicillins, cephalosporins, sulfonamides, tetracycline, quinine, polymyxin, isoniazid)
  - Anesthetic agents (curare)
  - Vasoactive agents (atropine, amphetamine, hydralazine)
  - Miscellaneous (bile salts, thiamine, dextran, deferoxamine)
- Drugs: mechanism unclear
  - Aspirin and other NSAIDs
- Hereditary angioedema
- Food allergies causing histamine release
  - Fruits, tomatoes, lobster, shrimp
- Physical agents
  - Dermatographia, cold, heat, pressure, vibration
- Idiopathic

Erythematous, Maculopapular (Morbilliform) Rashes
- Antibiotics (penicillin, ampicillin, sulfonamides, chloramphenicol)
  Erythematous maculopapular rashes are common in AIDS patients receiving sulfonamides and characteristically occur around day 10 of treatment for *Pneumocystis* pneumonia.
- Antihistamines
- Antidepressants (amitriptylline)
- Diuretics (thiazides)
- Oral hypoglycemics
- Anti-inflammatory drugs (gold, phenylbutazone)
- Sedatives (barbiturates)

Ampicillin commonly causes a generalized maculopapular eruption 2 to 4 weeks after administration of the first dose. Thus, it is important to check not only the current drugs the patient is receiving but also all recently discontinued drugs, since the eruption may appear several weeks after the drug has been stopped.

Vesicobullous Rashes
- Antibiotics (sulfonamides, dapsone)
- Anti-inflammatory drugs (penicillamine)
- Sedatives (barbiturates)
- Halogens (iodides, bromides)
- Herpes zoster
- Toxic epidermal necrolysis (sulfonamides, allopurinol)

Purpura
- Antibiotics (sulfonamides, chloramphenicol)
- Diuretics (thiazides)
- Anti-inflammatory drugs (phenylbutazone, indomethacin, salicylates)

Drug-induced thrombocytopenia causes nonpalpable purpura, whereas vasculitis causes palpable purpura.

Exfoliative Dermatitis (Erythroderma)
- Antibiotics (streptomycin)
- Anti-inflammatory drugs (gold, phenylbutazone)
- Antiepileptics (carbamazepine, phenytoin)

If a drug eruption is not recognized early and the drug is not discontinued, the patient may develop a generalized, dusky red, dry rash with profound scaling.

Fixed Drug Eruption
- Antibiotics (sulfonamides, metronidazole)
- Anti-inflammatory drugs (phenylbutazone)
- Analgesics (phenacetin)
- Sedatives (barbiturates, chlordiazepoxide)
- Laxatives (phenolphthalein)

Certain drugs may produce a skin lesion in a specific area. Repeat administration of the drug reproduces the skin lesion in the same location. The lesion is usually dusky red patches distributed over the trunk or proximal limbs.

MAJOR THREAT TO LIFE
- Anaphylactic shock

Urticarial skin rash may be a prodrome of *anaphylaxis*, whereas other types of skin rashes are not. Drugs and IV contrast material are the usual causes of anaphylactic shock in hospitalized patients—unless the allergic patient was unlucky enough to be stung by a wasp or to have eaten shrimp.

BEDSIDE
Quick Look Test

Does the patient look well (comfortable), sick (uncomfortable or distressed), or critical (about to die)?

The patient with an anaphylactic reaction looks apprehensive and, unless moribund, is usually SOB and sitting upright in bed.

Airway and Vital Signs

What is the BP?

Hypotension is an ominous sign in anaphylactic shock, and the patient requires immediate treatment. If anaphylaxis is suspected, insert a large-bore IV (size 16 when possible), if not already done, and run in NS as fast as possible.

What is the temperature?

Skin rashes are often more prominent when the patient is febrile.

Selective Physical Examination

Is there evidence of an impending anaphylactic reaction?

HEENT Pharyngeal, periorbital, or facial edema (anaphylaxis)
RESP   Weezing (anaphylaxis)
       If evidence of an impending anaphylactic reaction exists, refer to page 155 for immediate treatment.
SKIN   When an urticarial rash appearing as a manifestation of anaphylaxis has been ruled out, the remaining task is to describe the rash accurately to help you diagnose the lesion and perhaps to help someone else diagnose it if it disappears or changes by the morning.

Describe the location of the rash.

Is it *generalized*, *acral* (hands, feet), or *localized*? Remember always to examine the buttocks, a common site for the onset of drug eruptions.

Describe the color of the rash.

- Red, pink, brown, white

Describe the primary lesion (Fig. 25–1).

- *Macule*—flat (noticeable from the surrounding skin because of the color difference)
- *Patch*—a large macule
- *Papule*—solid, elevated, size < 1 cm
- *Plaque*—solid, elevated, size > 1 cm
- *Vesicle*—elevated, well circumscribed, size < 1 cm
- *Bulla*—elevated, well circumscribed, size > 1 cm
- *Nodule*—deep-seated mass, indistinct borders, size < 0.5 cm in both width and depth
- *Cyst*—nodule filled with expressible fluid or semisolid material
- *Wheal (hives)*—well circumscribed, flat-topped, firm elevation (papule, plaque, or dermal edema) ± central pallor, and irregular borders

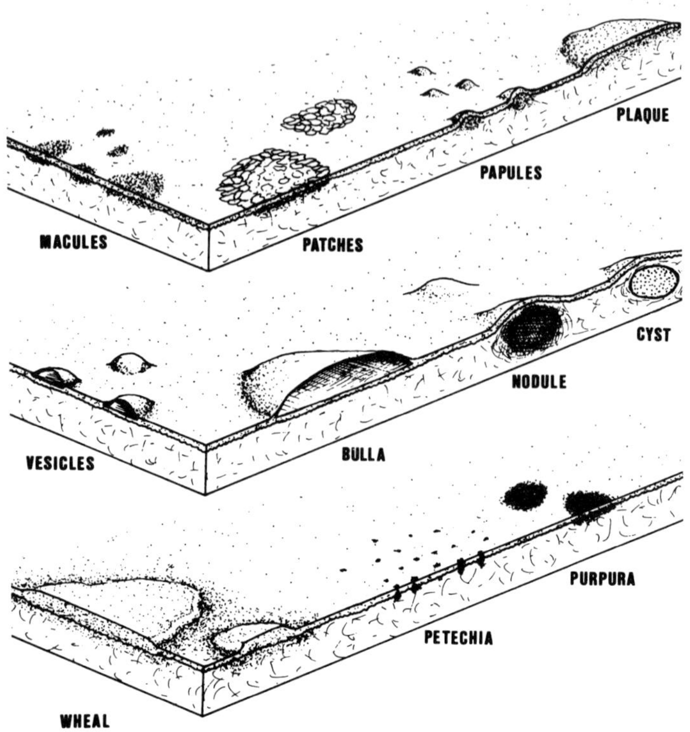

Figure 25–1 □ Primary skin lesions.

- *Petechia*—red/purple, nonblanchable macule, size < 3 mm
- *Purpura*—red/purple, nonblanchable macule or papule, size > 3 mm

Describe the secondary lesion (Fig. 25–2).
- *Scale*—dry, thin plate of thickened keratin layers (white color differentiates it from crust)
- *Lichenification*—dry, leathery thickening, shiny surface, accentuated skin markings
- *Pustule*—vesicle containing purulent exudate
- *Crust*—dried, yellow exudate of plasma (result of broken vesicle, bulla, or pustule)
- *Fissure*—linear, epidermal tear
- *Erosion*—wide, epidermal fissure, moist and well circumscribed
- *Ulcer*—erosion into the dermis

- *Scar*—flat, raised, or depressed area of fibrosis
- *Atrophy*—depression secondary to thinning of the skin

Describe the configuration of the rash.
- *Annular*—circular
- *Linear*—in lines
- *Grouped*—clusters, e.g., vesicular lesions of herpes zoster or herpes simplex

Selective History and Chart Review

- **How long has the rash been present?**
- **Does it itch?**
- **How has it been treated?**
- **Is this a new or a recurrent problem?**
- **Which drugs was the patient receiving before the rash started?**

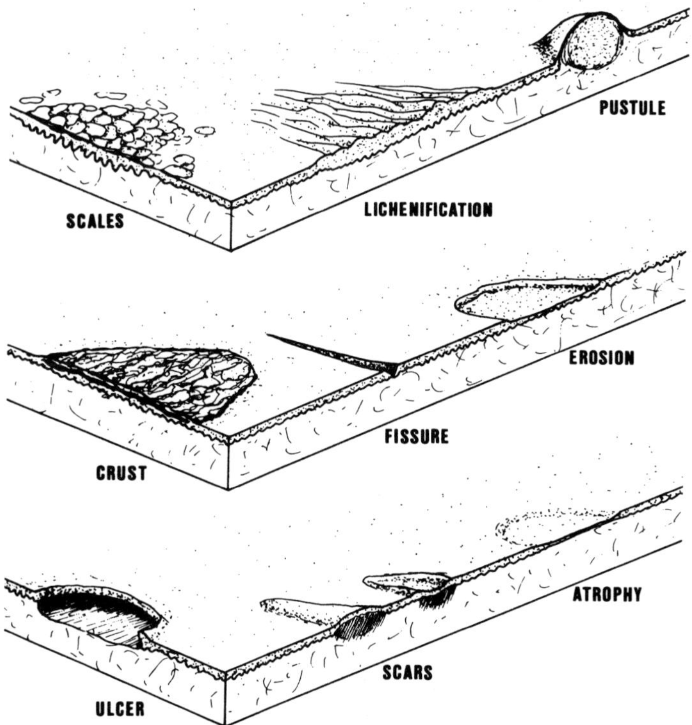

Figure 25–2 □ Secondary skin lesions.

Management

1. If the rash is associated with urticaria and thought to be secondary to a drug reaction, the drug should be withheld until confirmation of the diagnosis in the morning.
2. If the rash is nonurticarial and thought to be secondary to a drug reaction and the drug is deemed essential to the patient's management, the drug should be continued until confirmation of the diagnosis in the morning.
3. When the skin rash is not a drug eruption and the diagnosis is clear, the standard recommended treatment can be instituted. (Refer to a dermatology text for specific treatment.)
4. Often house staff have difficulty in diagnosing skin rashes with any degree of certainty. If uncertain, it is often sufficient to describe the lesion accurately and refer the patient to a dermatologist in the morning. Several important exceptions exist:
   a. A *petechial rash* suggests a disorder of platelet number or function. A *purpuric rash* may indicate a coagulation disorder. aPTT, PT, and platelet studies should be ordered where appropriate.
   b. *Herpes zoster* appearing in the immunocompromised patient (e.g., the patient with AIDS) may require urgent treatment because of the risk of systemic dissemination, especially to the CNS. If you suspect herpes zoster (initially erythematous macules and papules in a dermatomal distribution progressing to grouped vesicles and hemorrhagic crusts) in an immunocompromised patient, consult your resident or attending physician for consideration of beginning treatment with IV acyclovir.

26

SYNCOPE

Syncope is a brief loss of consciousness due to sudden reduction in cerebral blood flow. An additional term, "presyncope," has been coined referring to the situation in which there is reduction of cerebral blood flow sufficient to result in a sensation of impending loss of consciousness, although the patient does not actually pass out. Presyncope and syncope represent degrees of the same disorder and should be addressed as manifestations of the same underlying problem. Your task is to discover the *cause* of the syncopal attack.

PHONE CALL

1 **Did the patient actually lose consciousness?**
2 **Is the patient still unconscious?**
3 **What are the vital signs?**
4 **Was the patient recumbent, sitting, or standing when the episode occurred?**
   Syncope while the patient is in the recumbent position is almost always cardiac in origin.
5 **Was any seizurelike activity witnessed?**
6 **What is the admitting diagnosis?**
   An admitting diagnosis of seizure disorder, transient ischemic attack, or cardiac disease may help direct you to the cause of the syncopal attack.
7 **Has the patient sustained any evidence of injury?**

ORDERS

If the patient is still *unconscious*, order the following.
1. IV D5W TKVO immediately, if IV not already in place.
2. Turn the patient on the left side. This maneuver prevents the tongue from falling back into the throat, obstructing the upper airway, and also minimizes the risk of aspiration should vomiting occur.
3. Stat 12-lead ECG and rhythm strip. Although almost all patients with syncope will regain consciousness within a few minutes, you are more likely to be able to document a cardiac dysrhythmia early while the patient is still symptomatic.
4. If the patient has *regained consciousness*, if there is no evidence of head or neck injury, and if the vital signs are stable, do the following:
   a. To return the patient to bed, ask the RN to slowly raise the patient to a sitting position, then a standing position.

b. The patient should be placed back in bed, with instructions to remain there until you are able to assess the problem.
c. Order an ECG and rhythm strip.
d. Have the vital signs taken q15 min until you arrive at the bedside. Ask the RN to call you back immediately should the vital signs become unstable before you are able to assess the patient.

Inform RN

"Will arrive at bedside in . . . minutes."

Syncope requires you to see the patient immediately if the patient is still unconscious or if there are abnormalities in the HR or BP. If the patient is alert and conscious with normal vital signs (and if there are other more urgent problems to be assessed), the RN may observe the patient and call you if a problem arises before you are able to assess the patient.

ELEVATOR THOUGHTS (What causes syncope?)

1. Cardiac causes
   a. Dysrhythmias
      (1) Tachycardias
          (a) Ventricular tachycardia
          (b) Ventricular fibrillation
      (2) Bradycardias
          (a) Sinus bradycardia
          (b) Second- and third-degree AV block
          (c) SSS
   b. Pacemaker syncope
      (1) Pacemaker failure to capture
      (2) Pacemaker syndrome
   c. Syncope with exertion
      (1) Aortic stenosis
      (2) Pulmonic stenosis
      (3) Hypertrophic obstructive cardiomyopathy
      (4) Subclavian steal syndrome
2. Neurological causes
   a. Brainstem transient ischemic attack or stroke (drop attacks)
   b. Seizure
   c. Subarachnoid hemorrhage
   d. Cervical spondylosis
3. Vagal causes
   a. The common faint
   b. Valsalva's maneuver
   c. Cough syncope
   d. Micturition syncope

4. Carotid sinus syncope
5. Orthostatic hypotension
    a. Drug-induced
    b. Volume depletion
    c. Autonomic dysfunction
6. Miscellaneous
    a. Hyperventilation
    b. Anxiety attacks

MAJOR THREAT TO LIFE

If still unconscious, *aspiration*. If conscious, recurrence of potentially fatal cardiac *dysrhythmia*.

Since most patients recover from syncopal attacks within a few minutes, the actual loss of consciousness experienced by the patient is not the major problem. Of greater importance is that, while unconscious, the patient's tongue may block the oropharynx or the patient may aspirate oral or gastric contents into the lungs, an occurrence that may result in the development of aspiration pneumonia or ARDS. Therefore, in the unconscious patient, your primary goal is to protect the airway until the patient regains consciousness and the cough reflexes are once again effective.

Once the patient has regained consciousness, the major threat to life is the recurrence of an unrecognized potentially fatal cardiac dysrhythmia. This can be best identified and managed by transferring the patient to an ICU/CCU or other setting with ECG monitors if there is suspicion that a dysrhythmia was responsible for the syncopal episode.

BEDSIDE
Quick Look Test

Does the patient look well (comfortable), sick (uncomfortable or distressed), or critical (about to die)?

This simple observation helps determine the necessity of immediate intervention. Most patients who have had episodes of syncope and have regained consciousness look perfectly well.

Airway and Vital Signs

Airway

If the patient is still unconscious, ensure that the RN has placed him or her on the left side and that the patient's tongue has not fallen into the back of the throat. Most causes of syncope are very short lived, and by the time you arrive at the bedside, the patient will have regained consciousness. Look for abnormalities in the vital signs, which may help make your diagnosis of the specific cause of syncope much easier.

What is the heart rate?

Supraventricular or ventricular tachycardia should be documented on ECG tracings, and the patient should be treated immediately. (Refer to Chapter 15, p. 125, for treatment of supraventricular tachycardia and Chapter 15, p. 127, for treatment of ventricular tachycardia.)

Any patient with a transient or persistent supraventricular or ventricular tachycardia or its history when no other cause of syncope can be found should be transferred to the ICU/CCU or other setting with ECG monitoring for appropriate management.

What is the BP?

The patient with resting or orthostatic *hypotension* should be managed as outlined in Chapter 18. Remember that a massive internal hemorrhage (such as a GI bleed or a ruptured aortic aneurysm) can occasionally present with a syncopal attack.

Hypertension, if found in association with headache and neck stiffness, may indicate subarachnoid hemorrhage. A brief loss of consciousness is common at the onset of a subarachnoid hemorrhage and is often associated with dizziness, vertigo, or vomiting.

What is the temperature?

Patients with syncope are rarely febrile. If fever is present, it is usually due to a concomitant illness not related to the syncopal attack. However, especially if the syncopal attack was unwitnessed, be careful to exclude the possibility of a seizure secondary to meningitis, which may present as "fever + syncope."

Selective History and Chart Review

Has this ever happened before?

If it has, ask the patient if a diagnosis was made after the previous attack.

What does the patient or witnesses recall from the time immediately before the syncope?

- Syncope occurring while changing from the supine or sitting *position* to the standing position suggests orthostatic hypotension.
- An *aura*, though rare, is helpful in pointing to a seizure as the cause of syncope in an unwitnessed attack.
- *Palpitations* preceding an attack may suggest a cardiac dysrhythmia as a cause of syncope.
- Syncope during or immediately following performance of *Valsalva's maneuver*, a bout of *coughing*, or *micturition* may be due to mechanical reduction of venous return.
- Syncope after *turning the head to one side*, especially if one is

wearing a tight collar, may represent carotid sinus syncope. This condition is seen most often in elderly men.

- Numbness and tingling in the hands and feet are commonly experienced just before the presyncope or syncope due to hyperventilation or anxiety.

Is there any history of cardiac disease?

A patient with preexisting cardiac disease may have an increased risk of developing dysrhythmias.

Has the patient ever had a seizure?

An unwitnessed seizure may occur as a syncopal attack. Ask the patient if during the attack he bit his tongue or was incontinent of stool or urine. Either one is suggestive of seizure activity.

Has the patient ever had a stroke?

A patient with known cerebrovascular disease is a likely candidate for a brainstem TIA or stroke. However, remember that since atherosclerosis is a diffuse process, the patient with a history of stroke may also have coronary atherosclerosis that may result in cardiac dysrhythmias.

What does the patient remember on waking from the syncopal attack?

Headache, drowsiness, and mental confusion are common sequelae of seizures but not of cardiac causes of syncope.

What are the medications?

Check the chart to see what medications the patient is being given.

Digoxin, beta blockers, and calcium entry blockers may result in bradycardias. Digoxin, if present in toxic amounts, may also precipitate ventricular tachycardia.

Quinidine, procainamide, disopyramide, sotalol, amiodarone, tricyclic antidepressants, and phenothiazines may prolong the QT interval, leading to ventricular tachycardia (torsades de pointes) (Fig. 26–1a) or the prolonged QT interval syndrome (Fig. 26–1b).

Agents that reduce afterload (ACE inhibitors, hydralazine, prazosin) may cause syncope, especially in the elderly or volume depleted patient.

Phenothiazines and tricyclic antidepressants lower the seizure threshold and may result in seizure.

Selective Physical Examination

Your physical examination is directed toward finding a cause for the syncope. However, a search for evidence of injuries sustained if the patient fell during the syncopal attack is equally important at this time.

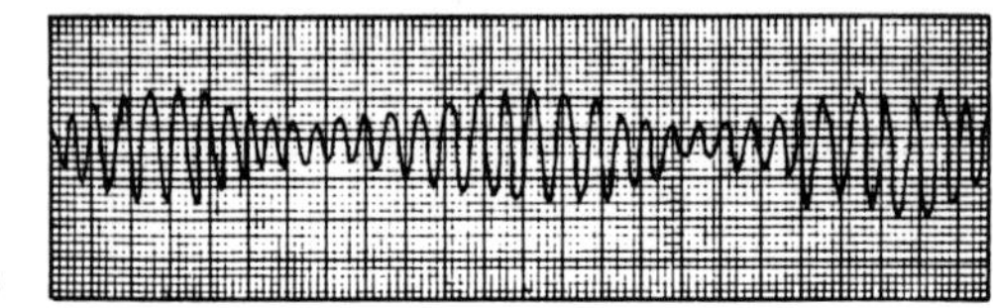

Figure 26–1 □ **A.** Torsades de pointes. **B.** Prolonged QT interval.

VITALS	Repeat now.
HEENT	Fundoscopy—Look for subhyaloid hemorrhages (SAH). Blood diffuses between the retinal fiber layer and the internal limiting membrane, forming a pocket of blood with sharp borders and often a fluid level.
	Tongue or check laceration (seizure disorder)
	Neck stiffness (meningitis leading to a seizure, SAH)
RESP	Crackles, wheezes (aspiration during the syncopal episodes)
CVS	Pacemaker (pacemaker syncope)
	Flat JVP (volume depletion)
	Atrial fibrillation (vertebrobasilar embolism)
	Systolic murmur (aortic stenosis, pulmonic stenosis, hypertrophic obstructive cardiomyopathy)
GU	Urinary incontinence (seizure disorder)
RECTAL	Incontinence of stool (seizure disorder)
MSS	Palpate bones for evidence of fracture that may have been sustained if patient fell.
NEURO	A complete neurological examination must be done, looking for evidence of residual localizing signs that may indicate a TIA, completed stroke, SAH, a space-occupying intracranial lesion, or Todd's paralysis. Vertebrobasilar TIAs or strokes are frequently accompanied by other evidence of brainstem dysfunction (e.g., cranial nerve

abnormalities, such as diplopia, nystagmus, facial paralysis, vertigo, dysphagia, dysarthria).

Management

An immediate cause for syncope frequently cannot be found. Because treatment of the various causes of syncope is so different, one must have *documented proof* of the cause of a syncopal episode before proceeding to definitive treatment. Investigations may take several days to complete. Your job, once you have assessed a patient with syncope, is to decide from the history, physical findings, and laboratory data what the most likely cause of syncope is and to arrange for further investigation, if necessary.

Cardiac Causes. If a cardiac cause of syncope is suspected, whether related to dysrhythmia, valvular, or pacemaker cause, the patient should be transferred to the CCU or to an intermediate care unit where continuous ECG monitoring is available. If there are no ECG monitored beds available and if there is no suspicion of ischemia-induced dysrhythmia, 24-hour Holter monitoring should be arranged for the patient first thing in the morning.

Always consider a silent MI with subsequent transient AV block, ventricular tachycardia, or ventricular fibrillation as the cause for syncope of cardiac origin.

Treatment of specific dysrhythmia, if still present at the time you are assessing the patient, is discussed in Chapter 15.

1. Tachycardias
   a. Ventricular tachycardia (p. 127)
   b. Supraventricular tachycardia (p. 125)
2. Bradycardias
   a. Sinus bradycardia (p. 133)
   b. AV blocks (p. 133)
   c. SSS (p. 133)

Pacemaker syncope will require cardiological consultation for reprogramming of the pacing rate or mode or for an upgrade to AV sequential pacing.

If *aortic stenosis, pulmonic stenosis,* or *hypertrophic obstructive cardiomyopathy* is thought to be responsible for exertional syncope, arrange for an echocardiogram in the morning to document the suspected cardiac lesion and ask for a cardiological consultation.

Neurological Causes. Suspected *brainstem TIA or stroke* should be evaluated by a CT scan of the head. Anticoagulation or platelet inhibitors should be started only after consultation with a neurologist.

If a *seizure* is suspected, you must first document the cause of the seizure, as outlined in Chapter 23, page 221.

If an SAH is suspected, arrange for an urgent noncontrast CT scan of the head, looking for evidence of aneurysm or blood in the subarachnoid space. A normal CT scan does not, however, exclude an SAH, and an LP may be required to look for xanthochromic cerebrospinal fluid. If such a lesion is identified, a neurosurgeon should be consulted for further investigation and management.

Vagal Causes.   Suspected vasovagal attacks can be managed without transfer to the ICU/CCU, as outlined in Chapter 18, page 153.

The definitive diagnosis of *carotid sinus syncope* requires potentially dangerous carotid sinus pressure, which must be done while the ECG is being monitored for cardiac dysrhythmia. Although the patient does not require ICU/CCU admission overnight, arrangements should be made in the morning to evaluate the cardiac rhythm during carotid sinus massage.

Orthostatic Hypotension.   Syncope due to *volume depletion* can be managed with IV fluid replacement, as outlined in Chapter 18, page 156.

Drug-induced orthostatic hypotension and *autonomic dysfunction* are complex treatment problems and, as long as the patient's volume status is normal, can be addressed in the morning through consultation with a neurologist or clinical pharmacologist.

Until the underlying problem responsible for orthostatic hypotension is corrected, instruct patients that if they must be out of bed during the night, they should (1) ask the RN for assistance and (2) move slowly from the supine to sitting position and then move slowly again from the sitting to standing position.

Miscellaneous.   Syncope due to *hyperventilation* or *anxiety states* can be alleviated by instructing the patient to breathe into a paper bag when he or she begins to feel anxious or presyncopal. This step will correct hypocapnia and thereby prevent a syncopal attack.

REMEMBER

1. In the elderly patient, the main hazard of a syncopal attack is not necessarily an underlying disease but rather a fracture or other injury sustained during a fall.
2. Except for the Stokes-Adams attack (third-degree AV block), true syncope rarely occurs when a patient is in the recumbent position.

27

TRANSFUSION REACTIONS

Blood transfusions are given around-the-clock in hospitals. Reactions to blood products may vary from severe to very mild. An organized approach will help you sort out both the nature of the reaction and what to do about it.

PHONE CALL
Questions

1 **What symptoms does the patient have?**
   Fever, chills, chest pain, back pain, diaphoresis, and SOB all can be manifestations of a transfusion reaction.
2 **What are the vital signs?**
3 **Which blood product is being transfused and how long ago was it started?**
4 **What was the reason for admission?**

Orders

1. Stop the transfusion immediately if the patient has any of the following symptoms.
   a. Sudden onset of hypotension
   b. Chest or back pain, tachypnea
   c. Any symptom (even fever, chills, or urticaria) occurring within minutes of the transfusion being started
   d. Fever in a patient who has never before received a blood transfusion or who has never been pregnant. This symptom may represent an acute hemolytic reaction.

   An acute hemolytic transfusion reaction can appear with any of the aforementioned symptoms. Acute hemolytic reactions, although very rare, are associated with an extremely high mortality rate, which is proportionate to the volume of blood infused. In previously pregnant or transfused patients, fever may be a nonhemolytic febrile reaction.
2. If the blood transfusion has been stopped, keep the IV open with NS.

Inform RN

"Will arrive at bedside in . . . minutes."

Any suspected hemolytic or anaphylactic transfusion reaction requires you to see the patient immediately.

ELEVATOR THOUGHTS (What causes transfusion reactions?)

Immune Hemolysis.   Mismatched RBCs (ABO incompatibility) are errors in either identification of the patient or labeling of the blood. Mismatched RBCs result in an *acute hemolytic reaction*. They are exceedingly rare and usually occur in emergency situations (i.e., in the postanesthetic, operating, or emergency room), when the usual precautions in identification of the patient or labeling of the blood are breached. *Delayed hemolytic reactions* develop as a consequence of prior exposure to foreign red cell antigens, i.e., pregnancy or previous transfusion. Reexposure to these antigens results in an anamnestic rise in alloantibodies that were not detectable at the time of the original crossmatch. Hemolysis occurs 3 to 14 days after transfusion and may be accompanied by fever, jaundice, and increasing anemia.

Nonimmune Hemolysis.   Nonimmune hemolysis may occur if the blood has been overheated or has undergone trauma. Trauma to blood products occurs either by excessive hand squeezing or pumping of the infusion bag during the rapid administration of blood in an emergency or by being delivered through too small a needle.

Anaphylaxis (IgG Response to IgA Antibodies).   Anaphylaxis may result from transmission of IgA antibodies from the donor's blood into a presensitized IgA-deficient patient.

Congenital IgA deficiency is a common (1:1000), asymptomatic disorder. The first transfusion that an IgA-deficient patient receives will contain IgA antibodies, which are recognized by the patient's immune system as foreign antigens. Thus, the IgA-deficient patient becomes sensitized and develops *anti-IgA antibodies*, which may result in anaphylaxis or urticaria with subsequent transfusions.

There are two known IgA *allotypes* (an allotype is simply a genetic variation in the structure of the immunoglobulin). Anaphylactic reactions are more common in patients who lack both allotypes of IgA, but they have been reported in patients who lack only one allotype. Individuals with IgA molecules of one allotype may develop antibodies against the other allotype, with subsequent transfusion reactions being exhibited as urticaria or, occasionally, anaphylaxis.

Urticaria.   Transmission of the following antigens from the donor's blood can cause urticaria.
1. Food allergens, e.g., shrimp (IgE response)
2. Other plasma protein allergens
3. IgA antibodies into an IgA-deficient patient (i.e., deficient

in one of the two allotypes). This is a very rare cause of urticaria.

Fever
1. Nonhemolytic febrile reaction. This is the most common cause of febrile transfusion reactions and does not require stopping the transfusion.
2. Early sign of acute hemolytic transfusion reaction. The patient's anti-HLA antibodies (from previous blood transfusions or pregnancies) react with the donor's WBCs, platelets, or both.
3. Pulmonary leukoagglutinin reaction. The donor's blood (usually from a multiparous woman) contains antibodies to the patient's WBCs, resulting in the agglutinated WBCs lodging in the pulmonary capillaries, causing noncardiogenic pulmonary edema.
4. Microbial contamination (very rare). Although many infectious agents can be transmitted via blood transfusions (e.g., non-A, non-B hepatitis, malaria, syphilis, CMV, infectious mononucleosis, rubella, Rocky Mountain spotted fever), they do not result in reactions during infusion of the blood product.

    Blood banks in North America screen for HIV and hepatitis B before blood is released for transfusion.

Pulmonary Edema
1. CHF. Volume overload may be induced in the patient with a history of CHF, since blood transfusions expand the intravascular volume.
2. Pulmonary leukoagglutinin reaction (see previous section).

MAJOR THREAT TO LIFE

- Anaphylaxis
- Acute hemolytic reaction

Both these reactions are very rare, but when they do occur, they can be fatal. *Anaphylaxis* may cause death either by severe laryngospasm or bronchospasm or by profound peripheral vasodilation and cardiovascular collapse. An *acute hemolytic reaction* is a medical emergency because of the possible development of renal failure, acute DIC, or both.

BEDSIDE
Quick Look Test

Does the patient look well (comfortable), sick (uncomfortable or distressed), or critical (about to die)?

The patient with impending anaphylaxis may look sick (agitated, restless, or SOB). Patients with pulmonary edema secondary to a transfusion reaction may look critical, with severe SOB.

Airway and Vital Signs

What is the BP?

Hypotension is an ominous sign—ensure that the transfusion has been stopped. It is seen in acute hemolytic reactions and in anaphylactic reactions. However, in the situation where the transfusion is being given for volume depletion, e.g., acute blood loss, hypotension may represent continued loss of intravascular volume from uncontrolled bleeding.

Tag and Wrist Band Check

Compare the identification tag on the blood with the patient's wrist band.

Selective Physical Examination

HEENT	Flushed face (hemolytic reaction or anaphylaxis)
	Pharyngeal, periorbital, or facial edema (anaphylaxis)
RESP	Wheezes (anaphylaxis)
NEURO	Decreased level of consciousness (anaphylaxis or hemolytic reaction)
SKIN	Heat along the vein being used for the transfusion (hemolytic reaction)
	Oozing from IV sites may be the only sign of hemolysis in the unconscious or anesthetized patient. DIC is a late manifestation of an acute hemolytic transfusion reaction.
URINE	Check the urine color. Free Hb will turn urine red or brown and is indicative of a hemolytic reaction.

If there is evidence of anaphylaxis or hemolysis, *stop the transfusion* and immediately begin emergency treatment (see below).

Selective History

Ask about symptoms that the patient may have developed since the initial phone call as follows.

- Fever or chills (nonhemolytic febrile reaction)
- Headache, chest pain, back pain, or diaphoresis (hemolytic reaction)
- SOB (volume overload or pulmonary leukoagglutinin reaction). A leukoagglutinin reaction occurring in the elderly patient is often misdiagnosed as cardiogenic pulmonary edema.

Has the patient had previous transfusion reactions? Chills and fever are most common in the patient who has received multiple transfusions or who has had several pregnancies.

Management

Anaphylaxis

1. Ensure that the transfusion has been stopped.
2. *Epinephrine* 3 to 5 ml (0.3 to 0.5 mg) of 1:10,000 solution IV by slow, direct injection; may repeat q5 min as necessary. If

epinephrine 1:10,000 solution is not immediately available, it can be made by adding 1 ml of a 1:1000 solution to 9 ml of NS.
3. NS 500 to 1000 ml IV to be given as fast as possible through a wide-open IV
4. *Oxygen* by bag and mask if necessary
5. *Diphenhydramine* (Benadryl) 50 mg IV by slow, direct injection
6. *Hydrocortisone* (Solu-Cortef) 250 mg IV by slow, direct injection
7. Intubation if necessary

Acute Hemolytic Reaction
1. Ensure that the transfusion has been stopped.
2. NS 500 ml IV to be given as fast as possible. Try to maintain the urine output over 100 ml/h with IV fluids and diuretics.
3. *Furosemide* (Lasix) 40 mg IV by slow, direct injection at a rate not faster than 4 mg/min or *mannitol* 25 g IV over 5 minutes (to promote diuresis).
4. Draw 20 ml of the patient's blood and send for the following:
   a. Repeat crossmatch
   b. Coombs' test, free Hb
   c. CBC, RBC morphology
   d. Platelets, PT, aPTT, FDP
   e. Urea, creatinine levels
   f. Unclotted blood for a stat spin
      Hemolysis is demonstrated when the plasma remains pink despite spinning for 5 minutes (i.e., hemoglobine- mia).
5. Obtain a urine sample for free Hb. In addition, urine can be tested with dipsticks. If there is hemoglobinuria, the dipstick results will be positive for Hb and negative for RBCs.
6. Send the donor's blood back to the blood bank for the following:
   a. Repeat crossmatch
   b. Coombs' test
7. If oliguria develops despite adequate IV fluids and appropriate diuretics, *acute renal failure* should be suspected. (For management of acute renal failure, see Chapter 9, p. 66.)

Urticaria
1. Do not stop the transfusion. Hives alone are rarely serious, but "hives and hypotension" is an anaphylactic reaction until proven otherwise.
2. *Diphenhydramine* (Benadryl) 50 mg PO or IV
3. Prior to future transfusions, the patient should be premedicated with *diphenhydramine* 50 mg PO or IV (*not* IM). If this fails to prevent urticarial reactions, washed RBCs should be given.

Fever
1. Do not stop the transfusion unless a hemolytic reaction is suspected. Fever developing within minutes of a blood transfusion being started is very likely to be a symptom of a hemolytic reaction.
2. Often no treatment is required. If the fever is high and the patient is distressed, however, an antipyretic drug, i.e., acetaminophen 650 mg PO, usually is effective.
3. If the patient has documented fever with two consecutive blood transfusions, premedication with an antipyretic before subsequent transfusions is indicated. If this step fails to prevent fever, washed RBCs can be given.

Pulmonary Edema
1. Stop the transfusion or slow the rate of transfusion, unless the patient urgently needs blood.
2. *Furosemide* (Lasix) 40 mg IV. If the patient is already receiving a diuretic or if there is renal insufficiency, a higher dose of furosemide may be required.
3. For the management of CHF refer to Chapter 24, page 237. Volume overload, with subsequent pulmonary edema, should be anticipated in a patient with a history of CHF. This problem may be prevented by administering a diuretic (e.g., furosemide 40 mg IV) during the transfusion.

LABORATORY-RELATED PROBLEMS: THE COMMON CALLS

28

ACID-BASE DISORDERS

Most cases of acidemia or alkalemia are first discovered by measurement of arterial pH.

■ ACIDEMIA (pH ≤ 7.35)

First decide whether the acidemia is a respiratory acidemia (i.e., due to hypoventilation) or a metabolic acidemia (i.e., due to acid gain or HCO_3 loss).

Respiratory Acidemia
- pH ≤7.35
- P_{CO_2} ↑
- HCO_3 normal or ↑

Metabolic Acidemia
- pH ≤7.35
- P_{CO_2} normal or ↓
- HCO_3 ↓

The normal response to respiratory acidemia is an increase in HCO_3. An immediate increase in HCO_3 occurs because the increase in P_{CO_2} results in the generation of HCO_3, according to the law of mass action.

$$CO_2 + H_2O \rightleftharpoons H + HCO_3$$

Later, renal tubular preservation of HCO_3 occurs to buffer the change in pH. The expected increase in HCO_3 in *acute respiratory acidemia* is 0.1 (ΔP_{CO_2}). The expected increase in HCO_3 in *chronic respiratory acidemia* is 0.4 (ΔP_{CO_2}). When the HCO_3 is less than expected, a mixed respiratory and metabolic acidemia should be suspected. An HCO_3 greater than expected suggests a combined respiratory acidemia and metabolic alkalemia.

The normal respiratory response to metabolic acidemia is hyperventilation, with a decrease in P_{CO_2}. The expected decrease in P_{CO_2} in uncomplicated metabolic acidemia is 1 to 1.5 (ΔHCO_3). When the P_{CO_2} is higher than this expected increase, a mixed metabolic and respiratory acidemia should be suspected. When the P_{CO_2} is lower than expected, a combined metabolic acidemia and respiratory alkalemia should be suspected.

■ *Respiratory Acidemia*
- pH ≤7.35
- P_{CO_2} ↑
- HCO_3 normal or ↑

Causes
1. CNS depression
   a. Drugs (e.g., morphine)
   b. Lesions of the respiratory center
2. Neuromuscular disorders
   a. Drugs (e.g., succinylcholine)
   b. Muscular disease
   c. Hypokalemia, hypophosphatemia
   d. Neuropathies
3. Respiratory disorders
   a. Acute airway obstruction
   b. Severe parenchymal lung disease
   c. Pleural effusion
   d. Pneumothorax
   e. Thoracic cage limitation

Manifestations
Respiratory acidemia occurs when there is a failure (either acute or chronic) in ventilation. The manifestations of respiratory acidemia are often overshadowed by those due to accompanying hypoxia. Symptoms and signs directly attributable to CO_2 retention are uncommon with P_{CO_2} <70 mm Hg but include the following:
- Bradypnea
- Drowsiness
- Confusion
- Papilledema
- Asterixis

Management

Assess the Severity
MILD.   pH 7.30–7.35. Patients with mild respiratory acidemia can be observed while reversible causes are searched for and corrected. Repeat ABGs should be obtained depending on the patient's clinical condition and course. The exception here is the patient with an acute asthmatic attack, in whom even a normal and certainly an elevated P_{CO_2} is a warning sign of impending respiratory failure.

MODERATE.   pH 7.20–7.29. The patient with moderate respiratory acidemia is in the gray zone. Further decrease in pH puts the patient at risk for life-threatening ventricular dysrhythmias. If a readily reversible cause can be found, the patient can be carefully monitored while treatment measures are instituted. Such a patient should not be left alone until it is determined that he or she is improving. Sequential determinations of pH should be guided by the patient's clinical condition and course.

SEVERE.   pH $\leq$7.19. This patient is at high risk for cessation of respiration, life-threatening ventricular dysrhythmias, or both. Call your resident for help now. This patient will most likely require transfer to the ICU for monitoring, intubation, and mechanical ventilation while reversible causes are searched for.

■ *Metabolic Acidemia*

- pH $\leq$7.35
- P_{CO_2} normal or $\downarrow$
- HCO_3 $\downarrow$

Causes

The metabolic acidemias are conveniently divided into *normal anion gap* and *high anion gap* varieties. The normal anion gap (Na + K) − (Cl + HCO_3) = 10 to 12 mmol/L. Remember that for every decline in serum albumin of 10 g/L, add 4 to the calculated anion gap. Failure to correct for hypoalbuminemia may lead to overlooking serious acidemias of the high anion gap type.

Normal Anion Gap Acidemia
1. Loss of HCO_3
   a. Diarrhea, ileus, fistula
   b. High output ileostomy
   c. Renal tubular acidosis
   d. Carbonic anhydrase inhibitors
2. Addition of H^+
   a. NH_4Cl
   b. HCl

High Anion Gap Acidemia
1. Lactic acidemia
2. Ketoacidosis (IDDM, alcohol, starvation)
3. Renal failure
4. Drugs (aspirin, ethylene glycol, methyl alcohol, paraldehyde)
5. High-flux dialysis acetate buffer

The change in anion gap should equal the change in HCO_3. Any deviation from this reveals a mixed acid-base disorder. Always remember to *calculate the osmolar gap* in high anion gap acidemias to determine if ingestions have contributed to the abnormalities.

Occasionally, the pH may be normal, but the presence of a wide anion gap may be a clue to underlying metabolic acidemia.

Manifestations

The signs and symptoms of metabolic acidemia are nonspecific, and include the following:

- Hyperventilation (in an effort to blow off CO_2)
- Fatigue
- Confusion→stupor→coma
- Decreased cardiac contractility
- Peripheral vasodilation→hypotension

Management

Assess the Severity

MILD. pH 7.30–7.35.

MODERATE. pH 7.20–7.29.

SEVERE. pH ≤7.19.

For all causes of metabolic acidemia, management involves reversing the underlying cause. In most cases of mild or moderate metabolic acidemia, the acid-base disorder can be treated effectively by reversing the underlying condition. However, in some conditions (e.g., chronic renal failure), the condition is not easily reversed. In this situation, mild or moderate metabolic acidemia does not require treatment. Severe metabolic acidemia from chronic renal failure can be treated with PO or IV $NaHCO_3$, being careful not to precipitate volume overload.

For other causes of metabolic acidemia it is occasionally necessary to raise the blood pH by administering $NaHCO_3$, but this usually is reserved for severe metabolic acidemias only. Several important precautions should be considered.

1. The amount of $NaHCO_3$ given depends on the pH and how effective and rapid therapy at reversing the underlying cause is going to be. For instance, a metabolic acidemia with a pH of 6.9 is a medical emergency and may require an initial dose of 150 mmol of IV $NaHCO_3$ while other resuscitation measures are employed. A metabolic acidemia with a pH of 7.10 in a patient with diabetic ketoacidosis may require only 50 mmol IV $NaHCO_3$ while insulin and fluids are administered.

An estimate of the amount of $NaHCO_3$ necessary to elevate the pH to the desired range can be made from the following equation.

$$HCO_3 \text{ deficit} = (\text{Wt in kg}) (0.4) (\text{desired } [HCO_3]) - \text{measured } [HCO_3]$$

where HCO_3 deficit = the amount of $NaHCO_3$ you need to administer, in mmol, Wt = the patient's weight in kg, and 0.4 = a correction factor to account for alkali neutralized by intracellular buffers.

It is not necessary (and may be dangerous) to administer enough $NaHCO_3$ to return the pH to normal. *The goal of $NaHCO_3$ therapy is to raise the pH above 7.2* while the underlying condition causing the acidemia is corrected. Enthusiastic administration of $NaHCO_3$ may result in serious metabolic alkalemia, with tetany, seizures, and ventricular dysrhythmias. Also, IV $NaHCO_3$ is a significant sodium load and may put the patient in CHF. Don't substitute one problem for another!

2. Unless given during the cardiac arrest situation, $NaHCO_3$ should always be diluted (50–150 mmol/L is achieved by adding one to three 50 mmol vials to 1 L of D5W) and be given slowly, as rapid direct infusion of undiluted $NaHCO_3$ can result in fatal ventricular dysrhythmias.

■ ALKALEMIA (pH ≥ 7.45)

First decide whether the patient has a respiratory or a metabolic alkalemia.

Respiratory Alkalemia
- pH ≥7.45
- P_{CO_2} ↓
- HCO_3 ↓

Metabolic Alkalemia
- pH ≥7.45
- P_{CO_2} normal or ↑
- HCO_3 ↑

The normal response to respiratory alkalemia is a decrease in HCO_3. An immediate decrease in HCO_3 occurs because the decrease in P_{CO_2} results in a reduction of HCO_3 according to the law of mass action.

$$CO_2 + H_2O \rightleftharpoons H + HCO_3$$

Later, renal tubular loss of HCO_3 occurs to buffer the change in pH. The expected decrease in HCO_3 in acute respiratory alkalemia is 0.2 (ΔP_{CO_2}). The expected decrease in HCO_3 in chronic respiratory alkalemia is 0.4 (ΔP_{CO_2}). When the HCO_3 is greater than expected, a combined respiratory and metabolic alkalemia should be suspected. When the HCO_3 is less than expected, a combined respiratory alkalemia and metabolic acidemia should be suspected.

The normal response to metabolic alkalemia is hypoventilation with an increase in the P_{CO_2}. The expected increase in uncomplicated metabolic alkalemia is 0.6 (ΔHCO_3). When the P_{CO_2} is greater than expected, a combined metabolic alkalemia and respiratory acidemia should be suspected. When the P_{CO_2} is less than expected, a combined metabolic and respiratory alkalemia should be suspected.

■ *Respiratory Alkalemia*

- pH ≥ 7.45
- $P_{CO_2} \downarrow$
- $HCO_3 \downarrow$

Causes

1. Physiologic conditions (pregnancy, high altitude)
2. CNS disorders (anxiety, pain, fever, tumor)
3. Drugs (aspirin, nicotine, progesterone)
4. Pulmonary disorders (CHF, pulmonary embolism, asthma, pneumonia)
5. Miscellaneous (hepatic failure, hyperthyroidism)

Manifestations

- Confusion
- Numbness, tingling, paresthesias (perioral, hands, feet)
- Lightheadedness
- Tetany in severe cases

Management

Assess the Severity

MILD.   pH 7.45–7.55.
MODERATE.   pH 7.56–7.69.
SEVERE.   pH ≥ 7.70.

Mild respiratory alkalemia is commonly seen in physiological conditions (pregnancy, high altitude) and in these cases requires no treatment. Any of the other causes listed may result in mild respiratory alkalemia, and many can be treated symptomatically—e.g., the febrile patient can be treated with antipyretics, the patient in pain can be treated with analgesics, and the anxious patient may be treated with reassurance or sedation. In addition to these measures, more pronounced degrees of respiratory alkalemia due to anxiety can be treated by rebreathing into a paper bag. The only effective treatment for the other causes listed is eliminating the underlying condition.

■ *Metabolic Alkalemia*

- pH ≥ 7.45
- P_{CO_2} normal or $\uparrow$
- $HCO_3 \uparrow$

Causes

1. With extracellular volume depletion and low (usually < 10 mEq/L) urinary Cl:
   a. GI losses
      (1) Vomiting

      (2) GI drainage (NG suction)
      (3) Chloride-wasting diarrhea
      (4) Villous adenoma
   b. Renal losses
      (1) Diuretic therapy
      (2) Posthypercapnea
      (3) Nonreabsorbable anions
      (4) Penicillin, carbenicillin, ticarcillin
      (5) Bartter's syndrome
2. With extracellular volume expansion and presence (usually > 20 mEq/L) of urinary Cl:
   a. Mineralocorticoid excess
      (1) Endogenous
         (a) Hyperaldosteronism
         (b) Cushing's syndrome
      (2) Exogenous
         (a) Glucocorticoids
         (b) Mineralocorticoids
         (c) Carbenoxolone
         (d) Licorice excess
      (3) Alkali ingestion
      (4) Poststarvation feeding

Manifestations

There are no specific signs or symptoms of metabolic alkalemia. Severe alkalemia may result in

- Apathy
- Confusion → stupor

Management

Assess the Severity
MILD.   pH 7.45—7.55
MODERATE.   pH 7.56–7.69.
SEVERE.   pH ≥7.70.

Beyond correcting the underlying cause, mild or moderate metabolic alkalemia rarely requires specific treatment. *Metabolic alkalemia associated with ECF volume depletion* usually responds to infusion of NS, which will enhance renal HCO_3 excretion.

Note that associated electrolyte abnormalities (particularly hypokalemia) may be more threatening to the patient's well-being than the metabolic alkalemia. Attention to concomitant electrolyte disorders is very important.

In *diuretic-induced alkalemia*, administration of KCl may improve the alkalemia.

If the patient is *volume overloaded* and has a metabolic alkalemia, *acetazolamide* 250 to 500 mg PO or IV q8h enhances the renal HCO_3 excretion and may be helpful.

In *Bartter's syndrome*, the alkalemia may respond to prostaglandin synthetase inhibitors, such as indomethacin.

It is very unusual to require acidifying agents, such as NH_4Cl or dilute HCl, even for severe metabolic alkalemia. Such agents should be given only under the direct guidance of your resident and the patient's attending physician.

29

ANEMIA

Serum hemoglobin (Hb) is one of the most common laboratory determinations made in hospitalized patients. Remember that Hb is a *concentration*, and its value can be modified by both a change in its *content* and a change in its *diluent* (plasma). For instance, a patient's Hb may be elevated (i.e., in the "normal" range) despite a sudden loss of intravascular volume, as is seen in an acute hemorrhage. Because of the possibility of transfusion-related illnesses, one must avoid the reflex administration of RBC transfusions to correct a low Hb level. *Remember to treat the patient, not the laboratory value.*

Causes

1. Blood loss
   a. Acute
      (1) GI hemorrhage
      (2) Trauma
      (3) Concealed hemorrhage
         (a) Ruptured aortic aneurysm
         (b) Ruptured ectopic pregnancy
         (c) Retroperitoneal hematoma
         (d) Postsurgical bleeding
   b. Chronic
      (1) GI bleeding
      (2) Uterine bleeding
2. Inadequate production of RBCs
   a. Anemia of chronic disease (chronic inflammation, uremia, endocrine failure, liver disease)
   b. Iron deficiency
   c. Megaloblastic anemias (vitamin B_{12} and folate deficiency, drugs, inherited)
   d. Sideroblastic anemias (drugs, alcohol, malignancy, RA, inherited)
3. Hemolysis
   a. Extrinsic factors (immune hemolysis, splenomegaly, mechanical trauma, infections)
   b. Membrane defects (e.g., hereditary spherocytosis, paroxysmal nocturnal hemoglobinuria)
   c. Internal RBC defects (e.g., thalassemia, sickle cell disease)

Manifestations

The manifestations of anemia depend on underlying medical conditions, the severity of the anemia, and the rapidity with which it develops. The body's reaction to an acute reduction in RBC mass is usually manifested by (compensatory) alterations in the cardiovascular and respiratory systems.

Acute anemias due to hemorrhage will result in symptoms and signs of intravascular volume depletion, including the following:

- Pallor, diaphoresis, tachypnea
- Cold, clammy extremities
- Hypotension, tachycardia
- Shock

Anemias that develop slowly over weeks or months are not usually accompanied by signs of intravascular volume depletion. In these cases, symptoms and signs often are not so obvious and may vary depending on disease in other organ systems.

Symptoms
- Fatigue, lethargy ⎫
- Dyspnea   ⎬   Common
- Palpitations ⎭
- Worsening of symptoms in patients with angina pectoris or claudication, or presentation with a TIA
- GI disturbances (due to shunting of blood from the splanchnic bed)—anorexia, nausea, bowel irregularity
- Abnormal menstrual patterns

Signs
- Pallor
- Tachypnea
- Tachycardia, wide pulse pressure, hyperdynamic precordium
- Jaundice/splenomegaly (in hemolytic anemias)

Management

Assess the Severity.   The severity of the situation should be determined according to the level of Hb, the patient's volume status, the rapidity with which the anemia developed, and the likelihood that the underlying process will continue unabated.

THE PATIENT WHO IS IN SHOCK OR WHO IS VOLUME DEPLETED.   An acute anemia due to blood loss (and, hence, intravascular volume depletion) will result in compensatory tachycardia and tachypnea. If full hemodynamic compensation is inadequate, hypotension or shock will result. Do not forget, in your assessment of the patient's volume status, to check for postural changes (Chapter 3, p. 10), which may be the earliest manifestation of an acute blood loss.

1. Notify your resident.
2. Ensure that at least one, and preferably two, large-bore (size 16 if possible) IVs are in place.
3. If there is evidence of active bleeding, ensure that there is blood on hold. If not, order stat crossmatch for 2, 4, or 6 units of packed RBCs, depending on your estimate of blood loss.
4. **Replenish intravascular volume** by giving IV fluids. The best immediate choice is a crystalloid (NS or Ringer's lactate), which will at least temporarily stay in the intravascular space. Albumin or banked plasma can be given but is expensive, carries a risk of hepatitis, and is not always available.
   The assumption here, when the association of a new, severe anemia with intravascular volume depletion is seen, is that blood has been lost from the intravascular space—hence, blood is ideally what needs to be replaced. If there is no blood on hold for the patient, a stat crossmatch usually will take 50 minutes. If blood is on hold, it should be available at the bedside in 30 minutes. In an emergency, O-negative blood may be given, although this practice is usually reserved for the acute trauma victim. Transfusion-related infections can be minimized by transfusing only when necessary. *Rule-of-thumb*: Maintain the Hb level at 90 to 100 g/L.
5. **Order the appropriate IV rate**, which will depend on the patient's volume status. *Shock* will require IV fluid wide open through at least two large-bore IV sites. Elevating the IV bag, squeezing the IV bag, or using IV pressure cuffs may help speed the rate of delivery of the solution. *Mild or moderate volume depletion* can be treated with 500 to 1000 ml of NS given as rapidly as possible, with serial determinations of volume status and assessment of cardiac status. If blood is not at the bedside within 30 minutes, delegate someone to find out why there has been a delay.
   Note: Aggressive volume depletion in a patient with a history of CHF may result in pulmonary edema. Do not overshoot the mark!
6. **Determine the site of hemorrhage.**
   a. **Look for obvious signs of external bleeding**—bleeding from IV sites, skin lesions, hematemesis, menstrual bleeding.
   b. **Examine for signs of occult blood loss.**
      (1) Perform a rectal examination to look for melena.
      (2) Swelling at biopsy or surgical sites (e.g., flank swelling after renal biopsy, ascites after liver biopsy; flank or periumbilical ecchymoses, which may indicate hemoperitoneum).
      (3) If the patient is a female in the childbearing years, a ruptured ectopic pregnancy must be considered. If in-

      dicated, a pelvic examination should be performed by an experienced physician.

      (4) If a ruptured thoracic or abdominal aortic aneurysm is likely, immediate surgical referral is necessary.

7. Review the chart for exacerbating factors that may contribute to ongoing hemorrhage, e.g., administration of **aspirin, heparin, warfarin, thrombolytic agents, or coagulopathies**, and for recent pertinent laboratory values (**aPTT, PT**, and **platelets**).

8. Request **surgical consultation** when appropriate.

THE PATIENT WHO IS NORMOVOLEMIC. Patients can tolerate even severe (Hb < 70 g/L) anemia if the anemia develops slowly. Mild (Hb 100–120 g/L) chronic anemias in the context of normal intravascular volume often do not alter the vital signs. If the patient is normovolemic, transfusion therapy is seldom warranted on an urgent basis. If you have excluded the presence of active hemorrhage, the anemia must be due to either (1) chronic blood loss, (2) inadequate production of RBCs, or (3) hemolysis.

1. An unexpected Hb of < 100 g/L merits a repeat measurement to exclude laboratory error while other assessment measures are taking place. Mild anemia (Hb 100–120 g/L) in an asymptomatic patient with normal vital signs usually can wait if other problems of higher priority exist. One must always keep in mind, however, that if active bleeding is responsible for the anemia, a stable patient may become unstable very quickly.

2. **What is the patient's usual Hb?** Look in the current or old chart to see if the anemia is a new finding. If the current Hb is more than 10 or 20 g/L lower than previous values, assume that the underlying cause of anemia has worsened or a second factor has developed (e.g., a patient with a chronic disease, such as SLE, may normally have an Hb of 90 g/L; a new value of 75 g/L may represent further marrow suppression, hemolysis, or new onset of bleeding).

3. If the patient is comfortable and has a normal cardiovascular examination, and your examination reveals no suspicion of active bleeding, further investigation can take place in the morning. Several baseline studies are helpful in pointing you in the right direction to diagnose the cause of the anemia.

    a. **Measurement of RBC cell volume.** The mean red cell volume (MCV) is useful in classifying the anemias due to decreased RBC production (microcytic, normocytic, macrocytic).

    b. **Examination of the blood smear** by an individual experienced in hematology often provides valuable clues helpful in diagnosing specific anemias (Fig. 29–1).

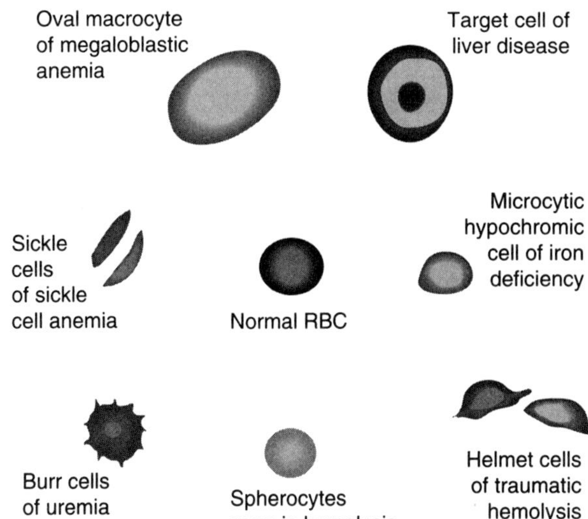

Figure 29–1 □ Blood smear demonstrating examples of helpful diagnostic features associated with specific anemias.

c. A **reticulocyte count** provides a measure of marrow erythropoiesis. An elevated reticulocyte count suggests hemolysis, recent hemorrhage, or a recently treated chronic anemia (e.g., recently treated vitamin B_{12} deficiency). An inappropriately low reticulocyte count suggests a failure to produce RBCs (e.g., untreated iron, vitamin B_{12}, or folate deficiency or anemia of chronic disease).

30

CALCIUM DISORDERS

■ HYPERCALCEMIA
Causes

1. Increased intake/absorption
   a. Vitamin D or A intoxication
   b. Excessive calcium supplementation
   c. Milk-alkali syndrome (excessive antacid ingestion)
   d. Sarcoidosis and other granulomatous disease
2. Increased production/mobilization from bone
   a. Primary hyperparathyroidism*
   b. Severe secondary hyperparathyroidism associated with renal failure
   c. Neoplasm.* There are four mechanisms for hypercalcemia of malignancy as follows:
      (1) Bony metastasis (prostate, thyroid, kidney, breast, lung)
      (2) PTH-like substance elaborated by tumor cells (lung, kidney, ovary, colon)
      (3) Prostaglandin E_2 increases bony resorption (multiple myeloma)
      (4) Osteoclast-activating factor (multiple myeloma, lymphoproliferative disorders)
   d. Paget's disease
   e. Immobilization
   f. Hyperthyroidism
   g. Adrenal insufficiency
   h. Acromegaly
   i. Sarcoidosis. In addition to sarcoidosis increasing absorption from the GI tract, there is an increased conversion of 25 (OH) vitamin D to the active form, $1,25(OH)_2$ vitamin D.
   j. Chronic lithium use
3. Decreased excretion
   a. Thiazide diuretics
   b. Familial hypocalciuric hypercalcemia

Manifestations

The manifestations of hypercalcemia are numerous and nonspecific, e.g., "bones, stones, and groans."

---

*Primary hyperparathyroidism and tumors account for 90% of cases of hypercalcemia.

HEENT	Corneal calcification (band keratopathy)
CVS	Short QT interval, prolonged PR interval (Fig. 30–1), dysrhythmias, digoxin sensitivity, hypertension
GI	Anorexia, nausea, vomiting, constipation, abdominal pain, pancreatitis ("groans")
GU	Polyuria, polydipsia, nephrolithiasis ("stones")
NEURO	Insomnia, restlessness, delirium, dementia, psychosis, lethargy, coma
MSS	Muscle weakness, hyporeflexia, bone pain, fractures ("bones")
MISC	Hyperchlorhydric metabolic acidosis

Management

Assess the Severity.   The severity of the situation should be determined according to the serum calcium concentration, the rate of progression, and the presence or absence of symptoms. It is important to recognize that most laboratories measure total serum calcium (ionized plus albumin bound), but the primary determinant of the physiological effect is the ionized component.

If the patient is hypoalbuminemic, a correction factor can be used to estimate the total calcium concentration. For every 10 g/L of hypoalbuminemia, add 0.2 mmol/L to the serum calcium value—e.g., if the measured serum calcium value is 2.6 mmol/L (the upper limit of normal) but the serum albumin value is low at 30 g/L (with an anticipated normal concentration of 40 g/L), the correct serum calcium value is 0.2 + 2.6 = 2.8 mmol/L (moderate elevation).

How high is the serum calcium?
- Normal range = 2.2 to 2.6 mmol/L
- Mild elevation = 2.6 to 2.9 mmol/L
- Moderate elevation = 2.9 to 3.2 mmol/L
- Severe elevation = > 3.2 mmol/L

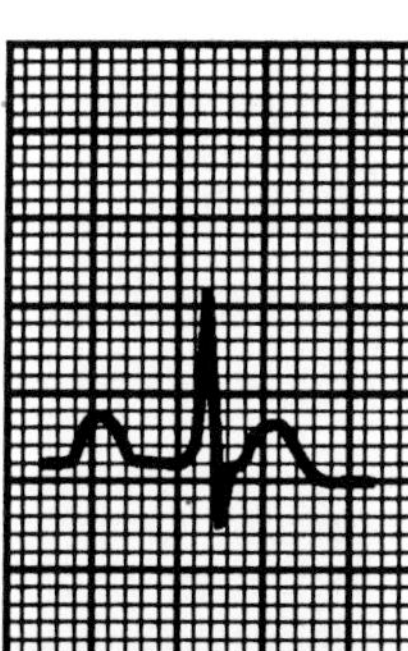

Figure 30–1 □ Hypercalcemia (short QT interval, prolonged PR interval).

Is there a progressive cause that is likely to result in further increases?

If the situation is progressive, the patient requires immediate treatment.

Is the patient symptomatic?

Any symptomatic patient requires immediate treatment.

Severe hypercalcemia (> 3.2 mmol/L) requires immediate treatment because of the danger of a fatal cardiac dysrhythmia.

1. *Correct volume depletion/expand extracellular volume.* Give NS IV 500 ml as fast as possible. Further NS boluses can be given dependent on the volume status. Titrate the NS IV maintenance rate to keep the patient slightly volume expanded. If the patient has a history of CHF, this volume expansion should be undertaken in the ICU/CCU, since close monitoring of the volume status will be required. A reduction in the serum calcium level will be expected because of hemodilution and because an increased urinary sodium excretion is accompanied by an increased calcium excretion.

2. *Establish diuresis* > *2500 ml/day.* In addition to maintaining volume expansion with NS, give *furosemide* (Lasix) 20 to 40 mg IV q2–4h to establish a diuresis of > 2500 ml/day. Care must be taken not to induce volume depletion with administration of furosemide. The patient may require 4 to 10 L of NS per day to maintain the volume expanded state. Furosemide inhibits the tubular reabsorption of calcium, thus increasing calcium excretion by the kidneys. Do not use thiazides to establish diuresis, since they elevate the serum calcium level.

3. *Dialysis.* Occasionally, when the serum calcium level is extremely high, e.g., > 4.5 mmol/L, hemodialysis or peritoneal dialysis may be required.

If *hypercalcemia is secondary to neoplasm*, in addition to the administration of NS and furosemide (as previously discussed), one of the following medications may be of value.

1. Corticosteroids. *Prednisone* 40 to 100 mg PO daily or *hydrocortisone* (Solu-Cortef) 200 to 500 mg IV daily in divided doses. Steroids antagonize the peripheral action of vitamin D (decreased absorption, decreased mobilization from bone, and decreased renal tubular reabsorption of calcium).

2. *Plicamycin* 15 to 25 μg/kg in 1 L of NS IV over 3 to 6 hours. Plicamycin inhibits bone resorption. The onset of action is 48 hours.

3. *Disodium etidronate* is an effective agent in the control of cancer-associated hypercalcemia. It is given in a dose of 7.5 mg/kg IV daily for 3 days. Each daily dose should be diluted in 250 ml NS or D5W and given IV over a period of at least 2 hours.

4. *Indomethacin* 50 mg PO q8h. Indomethacin inhibits the syn-

thesis of prostaglandin E_2, which is produced by some solid tumors, e.g., of the breast.

5. *Synthetic salmon calcitonin* may temporarily lower the serum calcium concentration but should not be initiated at night before first skin testing the patient for allergy (see package insert).

Moderate hypercalcemia or mild symptomatic hypercalcemia (2.9–3.2 mmol/L or lesser elevations in the presence of symptoms) should be managed as follows.

1. *Correct volume depletion* and expand extracellular fluid volume with NS 500 ml IV given over 1 to 2 hours. Further NS can be given at a rate to keep the patient slightly volume expanded.
2. *Establish diuresis > 2500/day* if volume expansion alone is unsuccessful in lowering the serum calcium.
3. *Oral phosphate* 0.5 to 3 g/day depending on GI tolerance (flatulence, diarrhea) may be given for patients with a low or normal serum phosphate level.
4. *Mild asymptomatic hypercalcemia* (2.6–2.9 mmol/L) does not require immediate treatment. The appropriate investigations may be ordered in the morning.

■ HYPOCALCEMIA

Causes

1. *Decreased intake/absorption*
   a. Malabsorption
   b. Intestinal bypass surgery
   c. Short bowel syndrome
   d. Vitamin D deficiency
2. *Decreased production/mobilization from bone*
   a. Hypoparathyroidism (following subtotal thyroidectomy or parathyroidectomy)
   b. Pseudohypoparathyroidism
   c. Vitamin D deficiency [decreased production of 25(OH) vitamin D or 1,25(OH)$_2$ vitamin D]
   d. Acute hyperphosphatemia (tumor lysis, acute renal failure, rhabdomyolysis)
   e. Acute pancreatitis
   f. Hypomagnesemia
   g. Alkalosis (hyperventilation, vomiting, fistulas)
   h. Neoplasm
      (1) Paradoxical hypocalcemia associated with osteoblastic metastasis (lung, breast, prostate)
      (2) Medullary carcinoma of the thyroid (calcitonin-producing tumor)
      (3) Rapid tumor lysis with phosphate release

3. *Increased excretion*
   a. Chronic renal failure
   b. Drugs (aminoglycosides, loop diuretics)

Manifestations

The earliest symptoms are paresthesias of the lips, fingers, and toes.

HEENT	Papilledema, diplopia
CVS	Prolonged QT interval without U-waves (Fig. 30–2)
GI	Abdominal cramps
NEURO	Confusion, irritability, depression
	Hyperactive tendon reflexes
	Carpopedal spasm, laryngospasm (stridor), tetany
	Generalized tonic-clonic seizures
	Paresthesias of lips, fingers, toes
	Special tests:
	Chvostek's sign (Fig. 30–3): Facial muscle spasm elicited by tapping the facial nerve immediately anterior to the ear lobe and below the zygomatic arch. (This is a normal finding in 10% of the population.)
	Trousseau's sign (Fig. 30–4): Carpal spasm elicited by occluding the arterial blood flow to the forearm for 3 to 5 minutes.

Management

Assess the Severity.   The severity of the situation should be determined according to the serum calcium and phosphate concentrations and the presence or absence of symptoms. If the serum albumin is not within the normal range, a correction factor can be used to estimate the total serum calcium (ionized plus albumin bound). See page 287 for a discussion of this correction factor.

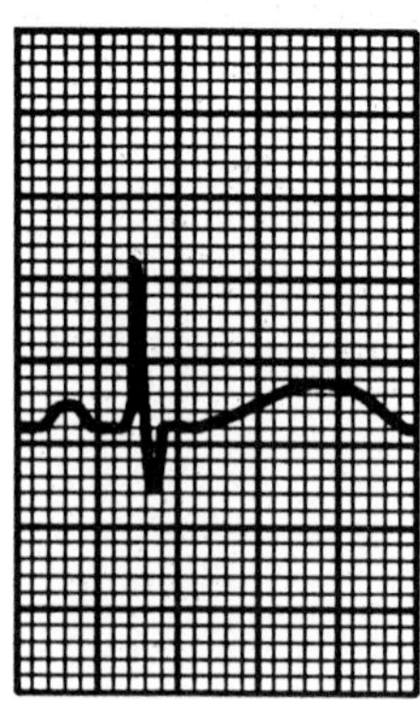

Figure 30–2 □ Hypocalcemia (long QT interval).

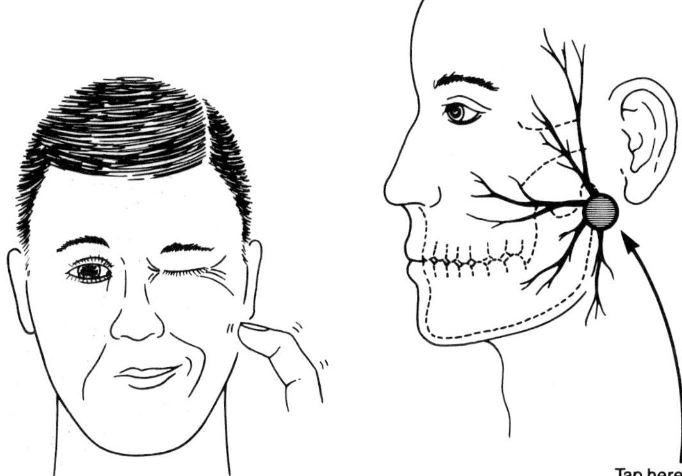

Figure 30–3 □ Chvostek's sign. Facial muscle spasm elicited by tapping the facial nerve immediately anterior to the earlobe and below the zygomatic arch.

How low is the serum calcium level?
- Normal range = 2.2 to 2.6 mmol/L
- Mild depletion = 1.9 to 2.2 mmol/L
- Moderate depletion = 1.5 to 1.9 mmol/L
- Severe depletion = < 1.5 mmol/L

What is the serum phosphate concentration?
If the serum phosphate concentration is markedly elevated (> 6 mmol/L) in severe hypocalcemia, correction of hyperphosphatemia must be carried out with IV glucose and insulin before calcium is given to avoid metastatic calcification.

Is the patient symptomatic?
Hypocalcemic patients who are asymptomatic do not require urgent correction with IV calcium.

Is the patient receiving digoxin?
Caution is required if the patient is receiving digoxin, since calcium potentiates the action of digoxin. Ideally, if IV calcium administration is required, the patient should have continuous ECG monitoring.

Severe, symptomatic hypocalcemia (< 1.5 mmol/L) requires im-

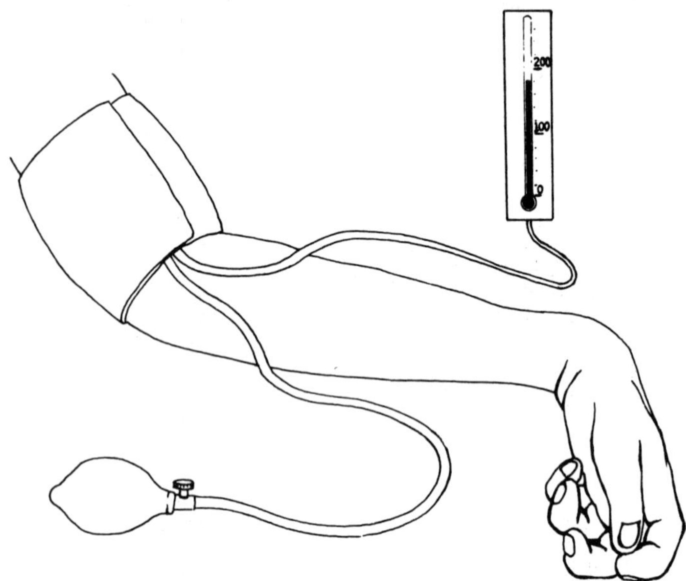

Figure 30–4 □ Trousseau's sign. Carpal spasm elicited by occluding the arterial blood flow to the forearm for 3 to 5 min.

mediate treatment because of the danger of respiratory failure from laryngospasm.

1. Provided the patient's PO_4 is normal or low, give 10 to 20 ml (1–2 g) of 10% solution of calcium gluconate IV in 100 ml D5W over 30 minutes. If the patient has evidence of tetany or laryngeal stridor, the same dose should be given over 2 minutes as a direct injection, i.e., calcium gluconate 10% solution 10 to 20 ml IV over 2 minutes. Oral calcium may be started immediately: 200 mg of elemental calcium q2h × 4 doses. If the corrected serum calcium value is < 1.9 mmol/L 6 hours after initiating this treatment, a calcium infusion is required. Add 10 ml (1 g) of a 10% calcium gluconate solution to 500 ml D5W and infuse over 6 hours. If the serum calcium value is not within the normal range after 6 hours of this infusion, 5 ml (500 mg) of calcium gluconate can be added to the initial infusion dose q6h until a satisfactory serum calcium level is achieved. The postparathyroidectomy patient may require 1 to 1.5 g calcium gluconate per hour. Add 100 ml (10 g) of a 10% calcium gluconate solution to 500 ml D5W and begin the infusion at 50 ml/h (1 g/h).

2. If the patient is hyperphosphatemic (PO_4 > 6 mmol/L), correction with glucose and insulin is required before adminis-

tration of IV calcium. Consult the nephrology service immediately.

Mild and moderate asymptomatic hypocalcemia does not require urgent IV calcium replacement. Oral calcium replacement with elemental calcium 1000 to 1500 mg/day may be started to achieve a corrected serum calcium level in the 2.2 to 2.6 mmol/L range. Long-term treatment with oral calcium or vitamin D depends on the etiology, which can be evaluated in the morning.

31

COAGULATION DISORDERS

You will be confronted on call by abnormal results of tests of hemostasis. These must always be interpreted in the clinical context in which the measurements were made. Bleeding is the commonest clinical manifestation of a coagulation disorder, and the type of bleeding can alert you to the probable type of disorder present.

Patients with *vessel or platelet abnormalities* may have petechiae, purpura, or easy bruisability. The bleeding characteristically occurs superficially (e.g., oozing from mucous membranes or IV sites). The bleeding of scurvy is seen only rarely in North America and is usually manifested by perifollicular hemorrhages, though gingival bleeding and intramuscular hematomas also may occur.

Bleeding due to *coagulation factor deficiencies* may occur spontaneously, in deeper organ sites, e.g., visceral hemorrhages and hemarthroses and tends to be delayed and prolonged. Bleeding associated with *thrombolytic agents* is usually manifested by continuous oozing from IV sites.

Three tests are in common use to assess hemostasis—the prothrombin time (PT), the activated partial thromboplastin time (aPTT), and the platelet count. A fourth test, the bleeding time, is used infrequently because it rarely helps make a specific diagnosis, and it carries the risk of accidental exposure to hepatitis and HIV. Laboratory features of the common coagulation disorders are listed in Table 31–1.

PROTHROMBIN TIME (PT)

Quide's one-stage prothrombin time (PT) tests the *extrinsic coagulation system* (Fig. 31–1). It is affected by deficiencies in factors I, II, V, VII, and X. However, antagonists of the extrinsic system, including heparin, activated antithrombin III, and fibrin degradation products, can prolong the PT.

Disorders Associated With PT Prolongation

- Coagulation factor abnormalities
- Oral anticoagulants
- Vitamin K deficiency
- Liver disease
- DIC
- Heparin (variable)

Table 31–1 □ LABORATORY FEATURES OF COMMON COAGULATION DISORDERS

Disorder	Diagnostic Laboratory Tests				
	aPTT	*PT*	*Platelets*	*Bleeding Time*	*Other*
Vessel Abnormalities					
Vasculitis	Normal	Normal	Normal	Normal or ↑	C3 C4 C1Q binding
Increased vascular fragility	Normal	Normal	Normal	↑	
Hereditary connective tissue disorders	Normal	Normal	Normal	↑	
Paraproteinemias	Normal	Normal	Normal	↑	
Coagulation Factor Abnormalities					
Heparin	↑	↑ or Normal	Normal or ↓	Normal or ↑	
Warfarin	Normal or ↑	↑	Normal	Normal	
Vitamin K deficiency	↑	↑	Normal	Normal	
DIC	↑	↑	↓	Normal or ↑ *	↑ Fibrin degradation products; ↓ fibrinogen
Factor VIII deficiency	↑	Normal	Normal	Normal	↓ Factor VIII assay
Factor IX deficiency	↑	Normal	Normal	Normal	Normal factor IX assay
Von Willebrand's disease	Normal or ↑	Normal	Normal	Normal or ↑	Normal or ↓ factor VIII assay ↓ Factor VIII antigen ↓ Ristocetin cofactor
Liver disease	↑	↑	Normal or ↓	Normal or ↑	
Platelet Disorders					
Thrombocytopenia	Normal	Normal	↓	Normal or ↑ *	
Impaired platelet function	Normal	Normal	Normal	↑	

*Depends on degree of thrombocytopenia.

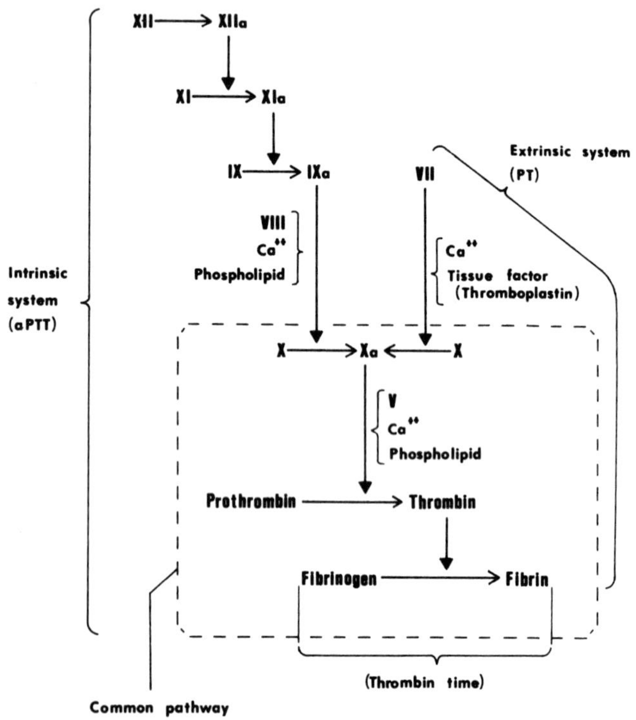

Figure 31–1 □ The coagulation cascade.

ACTIVATED PARTIAL THROMBOPLASTIN TIME (aPTT)

The activated partial thromboplastin time (aPTT) tests the *intrinsic coagulation system* (Fig. 31–1). It is most sensitive to deficiencies and abnormalities in the sequence of procoagulant activities that occur before factor X activation.

Disorders Associated With aPTT Prolongation

- Circulating anticoagulant
- Heparin
- Factor VIII, factor IX deficiency
- Von Willebrand's disease (variable)
- DIC
- Vitamin K deficiency
- Oral anticoagulants (variable)

A frequent benign cause of prolongation of aPTT in hospital is the presence of an acquired anticoagulant, such as the lupus erythematosus anticoagulant. This situation can be differentiated from a factor deficiency by demonstrating failure to normalize the aPTT when a sample of the plasma of a patient with an acquired anticoagulant is mixed with normal plasma 50:50.

PLATELET COUNT

The platelet count is a reflection of production and destruction (sequestration) of platelets.

Disorders Associated With Low Platelets
Decreased Marrow Production
- Marrow replacement by tumor, granuloma (e.g., TB, sarcoid), fibrous tissue
- Storage disease (e.g., Gaucher's disease)
- Marrow injury by drugs (e.g., sulfonamides, chloramphenicol)
- Defective maturation (e.g., vitamin B_{12} or folate deficiency)

Increased Peripheral Destruction
- Immune mediated
  - Drugs (e.g., quinine, quinidine, heparin)
  - Connective tissue disorders (e.g., SLE)
  - Lymphoproliferative disorders (e.g., CLL)
  - HIV infection
  - Idiopathic
  - Posttransfusion purpura
- Nonimmune mediated
  - Consumption (e.g., DIC, TTP, prosthetic valves)
  - Dilutional (e.g., massive transfusion)
- Sequestration (e.g., any cause of splenomegaly)

VESSEL OR PLATELET FUNCTION ABNORMALITIES

Bleeding can still occur in the face of a normal PT, aPTT, and platelet count. This may be a result of *vessel abnormalities* or *abnormal platelet function.*

Vessel Abnormalities (Vascular Factor)
Hereditary Disorders
- Hereditary hemorrhagic telangiectasia
- Ehlers-Danlos syndrome
- Marfan's syndrome
- Pseudoxanthoma elasticum
- Osteogenesis imperfecta

Acquired Disorders
- Vasculitis
  - Schonlein-Henoch purpura
  - Systemic lupus erythematosus
  - Polyarteritis nodosa
  - Rheumatoid arthritis
  - Cryoglobulinemia
- Increased vascular fragility
  - Senile purpura
  - Cushing's syndrome
  - Scurvy

Impaired Platelet Function

Hereditary Disorders
- Von Willebrand's disease
- Bernard-Soulier disease
- Glanzmann's thrombasthenia

Acquired Disorders
- Drugs (e.g., NSAIDs, aspirin, antibiotics, such as high-dose penicillin, cephalosporins, nitrofurantoin)
- Uremia
- Paraproteins (e.g., amyloidosis, multiple myeloma, Waldenstrom's macroglobulinemia)
- Myeloproliferative disease (e.g., CGL, essential thrombocytosis)

BLEEDING IN COAGULATION DISORDERS
Manifestations

Bleeding in the patient with a coagulation disorder is of concern for two reasons.

1. Progressive loss of intravascular volume, if uncorrected, may lead to hypovolemic shock, with inadequate perfusion of vital organs.
2. Hemorrhage into specific organ sites may produce local tissue or organ injury (e.g., intracerebral hemorrhage, epidural hemorrhage with spinal cord compression, hemarthrosis).

Thrombotic thrombocytopenic purpura characteristically occurs with a combination of hemolytic anemia, thrombocytopenia, fever, neurological disorders, and renal dysfunction. The *hemolytic uremic syndrome* has a presentation similar to that of TTP but without the neurological manifestations. These two syndromes can be distinguished from *disseminated intravascular coagulation* (DIC), in which prolonged aPTT and PT, reduced fibrinogen level, and elevated fibrin degradation products are seen. DIC most often occurs in the context of infection (e.g., gram-negative sepsis), obstetric catastrophes, malignancy (e.g., prostatic cancer), and tissue damage/shock.

Management

1. **Vessel abnormalities.** Treatment of bleeding due to vessel abnormalities is usually treatment of the underlying disorder.
   a. Serious bleeding due to *hereditary disorders of connective tissue* and to hereditary hemorrhagic telangiectasia most often requires local mechanical or surgical measures at the site of hemorrhage in order to control blood loss.
   b. In the *vasculitides,* control of bleeding is best achieved by use of corticosteroids, other immunosuppressive agents, or a combination of both.
   c. There is no good treatment for the increased vascular fragility that results in *senile purpura.* Purpura due to *Cushing's syndrome* is preventable with normalization of plasma cortisol levels. However, in the patient receiving therapeutic corticosteroids, the underlying indication for therapy often prevents significant reduction of steroid levels. Hemorrhages associated with *scurvy* will not recur following adequate dietary supplementation of ascorbic acid.
2. **Coagulation factor abnormalities.** Treatment of coagulation factor abnormalities is dependent on the specific factor deficiency or deficiencies.
   a. *Specific factor deficiencies* should always be treated in consultation with a hematologist. Factor VIII deficiency (hemophilia A) can be treated with factor VIII concentrate or cryoprecipitate. Nonblood products may also be of benefit, e.g., DDAVP, danazole. Factor IX deficiency (hemophilia B) may be treated with factor IX concentrate or banked plasma.
   b. *Liver disease.* Because patients with liver disease frequently are also vitamin K deficient, it is worthwhile to administer *vitamin K* 10 mg SC or IV daily for 3 days. IV vitamin K occasionally has caused anaphylactic reactions. If the patient does not respond to vitamin K, bleeding should be managed by fresh frozen plasma. Factor IX concentrates carry a risk of thromboembolism and are contraindicated in liver disease.
   c. *Vitamin K deficiency* may be treated in an identical manner to that subsequently outlined for correction of warfarin coagulopathy. Ideally, however, one should identify and treat the underlying cause of vitamin K deficiency.
   d. The treatment of *DIC* is both complicated and controversial. All medical authorities agree, however, that definitive management involves treating the underlying cause. Additionally, a patient with DIC often requires coagulation factor and platelet support in the form of fresh frozen plasma, cryoprecipitate, and platelet transfusions. The role of heparin in the treatment of DIC is controversial and should not be instituted before hematological consultation.

e. Bleeding due to *anticoagulant therapy* can be reversed slowly or rapidly depending on the clinical status of the patient and the site of bleeding.
  (1) *Heparin* has a half-life of only 1½ hours, and simply discontinuing a heparin infusion should normalize the aPTT and correct the heparin-induced coagulopathy in minor episodes of bleeding. Serious bleeding complications can be treated by discontinuing the heparin infusion and reversing the heparin effect with *protamine sulfate* 1 mg/100 units of heparin (approximately) IV slowly. Dosage is determined by estimating the amount of circulating heparin—e.g., for a patient on a maintenance infusion of heparin 1000 units IV/h, the heparin infusion should be stopped and enough protamine should be given to neutralize approximately one half of the preceding hour's dose, i.e., a total protamine dose of 5 mg. No more than 50 mg per single dose in a 10 minute period should be given. Side effects of protamine include hypotension, bradycardia, flushing, and bleeding.
  (2) Rapid reversal of *warfarin effect*, as may be required in life-threatening hemorrhages, can be achieved by administering *plasma* (e.g., 2 units at a time), with subsequent redetermination of PT. Although both fresh frozen plasma and banked plasma contain the vitamin K-dependent clotting factors, banked plasma is considerably less expensive and, hence, is the replacement solution of choice. Severe bleeding (e.g., intracranial hemorrhage) requires urgent hematological consultation. When prolonged reversal of anticoagulant effect is desired, *vitamin K* 10 mg PO, SC, or IV may be given daily for 3 days. Minor bleeding complications in patients on warfarin may require temporary discontinuation of this drug. IV vitamin K occasionally has caused anaphylactic reactions and, hence, should be given with caution.
f. *Bleeding due to thrombolytic agents.* Localized oozing at sites of invasive procedures often can be controlled by local pressure dressings or avoided in the first place by not doing invasive procedures. More serious hemorrhage requires discontinuation of the thrombolytic agent. Fibrinolytic agents that are not fibrin specific will cause systemic fibrinogenolysis, and, therefore, fresh frozen plasma may be required to replace fibrinogen. *Aminocaproic acid,* which is an inhibitor of plasminogen activator, has also been used (20–30 g/day) but should not be initiated before hematological consultation.

3. **Platelet abnormalities.** Treatment of bleeding in the thrombocytopenic patient varies depending on the presence of either an abnormality in platelet production or an increase in platelet destruction.
   a. *Decreased marrow production* of platelets is treated in the long term by identifying and, if possible, correcting the underlying cause (e.g., chemotherapy for tumor, removal of marrow toxins, vitamin B_{12} or folate supplementation when indicated). In the short term, however, a serious bleeding complication should be treated by platelet transfusion (e.g., 6–8 units at a time). One unit of platelets can be expected to increase the platelet count by 1000 in the patient with inadequate marrow production of platelets. Check the response to transfusion by ordering a 1 hour postplatelet transfusion count.
   b. *Increased peripheral destruction* of platelets is also best managed by identifying and correcting the underlying problem. Often this management involves the systemic use of corticosteroids or other immunosuppressive agents. The patient tends to have less serious bleeding manifestations than one with inadequate marrow production of platelets but may require platelet transfusion for life-threatening bleeding episodes. There are exceptions to platelet transfusion therapy in thrombocytopenia in the patient with TTP. In this situation, platelet transfusions should be avoided, since they actually may worsen the condition.
   c. *Dilutional thrombocytopenia* due to massive RBC transfusion and IV fluid therapy is treated with platelet transfusion as required. Dilutional thrombocytopenia can usually be prevented by remembering to transfuse 8 units of platelets for every 10 to 12 units of RBCs transfused.
   d. *Von Willebrand's disease* may be treated with cryoprecipitate or DDAVP.
   e. *Bleeding disorders resulting from acquired platelet dysfunction* are best managed by identification and correction of the underlying problem. Temporary treatment of bleeding disorders due to these conditions may involve platelet transfusion or other more specialized measures (e.g., cryoprecipitate, DDAVP, conjugated estrogens in uremia).

32

GLUCOSE DISORDERS

■ HYPERGLYCEMIA

Causes

Patients With Documented Diabetes Mellitus
- Poorly controlled IDDM or NIDDM
- Stress (surgery, infection, severe illness)
- Drugs (corticosteroids, thiazides)
- TPN administration

Patients Without Previously Documented Diabetes Mellitus
- New onset of diabetes mellitus
- Stress (surgery, infection, severe illness)
- Drugs (corticosteroids, thiazides)
- TPN administration

Acute Manifestations

Mild Hyperglycemia
(fasting blood glucose of 6.1 to 11.0 mmol/L)
- Polyuria, polydipsia, thirst

Moderate Hyperglycemia
(fasting blood glucose of 11.1 to 22.5 mmol/L)
- Volume depletion (tachycardia, decreased JVP, ± hypotension)
- Polyuria, polydipsia, thirst

Severe Hyperglycemia
(fasting blood glucose >22.5 mmol/L)
IDDM
- Musty odor on breath (ketone breath)
- Kussmaul's breathing (deep, pauseless respirations seen when pH is <7.2)
- Volume depletion (tachycardia, decreased JVP, ± hypotension)
- Anorexia, nausea, vomiting, abdominal pain (may mimic a surgical abdomen)
- Ileus, gastric dilatation
- Hyporeflexia, hypotonia, delirium, coma

NIDDM
- Polyuria, polydipsia
- Volume depletion
- Confusion, coma

Management

Many hyperglycemic patients will require SC or IV administration of insulin. Bovine, porcine, and human insulins are available, and each has different antigenicities. Bovine insulin is the most immunogenic, and human insulin is the least. Human insulin is associated with fewer adverse reactions (e.g., insulin allergy, antibody-mediated insulin resistance, lipoatrophy) and should be considered especially when treatment is intermittent. If the patient is already receiving bovine or porcine insulin without complications, it is fine to make dosage adjustments with the same preparation the patient is receiving.

Assess the Severity.   The severity of the situation should be determined according to the blood glucose level and the patient's symptoms (Table 32–1).

Mild, Asymptomatic Hyperglycemia.   This condition does not require urgent treatment. Order the following.
1. Fasting blood glucose in the morning: A fasting blood glucose of >7.8 mmol/L on more than one occasion confirms the diagnosis of diabetes mellitus. Make sure the patient is not receiving glucose-containing IV solutions that will make these results invalid. In addition, the diagnosis of diabetes mellitus cannot be made in the setting of stress (e.g., infection, surgery, severe illness). Any one of the following criteria is diagnostic for diabetes mellitus:
   a. Fasting blood sugar >7.8 mmol/L × 2 (venous plasma)
   b. Random blood sugar >11.1 mmol/L × 2 (venous plasma)
   c. A GTT with fasting blood glucose <7.8 mmol/L and a 2 hour PC ≥11.1 mmol/L (venous plasma)
2. Chemstrip or Glucometer readings before meals and at bedtime.

Table 32–1 □ BLOOD GLUCOSE LEVELS

	Fasting or AC Blood Glucose (mmol/L)	2 Hour PC Blood Glucose (mmol/L)
Normal range	3.5–6.0	<11.0
Mild hyperglycemia	6.1–11.0	11.1–16.5
Moderate hyperglycemia	11.1–22.5	16.6–27.5
Severe hyperglycemia	>22.5	>27.5

If the readings are >25 or <2.8 mmol/L, a stat blood glucose sample should be drawn and a physician informed.

Moderate Hyperglycemia. This condition may require an adjustment of the insulin being given. Examine the diabetic record for the past 3 days.

A sample adjustment in insulin dosage is given in Table 32–2. The Chemstrip or Glucometer readings are in millimoles per liter, and the SC insulin dose given is indicated in parentheses (e.g., 20/10 indicates that 20 units of NPH and 10 units of regular insulin have been given).

You have been called at night on August 3 because of a Chemstrip/Glucometer reading of 25 mmol/L. Order the following:

1. Stat random blood glucose to confirm the Chemstrip or Glucometer reading.
2. Regular insulin 5 to 10 units SC now. The main consideration now is not to devise a schedule that will achieve perfect blood glucose control for the rest of the patient's hospital stay. Short-term control of blood glucose levels has not been shown to decrease complications in the diabetic. When the blood glucose level is elevated at night, your aim is to prevent the development of ketoacidosis in the patient with IDDM or of the hyperosmolar state in the patient with NIDDM without producing symptomatic hypoglycemia with your treatment.
3. Determining the reason for poor control of blood glucose AC breakfast may aid in an ongoing adjustment of the patient's insulin. This can be achieved by ordering an 0300 h Chemstrip or Glucometer reading. Hypoglycemia documented at 0300 h would suggest that AC breakfast hyperglycemia is due to hyperglycemic rebound (the Somogyi effect), which is correctly managed by reducing the AC supper NPH insulin dose. Hyperglycemia documented at 0300 h would suggest that AC breakfast hyperglycemia is due to inadequate insulin coverage overnight. This is correctly managed by increasing the AC supper NPH insulin dose.

Table 32–2 □ SAMPLE INSULIN DOSAGE ADJUSTMENT

	AC Breakfast (NPH/REG)	AC Lunch (NPH/REG)	AC Supper (NPH/REG)	QHS (NPH/REG)
August 1	16.7* (20/10)†	13.9 (0/0)	16.7 (10/10)	18.1 (0/0)
August 2	13.9 (20/10)	16.7 (0/4)	8.3 (10/10)	19.4 (0/0)
August 3	16.7 (20/10)	15.2 (0/0)	13.1 (10/10)	25.0 (0/0)

*Chemstrip or Glucometer reading given in mmol/L.
†Indicates 20 units of NPH and 10 units of regular insulin.

Severe Hyperglycemia.   This condition requires urgent treatment.

1. **IDDM—Diabetic Ketoacidosis.** This complication may be seen in the patient with poorly controlled IDDM. It is due to an absolute insulin deficit, resulting in impaired resynthesis of long-chain fatty acids from acetate, with subsequent conversion to the acidic ketone bodies (ketosis).

   a. *Correct volume depletion.* Give 500 ml NS IV as fast as possible, with further IV rates guided by reassessment of volume status. If the patient has a history of CHF, weight <50 kg, or is ≥80 years of age, NS should be given cautiously to avoid iatrogenic CHF.

   b. *Begin an insulin infusion.* Give 5 to 10 units of IV regular insulin as a single dose by direct slow injection, followed by an infusion rate based on close monitoring of Chemstrip or Glucometer readings. Start the insulin infusion at 0.1 U/kg/h in NS. Regular insulin can bind to the plastic IV tubing. To ensure accurate insulin delivery, 30 to 50 ml of the infusion solution should be run through the IV tubing and discarded before connecting the IV tubing to the patient. Discontinue the standing order for SC insulin or oral hypoglycemics before beginning the insulin infusion.

   Monitor blood sugar hourly by Chemstrip or Glucometer. When the blood sugar has fallen to 14 mmol/L, continue the insulin infusion but switch the delivery solution from NS to D5W. Continue the insulin infusion until the blood sugars remain stable at 8 to 10 mmol/L. As the blood sugar falls, the rate of insulin infusion should be slowed (e.g., 0.025–0.05 U/kg/h). The rate of fall of blood sugar should be approximately 2.0 mmol/L/h. When the sugars have stabilized at 8 to 10 mmol/L, restart SC insulin, remembering that the insulin infusion must be continued for 1 to 2 hours after the injection of SC insulin, or ketogenesis will be reactivated. Continue to monitor the bedside sugars every 4 hours, adding supplemental regular insulin to keep blood sugars between 8 and 10 mmol/L.

   c. *Monitor blood glucose, serum electrolytes, and ABGs.* Hyperglycemic patients can have metabolic acidemia and hypokalemia. As NS and insulin are administered, the acidemia is corrected, and the potassium shifts into the cells from the extracellular fluid. This can result in worsening of the hypokalemia. Order baseline ABGs, electrolytes, urea, creatinine, and glucose levels. Repeat the ABGs and potassium level in 2 hours and thereafter as required. When hypokalemia is first noted, add KCl to the IV NS, provided the patient is passing urine and has normal urea and creatinine levels. If the patient is in renal failure, caution should be

taken in adding any potassium to the IV, to avoid iatrogenic hyperkalemia.
   d. *Search for the precipitating cause.* Common precipitating factors include the following.
      (1) Infection
      (2) Inadequate insulin dosage
      (3) Dietary indiscretion
      (4) Pancreatitis
2. **NIDDM—Hyperosmolar, Hyperglycemic, Nonketotic State.** This condition may be seen in a patient with poorly controlled NIDDM. Typically, the patient is 50 to 70 years old. Many have no prior histories of diabetes mellitus. The precipitating event is often stroke, infection, pancreatitis, or drugs. The blood glucose level is often very high (e.g., >55 mmol/L), but significant ketosis is absent.
   a. *Correct volume depletion and water deficit.* The objective of fluid therapy in the nonketotic hyperosmolar state is to both correct the volume deficit and resolve the hyperosmolarity. These can be achieved by giving 500 ml of NS IV over 2 hours, with further IV rates guided by reassessment of volume status. Once the volume deficit is corrected using NS, remaining water deficits, as indicated by persistent hypernatremia or hyperglycemia, are best corrected using hypotonic IV solutions, such as ½ NS.
   b. *Begin an insulin infusion.* See previous discussion of treatment of diabetic ketoacidosis. Rehydration alone often produces a substantial fall in blood glucose through renal excretion. As a result, patients with the hyperosmolar, hyperglycemic, nonketotic state generally require less insulin than the patient with IDDM and ketoacidosis.
   c. *Monitor blood glucose level and serum electrolytes.* Order baseline electrolytes, urea, creatinine, and glucose levels. Repeat the blood glucose level and the electrolytes determinations in 2 hours and thereafter as required.
   d. *Search for the precipitating cause.*
      (1) Infection
      (2) Inadequate fluid intake
      (3) Other acute illnesses (MI, stroke)

■ HYPOGLYCEMIA

Causes

Patients with Documented Diabetes Mellitus
- Excess insulin or oral hypoglycemic administration
- Decreased caloric intake
- Missed meals or missed snacks
- Increased exercise

Patients Without Documented Diabetes Mellitus

- Surreptitious intake of insulin or oral hypoglycemics
- Insulinoma
- Supervised 72-hour fasting for the investigation of hypoglycemia
- Drugs (ethanol, pentamidine, disopyramide, MAO inhibitors)
- Hepatic failure
- Adrenal insufficiency

Manifestations

Adrenergic Response   (i.e., catecholamine release due to a rapid decrease in glucose level). Diaphoresis, palpitations, tremulousness, tachycardia, hunger, acral and perioral numbness, anxiety, combativeness, confusion, coma.

CNS Response   (slow response may develop over 1 to 3 days). Headaches, diplopia, bizarre behavior, focal neurological deficits, confusion, seizures, and coma.

Patients receiving oral hypoglycemics may not experience the adrenergic response. Confusion and coma may develop solely because of hypoglycemia.

Management

Assess the Severity.   Any symptomatic patient with suspected hypoglycemia requires treatment. Symptoms may be precipitated by either a rapid fall in blood glucose level or an absolute low level of blood glucose.

1. *Draw 1 ml of blood* to be sent for blood glucose testing to confirm the diagnosis. If the cause of hypoglycemia is not clear, draw 10 ml, and ask the laboratory to save an aliquot for possible later insulin and C peptide measurement. Insulin produced endogenously includes the C peptide fragment, in contrast to commercial preparations of insulin. A high insulin level associated with a high C peptide fragment and hypoglycemia suggests endogenous production of excess insulin (e.g., insulinoma), whereas a high insulin level associated with a low C peptide level and hypoglycemia suggests surrepitious or therapeutic administration of exogenous insulin.

2. In the cooperative awake patient, oral glucose in the form of sweetened fruit juice may be given. If the patient is unable to take oral fluids or is unconscious, D50W 50 ml IV should be given by direct, slow injection. If there is no IV access and the patient is unable to take oral fluids (e.g., unconscious), *glucagon* 0.5 to 1.0 mg SC or IM should be given. Following glucagon administration, vomiting may develop, and so the patient who is not fully conscious should be monitored carefully to prevent aspiration.

3. If ongoing hypoglycemia is anticipated or if the patient's symptoms were severe (e.g., seizure, coma), begin a maintenance IV of D5W or D10W at a rate of 100 ml/h. Ask the RN to reassess the patient in 1 hour. In addition, remeasure the blood glucose level in 2 to 4 hours to ensure that hypoglycemic relapse has not occurred. Hypoglycemia due to oral hypoglycemics may require repeated doses of D50W because of the slow metabolism and excretion of these drugs.

33

POTASSIUM DISORDERS

■ HYPERKALEMIA
Causes

Excessive Intake
- Potassium supplements (PO or IV)
- Salt substitutes
- High-dose IV therapy with potassium salts of penicillin
- Blood transfusions

Decreased Excretion
- Renal failure (acute or chronic)
- Potassium-sparing diuretics (spironolactone, triamterene, amiloride)
- Addison's disease, hypoaldosteronism
- Distal tubular dysfunction (i.e., type IV RTA)

Shift from Intracellular to Extracellular Fluid
- Acidemia (especially nonanion gap)
- Insulin deficiency
- Tissue destruction (hemolysis, crush injuries, rhabdomyolysis, extensive burns, tumor lysis)
- Drugs (succinylcholine, digoxin, arginine, beta blockers)
- Hyperkalemic periodic paralysis

Factitious
- Prolonged tourniquet placement for venipuncture
- Blood sample hemolysis
- Leukocytosis
- Thrombocytosis

Manifestations

Cardiac
- Fatal ventricular dysrhythmias

The progressive ECG changes seen in hyperkalemia are peaked T waves → depressed ST segments → decreased amplitude of R waves → prolonged PR interval → small or absent P waves → wide QRS complexes → sine wave pattern (Fig. 33–1).

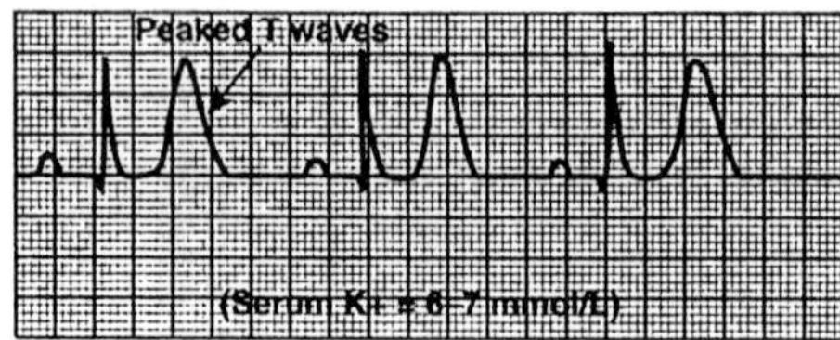

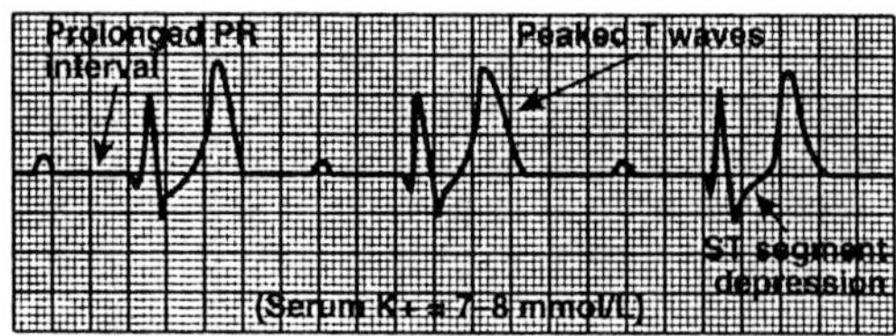

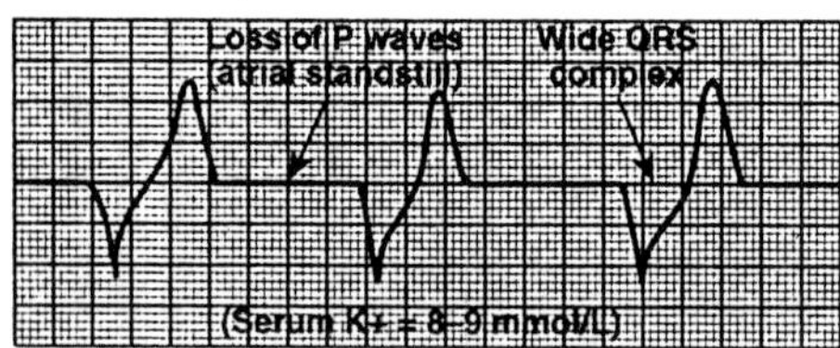

Figure 33–1 □ Progressive electrocardiographic manifestations of hyperkalemia.

Neuromuscular
- Weakness, often beginning in the lower extremities
- Paresthesias
- Depressed tendon reflexes

Management

ECG.   Fatal ventricular dysrhythmias can occur at any time during treatment; hence, continuous ECG monitoring is required if the potassium level is above 6.5 mmol/L.

Assess the Severity.   The severity of the situation should be determined according to the serum potassium concentration, the ECG findings, and whether or not the underlying cause is immediately remediable.

IF SEVERE
- Serum K^+ >8.0 mmol/L
- ECG findings more advanced than peaked T waves alone
- Cause not immediately remediable
1. Notify your resident.
2. Place the patient on continuous ECG monitoring.
3. Correct contributing factors (acidemia, hypovolemia).
4. Give one or more of the following:
   a. *Calcium gluconate* 5 to 10 ml of a 10% solution given IV over 2 minutes. This will temporarily antagonize the cardiac and neuromuscular effects of hyperkalemia. Calcium gluconate's onset is immediate, and its effect lasts 1 hour. It will not, however, reduce the serum concentration of potassium. *Caution:* Administration of calcium to the patient on digoxin may precipitate ventricular dysrhythmias due to the combined effects of digoxin and calcium.
   b. *D50W* 50 ml IV followed by *regular insulin* 5 to 10 units IV will shift potassium from the ECF to the ICF. Its effect is immediate and lasts 1 to 2 hours.
   c. *Sodium bicarbonate* 1 amp (44.6 mmol) IV will shift potassium from the ECF to the ICF. Its effect is immediate and lasts 1 to 2 hours.
   d. Give a *glucose-insulin-HCO$_3$ cocktail:* D10W 1000 ml with three ampules of NaHCO$_3$ and 20 units of regular insulin at 75 ml/h until more definitive measures are taken.
   e. *Sodium polystyrene sulfonate* (Kayexalate) 15 to 30 g (4–8 teaspoonfuls) in 50 to 100 ml of 20% sorbitol PO q3–4h or 50 g in 200 ml 20% sorbitol or D20W PR by retention enema for 30 to 60 minutes q4h. This is the only drug treatment that actually will remove potassium from the total body pool. Watch carefully for evidence of volume overload, as this resin works by exchanging Na for K^+.
5. *Hemodialysis* should be considered on an urgent basis if the aforementioned measures have failed or if the patient is in acute or chronic oliguric renal failure. *Peritoneal dialysis* may be preferable in the patient who is hemodynamically unstable.
6. Monitor the serum potassium concentration every 1 to 2 hours until it is below 6.5 mmol/L.

IF MODERATE
- Serum K^+ between 6.5 and 8.0 mmol/L
- ECG findings show peaked T waves only
- Cause is not progressive
1. Place the patient on continuous ECG monitoring.
2. Correct contributing factors (acidemia, hypovolemia).
3. Give one or more of the following in the dosages previously outlined.

    a. $NaHCO_3$
    b. Glucose and insulin
    c. Sodium polystyrene sulfonate
4. Monitor the serum potassium concentration every 1 to 2 hours until it is below 6.5 mmol/L.

IF MILD

- Serum K^+ <6.5 mmol/L
- ECG findings show peaked T waves only
- Cause is not progressive

1. Correct contributing factors (acidemia, hypovolemia).
2. Remeasure the serum potassium concentration 4 to 6 hours later, depending on the cause.

■ HYPOKALEMIA

Causes

Renal Losses (Urine K^+ >20 mmol/day)

- Diuretics, osmotic diuresis
- Antibiotics (carbenicillin, ticarcillin, nafcillin, amphotericin, aminoglycosides)
- RTA (classic type I)
- Hyperaldosteronism
- Glucocorticoid excess
- Magnesium deficiency
- Chronic metabolic alkalosis
- Bartter's syndrome
- Fanconi's syndrome
- Ureterosigmoidostomy
- Vomiting, NG suction. (Hydrogen ions are lost with vomiting and NG suction, inducing alkalosis that results in renal potassium wasting.)

Extrarenal Losses (Urine K^+ <20 mmol/day)

- Diarrhea
- Intestinal fistula

Inadequate Intake
Over 1 to 2 weeks

Shift from Extracellular to Intracellular Space

- Acute alkalosis
- Insulin therapy
- Vitamin B_{12} therapy
- Hypokalemic periodic paralysis
- Salbutamol
- Lithium

Manifestations

Cardiac
- Premature atrial contractions
- Premature ventricular contractions
- Digoxin toxicity
- ECG changes (Fig. 33–2)
  - T wave flattening
  - U waves
  - ST segment depression

Neuromuscular
- Weakness
- Depressed deep tendon reflexes
- Paresthesias
- Ileus

Miscellaneous
- Nephrogenic diabetes insipidus
- Metabolic alkalosis
- Worsening of hepatic encephalopathy

Management

If possible, correct the underlying cause.

Assess the Severity. The severity of the situation should be determined according to the serum potassium concentration, the ECG findings, and the clinical setting in which hypokalemia is occurring.

IF SEVERE
- Serum K^+ <3.0 mmol/L with PVCs in the setting of myocardial ischemia or with digoxin toxicity
  1. Notify your resident.
  2. Place the patient on continuous ECG monitoring.
  3. IV replacement therapy may be required, i.e., 10 mmol KCl

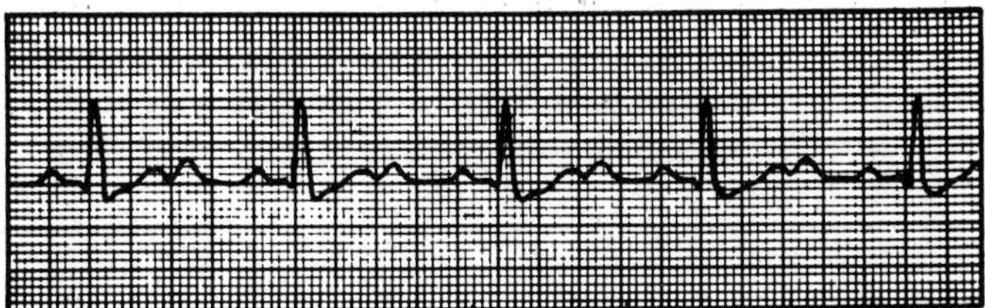

Figure 33–2 □ Electrocardiographic manifestations of hypokalemia.

in 100 ml D5W given IV over 1 hour. Repeat once or twice as necessary. KCl in small volumes should be given through central IV lines, since these high concentrations of potassium are sclerosing to peripheral veins. Further replacement can be achieved with maintenance therapy containing up to 40 to 60 mmol KCl/L of IV fluid at a maximum rate of 20 mmol/h. Potassium can also be given by administration of the liquid salt by NG tube or by oral supplementation.

4. Recheck serum potassium concentration after each 20 to 30 mmol IV KCl has been given.

IF MODERATE

- Serum K^+ ≤3.0 mmol/L with PACs but no (or infrequent) PVCs and no digoxin toxicity

1. Notify your resident.
2. Oral potassium supplementation is usually adequate, e.g., Slow-K = 8 mmol KCl per tablet, Kay Ciel Elixir = 20 mmol/15 ml, and K-Lyte = 25 mmol/packet.
3. IV replacement therapy in this situation should be reserved for patients with marked hypokalemia or patients who are unable to take oral supplements (see previous recommendations).
4. Recheck serum potassium concentration in the morning or sooner if clinically indicated.

IF MILD

- Serum K^+ between 3.1 and 3.5 mmol/L, no (or infrequent) PVCs, and patient asymptomatic

1. Oral supplementation usually is adequate (see previous recommendations).
2. Recheck serum potassium concentration in the morning or sooner if clinically indicated.

REMEMBER

1. Serious hyperkalemia has occurred as a result of potassium supplementation. Hence, serum potassium levels should be closely monitored during treatment. Be particularly cautious in patients with renal impairment.
2. Hypokalemia and hypocalcemia may coexist. Correction of hypokalemia without accompanying correction of hypocalcemia may increase the risk of ventricular dysrhythmias.
3. Hypokalemia and hypomagnesemia may coexist. Correction of hypokalemia may be unsuccessful unless hypomagnesemia is corrected simultaneously.

□ **34** □

SODIUM DISORDERS

■ HYPERNATREMIA
Causes
Inadequate Intake of Water
- Coma
- Hypothalamic dysfunction

Excessive Water Losses
- Renal Losses
  - Diabetes insipidus (nephrogenic or pituitary)
  - Osmotic diuresis (hyperglycemia, mannitol administration, urea)
- Extrarenal Losses
  - Vomiting, NG suction
  - Diarrhea
  - Sweating (e.g., febrile illnesses)
  - Insensible losses (e.g., tachypnea)

Excessive Sodium Gain
- Iatrogenic (excessive sodium administration)
- Primary hyperaldosteronism

Manifestations
Hypernatremia most often results from ECF volume depletion due to hypotonic fluid loss (e.g., vomiting, diarrhea, sweating, osmotic diuresis). Symptoms are dependent on the absolute increase in serum osmolality as well as the rate at which it develops. The manifestations of hypernatremia are due to acute brain cell shrinkage from an outward shift of intracellular water, which occurs as a result of increased ECF osmolality. They range from confusion and muscle irritability to seizures, respiratory paralysis, and death.

Management
1. **Assess the severity.** The severity of the situation should be determined according to the symptomatic state of the patient, the serum sodium concentration, the serum osmolality, and the ECF volume.
   a. Osmolality can be measured in the laboratory. However, sufficient information may be available to permit its cal-

culation from knowledge of the major osmotically active substances in the ECF.

$$\text{Osmolality (mmol/kg)} = 2\,\text{Na (mmol/L)} + \text{urea (mmol/L)} + \text{glucose (mmol/L)}$$

The normal range is 281 to 297 mmol/kg.

  b. Most patients with hypernatremia have an accompanying extracellular volume deficit that can compromise perfusion of vital organs. Assess the volume status of the patient (see Chapter 3).
  c. Most patients with hypernatremia have relatively few symptoms and are not at immediate risk of dying!
2. If possible, correct the cause, which is usually evident from the history and physical findings.
3. Correct volume and water deficits. The choice of fluid is dependent on the severity of the extracellular volume deficit.
  a. In patients who are volume depleted, hypernatremia can be corrected by giving IV NS until the patient is hemodynamically stable and then changing to ½ NS or D5W to correct the remaining water deficit.
  b. In patients who are not volume depleted, ½ NS or D5W can be used to correct the water deficit.
An estimation of the volume of water required can be calculated, remembering that the deficit is in *total body water*, which is approximately 60% of body weight.

$$\text{Water deficit} = \frac{[\text{Serum Na (observed)} - \text{serum Na (normal)}] \times 0.6\,\text{Wt (kg)}}{\text{Serum Na (normal)}}$$

EXAMPLE. A 65-year-old man is admitted to the hospital after being found in his apartment 2 days after falling and fracturing his hip. He is moderately volume depleted and has a serum sodium value of 156 mmol/L. His weight is 70 kg. To calculate the volume of water required to correct the serum sodium

$$\text{Free water deficit} = \frac{[156\,\text{mmol/L} - 140\,\text{mmol/L}] \times 0.6\,(70\,\text{L})}{140\,\text{mmol/L}} = 4.8\,\text{L}$$

Remember to correct the osmolality abnormality at a rate similar to the rate at which it developed. Biological systems are more responsive to rates of change than to absolute amounts of change. It is safest to correct half the deficit and then reevaluate. More rapid corrections than 1 to 2 mmol/L in serum sodium can lead to brain swelling, resulting in the development of confusion, seizures, or coma.

  c. In the occasional patient with hypernatremia who is volume overloaded, the hypernatremia can be corrected by initiating a diuresis using *furosemide* (Lasix) 20 to 40 mg IV and repeating at intervals of 2 to 4 hours as necessary. Once the extracellular volume has returned to normal, if the serum sodium level is still elevated, diuresis should be continued, with urinary volume losses replaced with D5W until the serum Na repeat level is again in the normal range.

■ HYPONATREMIA

Causes

1. Hyponatremia with Decreased ECF Volume
   a. Renal loss of sodium
      (1) Diuretic excess
      (2) Na-losing nephritis
      (3) Diuretic phase of acute tubular necrosis
      (4) Bartter's syndrome
      (5) Hypoaldosteronism
   b. Extrarenal losses of sodium
      (1) Vomiting, NG suction
      (2) Diarrhea
      (3) Sweating
      (4) Burns
      (5) Pancreatitis
2. Hyponatremia with ECF Volume Excess and Edema
   a. Renal failure
   b. Nephrotic syndrome
   c. CHF
   d. Cirrhosis of the liver
3. Hyponatremia with Normal Extracellular Fluid Volume
   a. SIADH
      (1) Tumors
         (a) Small cell carcinoma of the lung
         (b) Pancreatic carcinoma
         (c) Duodenal adenocarcinoma
      (2) CNS Disorders
         (a) Brain tumors
         (b) Brain trauma
         (c) Meningitis
         (d) Encephalitis
      (3) Pulmonary Disorders
         (a) Tuberculosis
         (b) Pneumonia
      (4) Drugs
         (a) Chlorpropamide
         (b) Clofibrate
         (c) Cyclophosphamide
         (d) Vincristine
         (e) Carbamazepine

        (f) Narcotics
        (g) Tricyclic antidepressants
        (h) Idiopathic
  b. Pseudohyponatremia
    (1) Hyponatremia with Normal Serum Osmolality
        (a) Hyperlipidemia
        (b) Hyperproteinemia
    (2) Hyponatremia with Increased Serum Osmolality
        (a) Excess urea
        (b) Hyperglycemia
        (c) Mannitol
        (d) Ethanol
        (e) Methanol
        (f) Ethylene glycol
        (g) Isopropyl alcohol
  c. Endocrine Disorders
    (1) Hypothyroidism
    (2) Addison's disease

Manifestations

Manifestations of hyponatremia depend on the absolute decrease in the serum osmolality, the rate of development of hyponatremia, and the volume status of the patient. When associated with a decreased serum osmolality, hyponatremia may cause the following.

- Confusion
- Lethargy
- Weakness
- Nausea and vomiting
- Seizures
- Coma

When hyponatremia develops gradually, a patient may tolerate a serum sodium concentration of less than 110 mmol/L with only moderate confusion or lethargy. However, a patient in whom the serum sodium concentration decreases rapidly from 140 to 115 mmol/L may experience a seizure.

Management

1. **Assess the severity.** The severity of the situation should be determined according to the symptomatic state of the patient, the serum sodium concentration, the serum osmolality, and the ECF.

    Remember that when attempting to correct disorders manifested by hyponatremia, brain cells try to maintain their volume in dilutional states by losing solutes (e.g., potassium). If the serum sodium level is corrected too rapidly (i.e., to levels greater than 120 to 125 mmol/L) the serum may become hypertonic relative to brain cells, resulting in an outward shift of water, with resultant CNS damage due to acute brain shrinkage.

2. If possible, correct the cause of the hyponatremia. Urinary electrolyte determination may be helpful in identifying the primary cause of hyponatremia when one or more possible etiologies exist. The renal response to salt and water loss differs depending on the cause of hyponatremia. When extrarenal losses of sodium and water occur through the skin (e.g., sweating, burns) or due to third-spacing (e.g., pancreatitis), the renal response is to conserve sodium (urine Na <20 mmol/L) and to conserve water through secretion of ADH (high urine osmolality). However, if volume loss is due to vomiting or NG suction, primarily HCl is lost from gastric secretions. The kidneys generate and excrete *Na*HCO$_3$ to maintain acid-base balance, resulting in a urine with a normal (>20 mmol/L) *Na* but a low (<20 mmol/L) Cl. If volume loss is due to diarrhea, primarily NaHCO$_3$ is lost in the stools. The kidneys generate and excrete NH$_4$*Cl* to maintain acid-base balance, resulting in a urine that is low in Na but not in *Cl*.

   Hyponatremia with ECF excess and edema may be accompanied by a low (<20 mmol/L) urinary Na (e.g., nephrotic syndrome, CHF, cirrhosis of the liver) or a normal urinary Na (renal failure).

3. Assess the volume status of the patient (see Chapter 3).

   a. If the patient is *volume depleted*, correct the ECF volume using NS. Aim for a JVP of 2 to 3 cm H$_2$O above the sternal angle. In this case, the amount of sodium required to improve the serum sodium concentration can be calculated using the following formula.

   $$\text{mmol Na} = [\text{serum Na(desired)} - \text{serum Na(observed)}] \times \text{TBW}$$

   where

   $$\text{TBW} = 0.6 \times \text{Wt in kg.}$$

   Remember that biological systems are more responsive to rates of change than to absolute amounts of change. Make corrections at a rate similar to the rate at which the abnormality developed. It is safest to correct half the deficit and reassess the situation.

   EXAMPLE. For a 70 kg man in whom you want to raise the serum sodium level from 120 to 135 mmol/L, the amount of Na required
   = (135 mmol/L − 120 mmol/L)(0.6 × 70 L)
   = (15 mmol/L)(42 L)
   = 630 mmol Na
   Since 1 L of NS contains 154 mmol of Na, you will require approximately 4 L of NS to raise the patient's serum level to 135 mmol/L.

b. If the patient has *extracellular volume excess and edema*, treat the volume excess and hyponatremia with water restriction and diuretics. Since most of these states are accompanied by secondary hyperaldosteronism, *spironolactone* is a reasonable choice of diuretic, as long as the patient is not hyperkalemic. Remember that the diuretic effect of spironolactone may be delayed for 3 to 4 days. The dose can range from 25 to 200 mg daily in adults and may be given once daily or in divided doses.

c. If the patient has a normal ECF volume, SIADH, pseudohyponatremia, or endocrine disorders should be considered.

■ *SIADH*

The *diagnosis* of SIADH requires that quite stringent criteria be met.

1. Hyponatremia with serum hypoosmolality
2. Urine that is less than maximally dilute when compared with serum osmolality (i.e., a simultaneous urine osmolality that is greater than the serum osmolality)
3. Inappropriately large amounts of urine Na (U_{Na} >20 mmol/L)
4. Normal renal function
5. Normal thyroid function
6. Normal adrenal function
7. Patient not on diuretics

Management

SIADH should be treated by

1. Correcting the underlying cause or contributory factors (e.g., drugs), if present.
2. Water restriction, usually to less than insensible losses (e.g., 500–1000 ml/day).
3. In addition to the first two measures, patients with severe symptomatic hyponatremia (serum Na of <115 mmol/L) may benefit from furosemide-induced diuresis, with hourly replacement of urinary sodium and potassium losses using NS. Very rarely, 3% saline will be required.

   Too rapid correction of hyponatremia can result in central pontine myelinolysis and other undesirable side effects. Correct the serum sodium level *slowly*. Once the serum sodium level is greater than 120 to 125 mmol/L, many of the symptoms of hyponatremia will begin to lessen.
4. *Demeclocycline* 300 to 600 mg PO BID occasionally is useful in patients with chronic symptomatic SIADH in whom water restriction has been unsuccessful.

■ *Pseudohyponatremia*

The diagnosis of pseudohyponatremia can be made by
1. Demonstrating a normal serum osmolality in the presence of hyperlipidemia or hyperproteinemia
2. Demonstrating a significant (>10 mmol/kg) osmolar gap, indicating the presence of additional osmotically active solutes, which can falsely lower the serum sodium level. This can be done by first having the laboratory *measure* serum osmolality. You should then *calculate* serum osmolality using the following formula.

$$\text{Serum osmolality (mmol/kg)} = 2\,\text{Na (mmol/L)} + \text{glucose (mmol/L)} + \text{urea (mmol/L)}$$

If the *measured* serum osmolality is more than 10 mmol/kg greater than the *calculated* serum osmolality, the hyponatremia is at least partially due to the presence of osmotically active solutes, such as excess lipids or plasma proteins.

Management

Treatment of pseudohyponatremia is restricted to correction of the underlying cause.

■ *Hyperglycemia*

In cases of hyperglycemia, the true serum sodium concentration can be estimated by the following formula.

$$\frac{(\text{Observed glucose} - \text{normal glucose})(1.4)}{\text{Normal glucose}} + \text{serum Na(observed)}$$

The factor 1.4 is an arithmetic approximation to account for the shift of water that follows glucose into the extracellular compartment, thereby diluting sodium.

EXAMPLE. A 35-year-old woman in diabetic ketoacidosis is admitted with the following laboratory results.
- Glucose = 83 mmol/L
- Sodium = 127 mmol/L
- Urea = 25 mmol/L
- Creatinine = 274 mmol/L

The true serum Na, where normal glucose is taken as 5 mmol/L,

$$= \frac{(83\ \text{mmol/L} - 5\ \text{mmol/L})(1.4)}{5} + 127\ \text{mmol/L}$$

$$= 22\ \text{mmol/L} + 127\ \text{mmol/L}$$

$$= 149\ \text{mmol/L}$$

■ *Endocrine Disorders*

Hypothyroidism and *Addison's disease* can be diagnosed by their typical clinical features in association with confirmatory laboratory studies. Hyponatremia in either of these two conditions responds to treatment of the underlying endocrine disorder.

APPENDIX

■ BLOOD PRODUCTS

The maximum time over which blood products can be administered is 4 hours for 1 unit because of the danger of bacterial infection and RBC hemolysis. For the same reasons, if the flow is interrupted for more than 30 minutes, the unit must be discarded.

PACKED RED BLOOD CELLS

- Volume: 300 ± 25 ml
- Maximum administration time: 4 hours
- Rate of infusion: Dependent on patient's clinical condition
- Administration: Standard blood set for each unit hung or Y-type set if blood is to be reconstituted
- Indications: Active bleeding with loss of ≥15% of total blood volume; anemia that is adversely influencing another medical disorder (e.g., unstable angina); symptomatic chronic anemia unrelated to nutritional deficiency
- Outcome measurement: Hb level within 24 hours

DELEUKOCYTED RBCs

- Volume: 300 ± 25 ml
- Maximum administration time: 4 hours
- Rate of infusion: Dependent on the patient's clinical condition
- Administration: Standard blood set for each unit hung plus a filter (filter not required if RBCs are washed)
- Indications: Clinically significant transfusion reactions; to reduce sensitization to histocompatibility antigens

FROZEN RBCs (DEGLYCEROLIZED)

- Volume: Approximately 200 ml
- Maximum administration time: 4 hours
- Rate of infusion: Dependent on the patient's clinical condition
- Administration: Standard blood set for each unit hung
- Indications: Storing of rare blood groups and autotransfusion
- *Note:* Use only in special situations

PLASMA

- Volume: Approximately 200 ml
- Maximum administration time: 4 hours
- Rate of infusion: Dependent on patient's clinical condition
- Administration: Standard blood set
- Indications: Plasma is indicated as a source of coagulation factors. *Frozen plasma* is frozen within 24 hours of collection and contains higher levels of labile coagulation factors (V and VIII). Nonlabile factors are well maintained in both frozen and *stored (banked) plasma.* Plasma may be used for

- Significant hemorrhage due to a deficiency of coagulation factors
- Immediate hemostasis in a patient on warfarin
- A patient with severe liver disease or massive transfusion (whole blood volume replaced within 24 hours) with abnormal clotting tests and active bleeding
- TTP
- Prophylaxis before an invasive procedure associated with a significant bleeding risk
- Outcome measurement: PT or aPTT or both within 4 hours of transfusion

PLATELETS

- Volume: Approximately 50 ml
- Rate of infusion: As rapidly as is tolerated by the patient
- Administration: Blood components recipient set
- Indications: The therapeutic aim of platelet transfusions is to improve hemostasis. Their use should be considered in the following situations.
  - Patients with platelet counts of less than 20 g/L on the basis of decreased platelet production
  - Patients with consumptive thrombocytopenia (e.g., immune thrombocytopenia, DIC) only when there is significant bleeding
  - Patients with significant platelet dysfunction
- Outcome measurement: Platelet count 1 hour posttransfusion
- *Note:* Platelet transfusion reactions are common. In patients with a history of reactions, the use of acetaminophen 650 mg PO and diphenhydramine (Benadryl) 50 mg IV may prevent reactions. Narcotics (morphine 5–10 mg IV) or steroids (hydrocortisone 100 mg IV) also may be helpful. If these measures fail, deleukocyted platelets are recommended.
  In patients who are unresponsive to random donor platelets (defined by less than a 5 g/L increment in platelets 1 hour posttransfusion on two successive transfusions), platelets collected from a single donor by apheresis should be considered.

CRYOPRECIPITATE

- Volume: 5 to 10 ml
- Rate of infusion: As rapidly as possible
- Administration: Blood component recipient set
- Indications: Cryoprecipitate contains significant amounts of factor VIII (100 units per unit of cryoprecipitate), fibrinogen (250 mg per unit), and von Willebrand's factor. It is, therefore, useful in the treatment of mild hemophilia A and von Willebrand's disease and in the repletion of fibrinogen (e.g., DIC, dilutional coagulopathy). The dose is dependent on body mass, the indication for use, and the severity of the preexisting deficiency.

BLOOD TUBES

Lavender Top (EDTA)
CBC and differential   Sickle cell
Reticulocyte count   Malaria stain
Direct Coombs' test   ACTH
G-6-PD

Red/Gray ("Tiger Top")
SMAC (glucose)*   C3, C4, cryo-
                     globulins
Cardiac enzymes   Osmolality
Liver enzymes   Pregnancy test
Drug concentrations (alcohol, digoxin,
   gentamicin, and so forth)
C peptide/insulin
Protein electrophoresis

Red Top
Crossmatch   RA latex
Haptoglobin   ANA
TCA concentrations

Green Top
Lactate*   Ammonia*

Blue Top (Citrate)
PT, aPTT   Fibrinogen
Circulating anticoagulants
Coagulation factor assays

Blue Top (for FDP only)
Fibrin degradation products

*These specimens must be delivered to the laboratory immediately or else put on ice for transportation.

- Outcome measurement: Factor VIII level and aPTT (hemophilia A); von Willebrand's factor antigen level, bleeding time, or both (von Willebrand's disease); fibrinogen level (DIC, dilutional coagulopathy)—within 4 hours of transfusion

FACTOR VIII CONCENTRATE

- Lyophilized, fractionated plasma product
- Specific activity and storage conditions stated on label
- Must be reconstituted before use
- Indications: Moderate to severe factor VIII deficiency and low titer of factor VIII inhibitors
- *Note:* Not for use in von Willebrand's disease. Consult with hematologist before administration.

FACTOR IX COMPLEX

- Lyophilized, fractionated plasma product
- Factor IX content and storage conditions stated on labels
- Must be reconstituted before use
- Indications: Factor IX deficiency. Consult with hematologist before administration

NORMAL SERUM ALBUMIN

- Concentrates of 25% in vials of 100 ml and 5% in vials of 250 and 500 ml
- Sodium content approximately 145 mmol/L
- Indications: Hypoproteinemia with peripheral edema (give 25%); volume depletion where IV NS is contraindicated (give 5%); *not indicated* in the asymptomatic hypoproteinemic patient

■ READING ECGS
RATE

Multiply the number of QRS complexes in a 6-second period (30 large squares) (between the two large dots) by 10 = beats/min (Fig. A–1).

- Normal = 60 to 100 beats/min
- Tachycardia = >100 beats/min
- Bradycardia = <60 beats/min

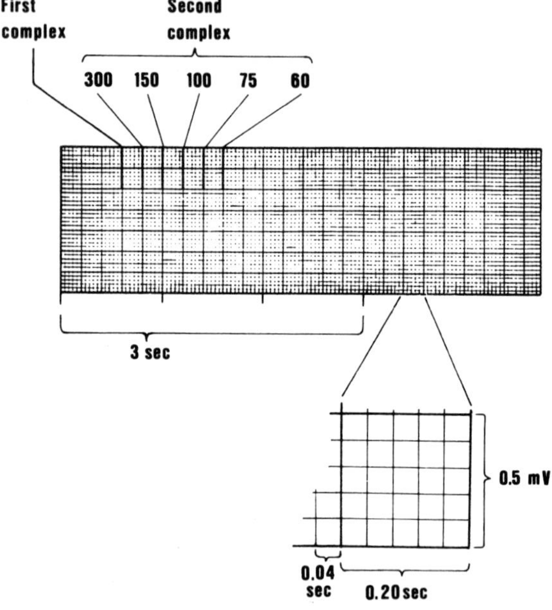

Figure A–1 □ Reading ECGs. Rate.

RHYTHM

Is the rhythm regular?

Is there a P wave preceding every QRS complex? Is there a QRS complex following every P wave?

1. Yes = sinus rhythm.
2. No P waves with irregular rhythm = atrial fibrillation.
3. No P waves with regular rhythm = junctional rhythm. Look for retrograde P waves in all leads.

AXIS

See Figure A–2.

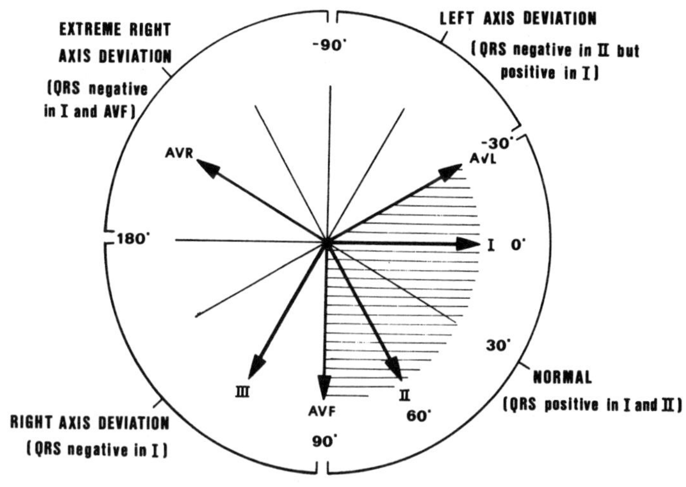

Figure A–2 □ Axis.

P WAVE CONFIGURATION

Normal P wave. Look at all leads (Fig. A–3A).

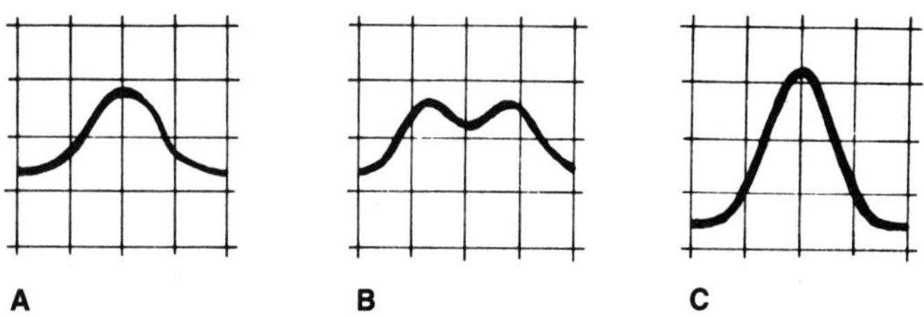

Figure A–3 □ Reading ECGs. P wave configuration in lead II. **A.** Normal P wave. **B.** Left atrial enlargement. **C.** Right atrial enlargement.

Left Atrial Enlargement (Fig. A–3B)

- Duration: 120 msec (three small squares in lead II) Often notched = P mitrale.
- Amplitude: Negative terminal P wave in lead V_1 >1 mm in depth *and* >40 msec (one small square).

Right Atrial Enlargement (Fig. A–3C)

- Amplitude: 2.5 mm in leads II, III, or aVF (i.e., tall peaked P wave of P pulmonale); 1.5 mm in the initial positive deflection of the P wave in lead V_1 or V_2.

QRS CONFIGURATION
Left Ventricular Hypertrophy

1. Increased QRS voltage (S in V_1 or V_2 plus R in V_5 >35 mm or R in aVL $\geq$11 mm)
2. Left atrial enlargement
3. ST segment depression and negative T wave in left lateral leads

Right Ventricular Hypertrophy

1. R >S in V_1
2. Right axis deviation (> + 90°)
3. ST segment depression and negative T wave in right precordial leads

CONDUCTION ABNORMALITIES
First Degree Block

- PR interval $\geq$0.20 second ($\geq$1 large square)

Second Degree Block

Occasional absence of QRS and T after a P of sinus origin.

1. Type I (Wenckebach's): Progressive prolongation of the PR interval before the missed QRS complex (Fig. 15–22)
2. Type II: Absence of progressive prolongation of the PR interval before the missed QRS complex (Fig. 15–23)

Third Degree Block

Absence of any relationship between P waves of sinus origin and QRS complexes (Fig. 15–25)

Left Anterior Hemiblock

Left axis deviation, Q in I and aVL; a small R in III, in the absence of left ventricular hypertrophy.

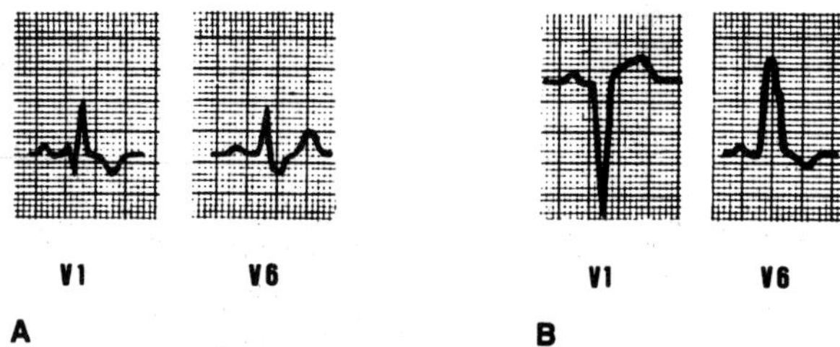

Figure A–4 □ Reading ECGs. QRS configuration. **A.** Complete right bundle branch block. **B.** Complete left bundle branch block.

Left Posterior Hemiblock

Right axis deviation, a small R in I and a small Q in III, in the absence of right ventricular hypertrophy.

Complete Right Bundle Branch Block

See Figure A–4A.

Complete Left Bundle Branch Block

See Figure A–4B.

Ventricular Preexcitation

1. PR interval <0.11 second with widened QRS (>0.12 second) due to a delta wave = Wolff-Parkinson-White syndrome.
2. PR interval <0.11 second with a normal QRS complex = Lown-Ganong-Levine syndrome.

MYOCARDIAL INFARCTION PATTERNS

Type of Infarct	Patterns of Changes (Q Waves, ST Elevation or Depression, T Wave Inversion)*
Inferior	Q in II, III, aVF
Inferoposterior	Q in II, III, aVF, and V_6
	R > S and positive T in V_1
Anteroseptal	V_1 to V_4
Anterolateral to posterolateral	V_1 to V_5; Q in I, aVL, and V_6
Posterior	R > S in V_1, positive T, and Q in V_6

*A significant Q wave is > 40 msec wide or > one-third of the QRS height. ST segment or T wave changes in the absence of significant Q waves may represent a non-Q wave infarct.

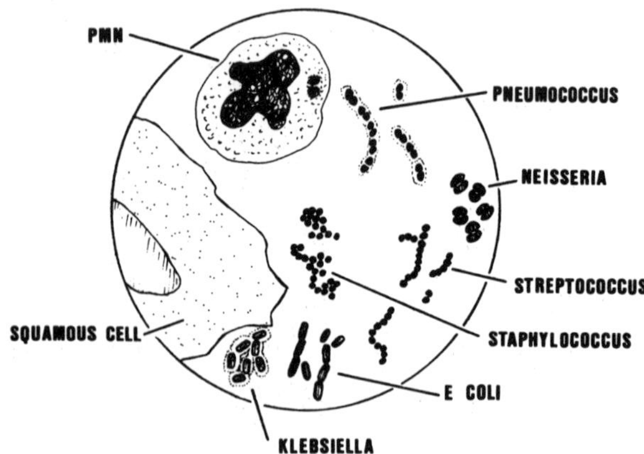

Figure A–5 □ Sputum Gram's stain. A useful sputum specimen for identification of the bacterial cause of pneumonia should have ≥25 PMNs and fewer than 10 squamous cells per low power field.

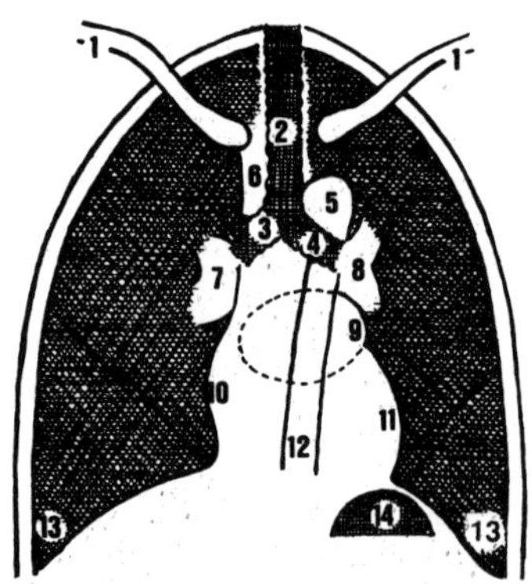

Figure A–6 □ Posteroanterior chest x-ray.

1. Clavicles
2. Trachea
3. Right mainstem bronchus
4. Left mainstem bronchus
5. Aortic knuckle
6. Superior vena cava
7. Right pulmonary artery
8. Left pulmonary artery
9. Left atrium
10. Right atrium
11. Left ventricle
12. Aortic stripe
13. Costophrenic angles
14. Gastric bubble

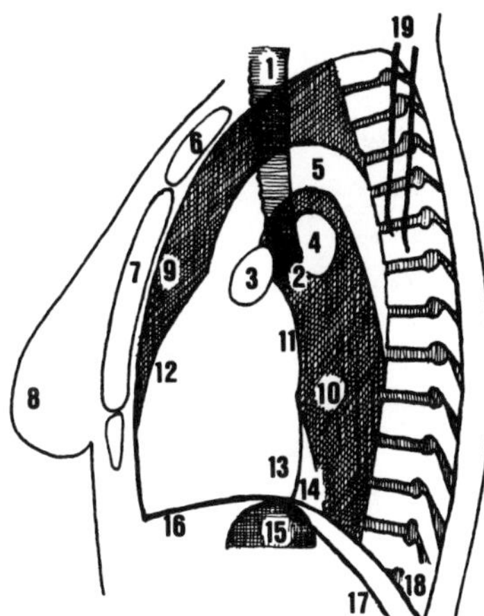

Figure A–7 □ Lateral chest x-ray.
1. Trachea
2. Left mainstem bronchus
3. Right pulmonary artery
4. Left pulmonary artery
5. Aortic arch
6. Manubrium
7. Sternum
8. Breast shadow
9. Retrosternal space
10. Retrocardiac space
11. Left atrium
12. Right ventricle
13. Left ventricle
14. Inferior vena cava
15. Gastric air bubble
16. Left hemidiaphragm
17. Right hemidiaphragm
18. Costophrenic angle
19. Scapular shadows

■ CARDIAC ARREST PROTOCOLS

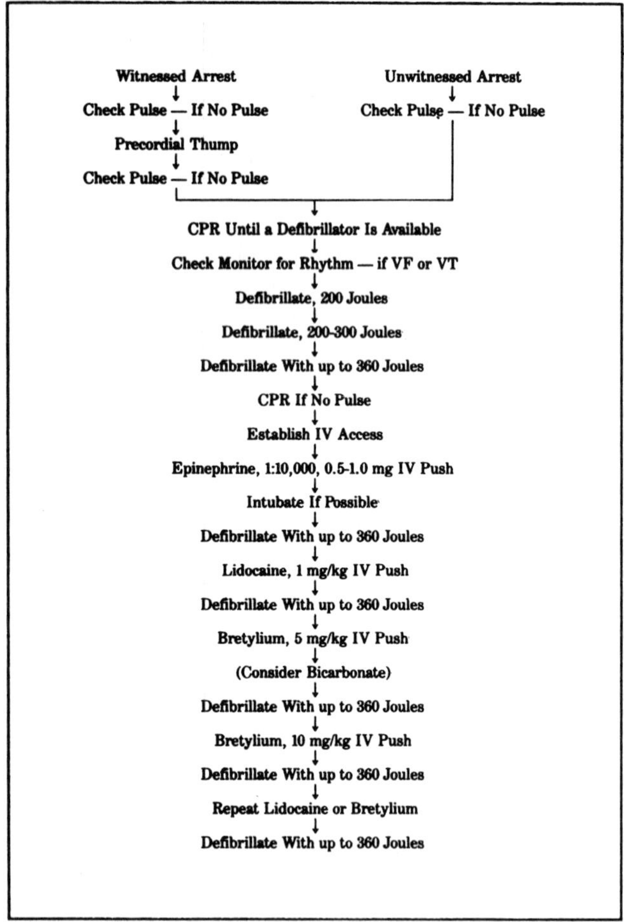

Treatment Algorithm for Ventricular Fibrillation (VF) and Pulseless Ventricular Tachycardia. The pulse and rhythm should be checked after each electric shock. If VF recurs after transient conversion, the previously successful energy level should be used for defibrillation. If intubation can be performed simultaneously with other interventions, the patient should be intubated as early in the sequence as possible. However, defibrillation and epinephrine are more important initially if the patient can be ventilated without intubation. Epinephrine (in the indicated doses) should be administered every 5 minutes. Lidocaine hydrochloride 0.5 mg/kg every 8 minutes for a total dose of 3 mg/kg is an acceptable alternative to bretylium tosylate 5 mg/kg or 10 mg/kg. If sodium bicarbonate is given, a dose of 1 mmol/L followed by 0.5 mg/kg every 10 minutes may be used. (Reproduced with permission. *JAMA*. American Heart Association.)

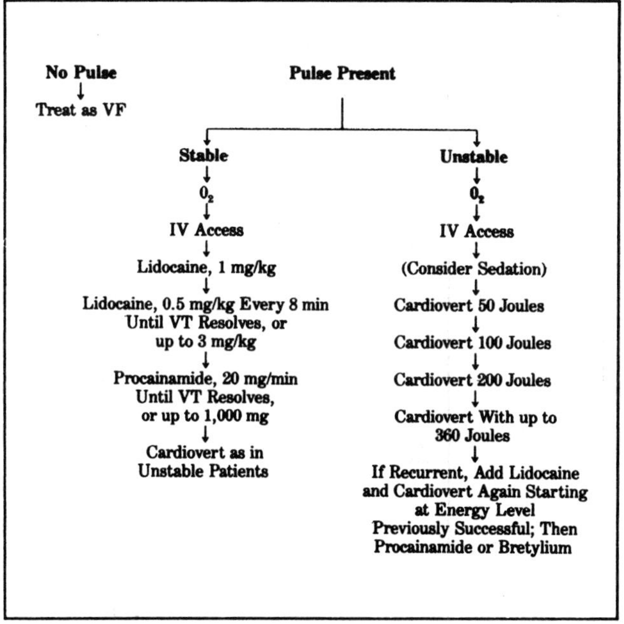

Treatment Algorithm for Sustained Ventricular Tachycardia (VT) with Pulse.   The unstable arm of the algorithm should be followed for stable patients who become unstable. Sedation before cardioversion should be considered for all patients except those with hemodynamic instability (e.g., hypotension, pulmonary edema, unconsciousness). For patients who are hemodynamically unstable, unsynchronized cardioversion is indicated to avoid delays associated with synchronization. A precordial thump may be used before cardioversion in hemodynamically stable patients. (Reproduced with permission. *JAMA*. American Heart Association.)

If Rhythm Is Unclear and Possibly Ventricular
Fibrillation, Defibrillate as for VF. If Asystole is Present
↓
Continue CPR·
↓
Establish IV Access
↓
Epinephrine, 1:10,000, 0.5 - 1.0 mg IV Push
↓
Intubate When Possible
↓
Atropine, 1.0 mg IV Push (Repeated in 5 min)
↓
(Consider Bicarbonate)
↓
Consider Pacing

Treatment Algorithm for Asystole. Intubation is recommended early in the sequence if it can be accomplished simultaneously with other interventions. However, CPR and epinephrine are more important initially if the patient can be ventilated without intubation. Epinephrine should be given every 5 minutes. The endotracheal route may be used. The value of sodium bicarbonate in this sequence is unproved, and routine use is not recommended. If sodium bicarbonate is given, a dose of 1 mmol/ L followed by 0.5 mmol/L every 10 minutes may be used. (Reproduced with permission. *JAMA*. American Heart Association.)

Continue CPR
↓
Establish IV Access
↓
Epinephrine, 1:10,000, 0.5 - 1.0 mg IV Push
↓
Intubate When Possible
↓
(Consider Bicarbonate)
↓
Consider Hypovolemia,
Cardiac Tamponade,
Tension Pneumothorax,
Hypoxemia,
Acidosis,
Pulmonary Embolism

Treatment Algorithm for Electromechanical Dissociation. Intubation is recommended early in the sequence if it can be accomplished simultaneously with other interventions. However, epinephrine is more important initially if the patient can be ventilated without intubation. Epinephrine should be administered every 5 minutes. The value of sodium bicarbonate in this sequence is unproved, and routine use is not recommended. If sodium bicarbonate is given, a dose of 1 mmol/L followed by 0.5 mmol/L every 10 minutes may be used. (Reproduced with permission. *JAMA*. American Heart Association.)

Unstable	Stable
↓	↓
Synchronous Cardioversion 75-100 Joules	Vagal Maneuvers
↓	↓
Synchronous Cardioversion 200 Joules	Verapamil, 5 mg IV
↓	↓
Synchronous Cardioversion 360 Joules	Verapamil, 10 mg IV (in 15-20 min)
↓	↓
Correct Underlying Abnormalities	Cardioversion, Digoxin, β-Blockers, Pacing as Indicated (See Text)
↓	
Pharmacological Therapy + Cardioversion	

If conversion occurs but PSVT recurs, repeated electrical cardioversion is *not* indicated. Sedation should be used as time permits.

Paroxysmal supraventricular tachycardia (PSVT). This sequence was developed to assist in teaching how to treat a broad range of patients with sustained PSVT. Some patients may require care not specified herein. This algorithm should not be construed as prohibiting such flexibility. Flow of algorithm presumes PSVT is continuing.

Treatment Algorithm for Paroxysmal Supraventricular Tachycardia (PSVT). If PSVT recurs after successful cardioversion, repeated electric cardioversion is not indicated. Sedation should be used as time permits. (Reproduced with permission. *JAMA*. American Heart Association.)

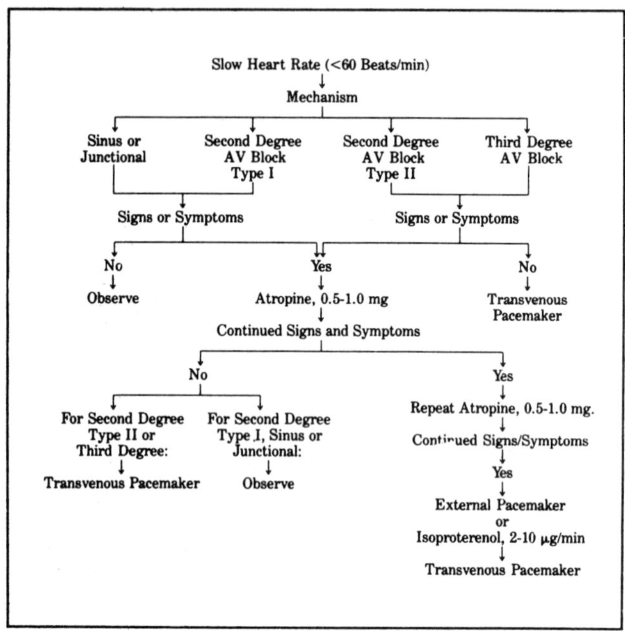

Treatment Algorithm for Bradycardia.   A single chest thump or cough may stimulate cardiac electrical activity and improve cardiac output. These maneuvers may be tried initially. Use of isoproterenol or an external pacemaker for patients who do not respond to atropine is a temporizing measure. (Reproduced with permission. *JAMA*. American Heart Association.)

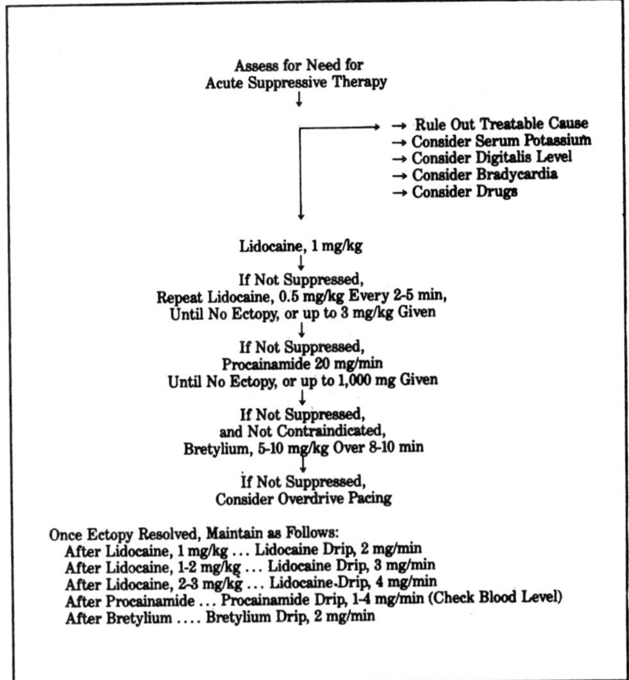

Treatment Algorithm for Ventricular Ectopy: Acute Suppressive Therapy.   If ventricular ectopy persists following correction of treatable causes, an antidysrhythmic, such as lidocaine, procainamide, or bretylium, may be required. (Reproduced with permission. *JAMA.* American Heart Association.)

■ EMPIRIC AMINOGLYCOSIDE DOSING GUIDELINES FOR GENTAMICIN AND TOBRAMYCIN

- Loading dose: 2.0 to 2.5 mg/kg (IBW)
- Maintenance dose: 1.5 mg/kg (IBW) per dosing interval as suggested subsequently

Estimated Creatinine Clearance (CrCl)	Dosing Intervals
>1.25	q8h
0.8–1.25	q12h
0.7–0.8	q16h
0.6–0.7	q18h
0.4–0.6	q24h
0.3–0.4	q30h
0.25–0.3	q36h
0.2–0.25	q48h
<0.2	Once

CALCULATION OF CrCl

$$\text{CrCl (ml/sec)} = \frac{(140 - \text{age in years}) \times 1.5}{\text{Serum creatinine } (\mu mol/L)} (\times\ 0.85 \text{ in female})$$

■ CALCULATION OF THE ALVEOLAR-ARTERIAL OXYGEN GRADIENT $P(A\text{-}a)_{O_2}$

The $P(A\text{-}a)_{O_2}$ can be calculated easily from the ABG results. It is useful in confirming the presence of a shunt.

$$P(A\text{-}a)_{O_2} = P_{A O_2} - P_{a O_2}$$

- $P_{A O_2}$ = the alveolar oxygen tension calculated as shown subsequently.
- $P_{a O_2}$ = the arterial oxygen tension measured by ABG determination.

$P_{a O_2}$ can be calculated by the following formula.

$$P_{A O_2} = (PB - PH_2O)(F_{IO_2}) - P_{a CO_2}/R$$

- PB = barometric pressure (760 mm Hg at sea level)
- PH_2O = 47 mm Hg
- F_{IO_2} = the fraction of O_2 in inspired gas
- $P_{a CO_2}$ = the arterial CO_2 tension measured by ABG determination
- R = the respiratory quotient (0.8)

Normal $P(A\text{-}a)_{O_2}$ is 12 mm Hg in the young adult to 20 mm Hg at age 70.

In pure ventilatory failure, the $P(A\text{-}a)_{O_2}$ will remain 12 to 20 mm Hg. In oxygenation failure, it will increase.

GUIDELINES FOR DRUG THERAPY IN CARDIOPULMONARY RESUSCITATION OF ADULTS*

Drug	Indication	Dose	Frequency	Dilution	Comments
Drugs To Increase Blood Pressure or Cardiac Output					
Epinephrine hydrochloride	Degenerative rhythms (asystole, VF, bradycardia with hypotension, EMD)	0.5–1.0 mg IV, ET or 1–4 μg/min IV; titrate BP	Every 5 min or as needed	1 mg in 10 ml of 1:10,000 solution	Vasopressor. Do not delay administration. Do not mix with sodium bicarbonate. Intracardiac injection is last resort. Infusion may be used. Monitor systolic and diastolic blood pressure.
Dopamine hydrochloride	Hypotension	Titrate BP, IV	Continuous infusion. Begin at 10 μg/kg/min for hypotension	Use hospital's standard dilution	Doses of 2–10 μg/kg/min have predominantly inotropic effect. Doses $>$ 10 μg/kg/min have vasoconstrictor effect. May decrease renal, mesenteric blood flow at high doses or produce arrhythmias. Monitor ECG, BP, and organ perfusion.

D5W, 5% dextrose injection; EMD, electromechanical dissociation; ET, endotracheal; VT, ventricular tachycardia; VF, ventricular fibrillation; BP, blood pressure.
*Incorporates American Heart Association and National Academy of Sciences—National Research Council 1985 national conference recommendations and the source author's experience. These guidelines should be coupled with prudent independent clinical judgment. Other drugs that may prove useful include morphine sulfate, β-blocking agents, amrinone, nitroglycerin, and sodium nitroprusside. (Reproduced with permission. *Clin. Pharm.* vol. 6, Feb. 1987.)

Continued.

GUIDELINES FOR DRUG THERAPY IN CARDIOPULMONARY RESUSCITATION OF ADULTS* *Continued*

Drug	Indication	Dose	Frequency	Dilution	Comments
Metaraminol bitartrate	Hypotension	Initial dose 5 mg IV ET; titrate BP	Continuous infusion. Begin at 5 μg/min	ET: 5 mg in 5–10 ml. IV infusions: 100 mg/250 ml D5W	May begin therapy with 5 mg (IV push or ET). Monitor BP, heart rate, urine output, organ perfusion.
Norepinephrine (levarterenol bitartrate)	Hypotension and low total peripheral resistance	Titrate BP, IV; must dilute	Continuous infusion. Begin at 1–2 μg/min	4 mg (base)/250 ml D5W	Avoid extravasation. Titrate BP. Monitor urine output and organ perfusion. (Treat extravasation with 5–10 mg phentolamine mesylate in 10–15 ml 0.9% sodium chloride injection infiltration.)
Methoxamine hydrochloride	Hypotension	Initial dose: 3–5 mg IV push; titrate BP	Continuous infusion. Begin at 5 μg/min	40 mg/250 ml D5W	May give ET. May cause bradycardia. Monitor BP, urine output, heart rate.
Phenylephrine hydrochloride	Hypotension	0.1–0.5 mg IV; titrate BP	Every 10–15 min; titrate BP	10 mg/250 ml D5W	Slow IV injection. Consider infusion.
Intropic Agent					
Dobutamine hydrochloride	Inotropic agent (not vasoconstriction) Cardiogenic shock	Usually 2.5–10 μg/kg/min IV	Continuous infusion	250 mg/250 ml D5W	Used to improve cardiac output. May increase heart rate. Monitor BP, heart rate, organ perfusion.

Drugs To Control Heart Rhythm and Rate

Atropine sulfate	Symptomatic bradycardia Temporary treatment of symptomatic 2nd- and 3rd-degree heart block Slow idioventricular rhythm Asystole	0.5–1.0 mg IV, ET	Every 5 min	Undiluted (1 mg/ 10 ml syringe)	Maximum total dose 2 mg. Doses less than 0.5 mg may cause bradycardia. May increase infarct size.
Isoproterenol hydrochloride	Hemodynamically important bradycardia unresponsive to atropine (not cardiac arrest)	Titrate heart rate, IV	Continuous infusion 0.5–10 μg/min	1 mg/250 ml D5W	May begin therapy with small (0.2–0.5 mg) IV dose; then begin IV infusion. Avoid excessive heart rate, especially in acute MI. Vasodilatation with decrease in blood pressure. Alert pacer team.
Lidocaine hydrochloride	Ventricular arrhythmias. Follow successful cardioversion of VF. First-line drug for ventricular ectopy, VT, VF	Initial dose of 1 mg/ kg, then 0.5 mg/ kg up to 3 mg/kg IV, ET	Continuous infusion (2–4 mg/ min). May repeat bolus	ET and IV push undiluted. Infusion: 1 g/250 ml D5W	Give IV push over 2–3 min. Begin infusion when feasible. Adjust maintenance infusion based on age, weight, and cardiac and hepatic function.

Continued.

GUIDELINES FOR DRUG THERAPY IN CARDIOPULMONARY RESUSCITATION OF ADULTS* *Continued*

Drug	Indication	Dose	Frequency	Dilution	Comments
Procainamide hydrochloride	Ventricular ectopy after lidocaine has failed	Loading dose of 1.0–1.25 g infused over 1–1.5 h or 50 mg IV every 5 min	Continuous infusion (1–4 mg/min)	1g/250 ml D5W	Observe closely for cardiac depression while loading. Begin IV loading infusion at no faster than 20 mg/min. Monitor BP every 2–3 min until total infusion loading dose of 1–1.25 g infused. Maintenance infusion reduced in renal failure. Monitor ECG (QRS and QT interval.)
Bretylium tosylate	Resistant VF, VT (lidocaine, defibrillation, procainamide failures)	Initial dose: 5–10 mg/kg IV. Repeat PRN up to 30 mg/kg	Bolus every 15–30 min. Infusion 1–2 mg/min	Undiluted for life-threatening arrhythmia. Infusion: 1 g/250 ml	Monitor for biphasic effect; Phase 1: transient hypertensive response and worsening of arrhythmia; Phase 2: antiarrhythmic effect, hypotension. Severe nausea and vomiting. Avoid in patients with increased intracranial pressure.

Verapamil hydro-chloride	Supraventricular tachyar-rhythmias if carotid sinus massage unsuccessful	Initial dose: 5 mg (0.075–0.15 mg/kg) IV. Repeat dose: 10 mg	Separate first and second bolus by $\geq$ 10 min	Undiluted	May produce hypotension, sinus bradycardia, and AV block. Administer with caution to patients who receive IV propranolol or who are on high doses of oral β blockers. May worsen severe heart failure.

Miscellaneous Indications

Oxygen	Hypoxemia; all cardiopulmonary arrests	Highest possible initially; FIO_2 100%	Continuous	. . .	Critical to improve oxygenation to the tissues.
Sodium bicarbonate	Documented metabolic acidosis. Use after defibrillation, CPR, intubation, epinephrine, antiarrhythmics fail (i.e., usually after 10 min of routine cardiac arrest sequence)	Initial dose 1 mmol/L/kg IV; subsequent doses decrease by half	Per ABGs or every 10–15 min	Undiluted 44.6 mmol/L or 50 mmol/L in 50 ml	Must have effective ventilation. May cause hyperosmolar, hypernatremic state and impair CNS recovery. Inactivates catecholamines. Use 3-way stopcock to ease administration. Do not mix with other drugs.
Calcium salts	Only for life-threatening hyperkalemia, prearrest hypocalcemia, verapamil toxicity	10% calcium chloride: 2 ml IV Slow push	Limit use	Undiluted	Efficacy in treating asystole not proved. Avoid administration in digitalized patients. Give slowly (over at least 2 min IV). IV push with ECG monitoring.

ANTIBIOTIC SUSCEPTIBILITY GUIDELINES (SENSITIVITIES MUST BE CHECKED)

Drug + + Drug of Choice + Effective − Not Effective ± Depends on Sensitivities ? Clinical Efficacy Not Proven	Aerobes								Anaerobes	
	Pneumococci	Staphylococcus aureus (penicillin resistant)	Haemophilus Influenzae	H. influenzae, (ampicillin resistant)	Escherichia coli (community acquired)	Klebsiella	Pseudomonas	Coliforms	Above Diaphragm Excluding Bacillus fragilis	B. fragilis
Amikacin	−	?	−	−	+	+	+	+	−	−
Ampicillin/Amoxicillin	+	−	+ +	−	+ +	−	−	±	+	−
Cefazolin	+	+	−	−	+	+	−	±	+	−
Cefotaxime	+	?	+	+	+	+	−	±	?	−
Cefoxitin	+	+	−	−	+	+	−	±	+	−
Ceftazidime	?	?	+	+	+	+	+	±	+	+
Ceftriaxone	+	?	+	+	+	+	−	±	?	−

Cefuroxime	+	+	+	+	+	+	−	±	+	−
Chloramphenicol	+	+	+	+	+	+	−	±	+	+
Ciprofloxacin	−	+	+	+	+	+	+	±	−	−
Clindamycin	+	+	−	−	−	−	−	−	+	+
Cloxacillin	+	+ +	−	−	−	−	−	−	−	−
Co-trimoxazole	±	±	+	+	+	−	−	−	−	−
Erythromycin	+	+	?	?	−	−	−	−	?	?
Gentamicin	−	?	−	−	+	+	+	+	−	−
Imipenem	+	+	+	+	+	+	+	+	+	+
Metronidazole	−	−	−	−	−	−	−	−	+	+ +
Penicillin	+ +	−	−	−	−	−	−	−	+ +	−
Piperacillin	+	−	+	−	+	+	+	+	+	+
Tetracycline	±	+	+	±	±	±	±	±	±	+
Tobramycin	−	?	−	−	+	+	+ +	+	−	−
Vancomycin	+	+	−	−	−	−	−	−	−	−

Courtesy of St. Paul's Formulary, St. Paul's Hospital, Vancouver, British Columbia.

ANTIBIOTIC STANDARD DOSES FOR PATIENTS WITH NORMAL RENAL FUNCTION

Drug	Dosage Range (g/day) IV/IM*	Usual Dosage (g/dosing interval) IV/IM*	Special Comments Regarding Uses
Amikacin	15 mg/kg	7.5 mg/kg q12h	For infections due to gram-negative rods resistant to gentamicin and tobramycin
Amoxicillin	1–6	0.5–1.0 q8h	
Ampicillin	2–12	1 q6h	
Cefazolin	3–6	1 q8h	Useful first generation cephalosporin for gram-positive aerobes
Cefotaxime	3–12	a. 1 q8h	a. For susceptible bacteria resistant to less expensive agents
		b. 2 q4h	b. Mengingitis due to gram-negative rods resistant to ampicillin
Cefoxitin	3–8	1 q6h	As a single agent in mixed infections including *Bacillus fragilis*
Ceftazidime	3–8	1 q8h	For *Pseudomonas aeruginosa* when aminoglycosides inappropriate
Ceftriaxone	1–4	1–2 q12–24h	a. For susceptible bacteria resistant to less expensive agents
			b. Mengingitis due to gram-negative rods resistant to ampicillin
Cefuroxime	2.25–4.5	0.75 q8h	a. Mixed lung infections in penicillin-allergic patients
			b. *Haemophilus influenzae* resistant to ampicillin
Chloramphenicol	2–6	1 q6h	Rarely indicated (irreversible aplastic anemia 1/25,000)

Drug	Daily Dose*	Individual Dose	Comments
Clindamycin	0.6–2.4	a. 0.6 q8h	a. *B. fragilis*
		b. 0.3 q6h	b. Other susceptible bacteria
Cloxacillin/ Methicillin	2–12	1 q6h	Effective for *Staphylococcus aureus* (penicillin sensitive), but penicillin is drug of choice
Co-trimoxazole†	—	—	
Erythromycin	1–4	0.5 q6h	IV drug of choice for *Legionella*
Gentamicin	3–5 mg/kg	1.5 mg/kg q8h	Initially for serious aerobic gram-negative rod infections
Imipenem	1–2	0.5 q6h	For susceptible bacteria resistant to less expensive agent
Metronidazole	1–2	0.5 q8h	Well absorbed orally
			Useful for *Clostridium difficile* pseudomembranous colitis
Penicillin	mu‡ 2–20	mu 1 q6h	
Piperacillin	a. 6–12	a. 1.5 q4h	a. For susceptible bacteria resistant to less expensive agents
	b. 8–18	b. 2.0 q4h	b. With an aminoglycoside for leukopenic patients with *P. aeruginosa*
Tetracycline	1–2	0.5 q6h	
Tobramycin	3–5 mg/kg	1.5 mg/kg q8h	Better than gentamicin only for *P. aeruginosa*
Vancomycin	1–2	1 q12h	For cloxacillin-resistant staphylococci

*Unless otherwise specified.

†Trimethoprim and sulfamethoxazole.

‡Million units.

Courtesy of St. Paul's Formulary, St. Paul's Hospital, Vancouver, British Columbia.

ANTIBIOTIC DOSAGE ADJUSTMENTS RELATIVE TO RENAL FUNCTION

Drug	Creatine Clearance		
	>0.8 ml/s >50 ml/min	0.8–0.4 ml/s 50–25 ml/min	<0.4 ml/s <25 ml/min
Parenteral Therapy			
Acyclovir	5–10 mg/kg q8h	5–10 mg/kg q12h	5–10 mg/kg q24h
Amikacin			
Ampicillin	1–2 g q6h	1–2 g q6–12h	1–2 g q12–16h
Cefazolin	1–2 g q8h	1–2 g q12h	1–2 g q12–24h
Cefotaxime	1–2 g q6–8h	1–2 g q6–8h	1–2 g q12h
Cefoxitin	1–2 g q6h	1–2 g q8–12h	1–2 g q12–24h
Ceftazidime	1–2 g q8h	1–2 g q12h	1–2 g q12–24h
Ceftriaxone	1–2 g q24h	1–2 g q24h	1–2 g q24h
Cefuroxime	750–1500 mg q8h	750–1500 mg q8–12h	750–1500 mg q12–24h
Clindamycin	600 mg q8h	NDN*	NDN
Cloxacillin	250–1000 mg q4–6h	NDN	NDN
Gentamicin†			
Imipenem	500 mg q6–8h	500 mg q8h	500 mg q12h
Metronidazole	500 mg q8h	500 mg q8–12h	250–500 mg q12h
Piperacillin	2–4 g q4–6h	2–4 g q6–12h	2–4 g q12h
Oral Therapy			
Acyclovir	NDN*	NDN	Increase to q12h
Amoxicillin	NDN	NDN	Increase to q12h
Ampicillin	NDN	NDN	Increase to q12h
Cephalexin	NDN	NDN	Increase to q12h
Cloxacillin	NDN	NDN	NDN
Clindamycin	NDN	NDN	NDN
Co-trimoxazole	NDN	NDN	Decrease by 50%
Doxycycline	NDN	NDN	Increase to q24h
Erythromycin	NDN	NDN	Decrease by 50%
Ketoconazole	NDN	NDN	NDN
Metronidazole	NDN	NDN	Increase to q12h
Nitrofurantoin	NDN	Avoid	Avoid
Norfloxacin	NDN	NDN	Increase to q24h
Tetracycline	NDN	Avoid	Avoid

*NDN, no dosage adjustment needed.
†See page 339.
Courtesy of St. Paul's Formulary, St. Paul's Hospital, Vancouver, British Columbia.

SI UNITS CONVERSION TABLE

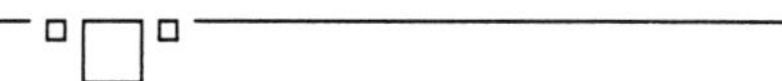

SI units is the abbreviation for *le Systeme International d'Unites.* The SI is an outgrowth of the metric system and provides a uniform system of reporting laboratory data between nations. Most laboratory values in *On Call* are presented in SI units. As some laboratories have not yet converted to this system of reporting, a conversion table for commonly measured laboratory parameters is provided.

Laboratory Test	Previous Reference Intervals	Previous Unit	Conversion Factor	SI Reference Intervals	SI Unit Symbol
Erythrocyte count					
Female	3.5–5.0	$10^6/mm^3$	1	3.5–5.0	$10^{12}/L$
Male	4.3–5.9	$10^6/mm^3$	1	4.3–5.9	$10^{12}/L$
Erythrocyte sedimentation rate (ESR)					
Female	0–30	mm/h	1	0–30	mm/h
Male	0–20	mm/h	1	0–20	mm/h
Hemoglobin					
Female	12.0–15.0	g/dl	10	120–150	g/L
Male	13.6–17.2	g/dl	10	136–172	g/L
Leukocyte count					
Number fraction (differential)		%	0.01		1
Platelet count	130–400	$10^3/mm^3$	1	130–400	$10^9/L$
Reticulocyte count	10,000–75,000	mm^3	0.001	10–75	$10^9/L$
Number fraction	1–24	Number per 1000 RBCs	0.001	0.001–0.024	1
	0.1–2.4	%	0.001	0.001–0.024	1
Albumin (serum)	4.0–6.0	g/dl	10.0	40–60	g/L
Alkaline phosphatase	30–120	U/L	0.01667	0.5–2.0	μkat/L
Amylase (serum)	0–130	U/L	0.01667	0–2.17	μkat/L
Aspartate aminotransferase (AST)	0–35	U/L	0.01667	0–0.58	μkat/L

Analyte					
Bilirubin					
Total	0.1–1.0	mg/dl	17.10	2–18	μmol/L
Conjugated	0–0.2	mg/dl	17.10	0–4	μmol/L
Calcium (serum)					
Male	8.8–10.3	mg/dl	0.2495	2.20–2.58	mmol/L
Female (<50 years)	8.8–10.0	mg/dl	0.2495	2.20–2.50	mmol/L
Female (>50 years)	8.8–10.2	mg/dl	0.2495	2.20–2.56	mmol/L
	4.4–5.1	mEq/L	0.500	2.20–2.56	mmol/L
Calcium ion (serum)	2.00–2.30	mEq/L	0.500	1.00–1.15	mmol/L
CO_2 content (= HCO_3 + CO_2)	22–28	mEq/L	1.00	22–28	mmol/L
CO (proportion of Hb that is COHb)	<15	%	0.01	<0.15	1
Chloride (serum)	95–105	mEq/L	1.00	95–105	mmol/L
Cholesterol (plasma)					
<29 years	<200	mg/dl	0.02586	<5.20	mmol/L
30–39 years	<225	mg/dl	0.02586	<5.85	mmol/L
40–49 years	<245	mg/dl	0.02586	<6.35	mmol/L
>50 years	<265	mg/dl	0.02586	<6.85	mmol/L
Complement (serum)					
C3	70–160	mg/dl	0.01	0.7–1.6	g/L
C4	20–40	mg/dl	0.01	0.2–0.4	g/L

Continued.

Laboratory Test	Previous Reference Intervals	Previous Unit	Conversion Factor	SI Reference Intervals	SI Unit Symbol
Creatine kinase (CPK) (serum)	0–130	U/L	0.01667	0–2.16	μkat/L
MB fraction	>5 in MI	%	0.01	>0.05	1
Creatinine					
Serum	0.6–1.2	mg/dl	88.40	50–110	μmol/L
Urine	Variable	g/24 h	8.840	Variable	mmol/d
Creatinine clearance	75–125	ml/min	0.01667	1.24–2.08	ml/s
Digoxin (plasma)					
Therapeutic	0.5–2.2	ng/ml	1.281	0.6–2.8	nmol/L
	0.5–2.2	μg/L	1.281	0.6–2.8	nmol/L
Toxic	>2.5	ng/ml	1.281	>3.2	nmol/L
Electrophoresis, serum protein					
Albumin	60–65	%	0.01	0.60–0.65	1
Alpha$_1$ globulin	1.7–5.0	%	0.01	0.02–0.05	1
Alpha$_2$ globulin	6.7–12.5	%	0.01	0.07–0.13	1
Beta globulin	8.3–16.3	%	0.01	0.08–0.16	1
Gamma globulin	10.7–20.0	%	0.01	0.11–0.20	1
Albumin	3.6–5.2	g/dl	10.0	36–52	g/L
Alpha$_1$ globulin	0.1–0.4	g/dl	10.0	1–4	g/L
Alpha$_2$ globulin	0.4–1.0	g/dl	10.0	4–10	g/L
Beta globulin	0.5–1.2	g/dl	10.0	5–12	g/L
Gamma globulin	0.6–1.6	g/dl	10.0	6–16	g/L

Ethanol (plasma)					
Legal limit [driving]	<80	mg/dl	0.2171	<17	mmol/L
Toxic	>100	mg/dl	0.2171	>22	mmol/L
Ferritin (serum)	18–300	ng/ml	1.00	18–300	μg/L
Fibrinogen (plasma)	200–400	mg/dl	0.01	2.0–4.0	g/L
Folate					
Serum	2–10	ng/ml	2.266	4–22	nmol/L
RBC	140–960	ng/ml	2.266	550–2200	nmol/L
Gases (arterial blood)					
P_{O_2}	75–105	mm Hg (= Torr)	0.1333	10.0–14.0	kPa
P_{CO_2}	33–44	mm Hg (= Torr)	0.1333	4.4–5.9	kPa
Gamma-glutamyltransferase (GGT) (serum)	0–30	U/L	0.01667	0–0.50	μkat/L
Glucose					
Serum (fasting)	70–110	mg/dl	0.05551	3.9–6.1	mmol/L
Spinal fluid	50–80	mg/dl	0.05551	2.8–4.4	mmol/L
Haptoglobin (serum)	50–220	mg/dl	0.01	0.50–2.20	g/L
Hemoglobin (blood)					
Male	14.0–18.0	g/dl	10.0	140–180	g/L
Female	11.5–15.5	g/dl	10.0	115–155	g/L
Iron (serum)					
Male	80–180	μg/dl	0.1791	14–32	μmol/L
Female	60–160	μg/dl	0.1791	11–29	μmol/L
Iron binding capacity (serum)	250–460	μg/dl	0.1791	45–82	μmol/L
Lactate dehydrogenase (LDH) (serum)	50–150	U/L	0.01667	0.82–2.66	μkat/L

Continued.

Laboratory Test	Previous Reference Intervals	Previous Unit	Conversion Factor	SI Reference Intervals	SI Unit Symbol
LD1	15–40	%	0.01	0.15–0.40	1
LD2	20–45	%	0.01	0.20–0.45	1
LD3	15–30	%	0.01	0.15–0.30	1
LD4	5–20	%	0.01	0.05–0.20	1
LD5	5–20	%	0.01	0.05–0.20	1
LD1	10–60	U/L	0.01667	0.16–1.00	μkat/L
LD2	20–70	U/L	0.01667	0.32–1.16	μkat/L
LD3	10–45	U/L	0.01667	0.22–0.76	μkat/L
LD4	5–30	U/L	0.01667	0.08–0.50	μkat/L
LD5	5–30	U/L	0.01667	0.02–0.50	μkat/L
Lipase (serum)	0–160	U/L	0.01667	0–2.66	μkat/L
Lithium ion (serum)	0.50–1.50	mEq/L	1.00	0.50–1.50	mmol/L
(therapeutic)		μg/L	0.001441		mmol/L
		mg/dl	1.441		mmol/L
Magnesium (serum)	1.8–3.0	mg/dl	0.4114	0.80–1.20	mmol/L
	1.6–2.4	mEq/L	0.500	0.80–1.20	mmol/L
Osmolality					
Plasma	280–300	mOsm/kg	1.00	280–300	mmol/kg
Urine	50–1200	mOsm/kg	1.00	50–1200	mmol/kg
Phosphate (serum)	2.5–5.0	mg/dl	0.3229	0.80–1.60	mmol/L
Potassium ion					
Serum	3.5–5.0	mEq/L	1.00	3.5–5.0	mmol/L
Urine (diet dependent)	25–100	mEq/24 h	1.00	25–100	mmol/d

Protein, total					
Serum	6.0–8.0	g/dl	10.0	60–80	g/L
Urine	<150	mg/24 h	0.001	<0.15	g/d
Sodium ion					
Serum	135–147	mEq/L	1.00	135–147	mmol/L
Urine	Diet dependent	mEq/24 h	1.00	Diet dependent	mmol/d
Theophylline (plasma)					
Therapeutic	10.0–20.0	mg/L	5.550	55–110	μmol/L
Thyroid tests (serum)					
TSH	2–11	μU/ml	1.00	2–11	mU/L
T_4	4.0–11.0	μg/dl	12.87	51–142	nmol/L
TBG	12.0–28.0	μg/dl	12.87	150–360	nmol/L
Free T_4	0.8–2.8	ng/dl	12.87	10–36	pmol/L
T_3	75–220	ng/dl	0.01536	1.2–3.4	nmol/L
T_3 uptake	25–35	%	0.01	0.25–0.35	1
Transferrin (serum)	170–370	mg/dl	0.01	1.70–3.70	g/L
Triglycerides (plasma)	<160	mg/dl	0.01129	<1.80	mmol/L
Urate (as uric acid)					
Serum	2.0–7.0	mg/dl	59.48	120–420	μmol/L
Urine	Diet dependent	g/24 h	5.948	Diet dependent	mmol/d
Urea (serum)	8–18	mg/dl	0.3570	3.0–6.5	mmol/L
Vitamin B_{12}	200–1000	pg/ml	0.7378	150–750	pmol/L
(plasma or serum)		ng/dl	7.378		pmol/L

ON CALL FORMULARY: COMMONLY PRESCRIBED MEDICATIONS

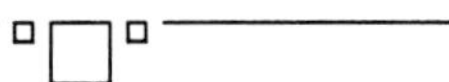

The On Call Formulary is a quick reference for information on medications that are commonly encountered or prescribed by the student or resident on call.

Antibacterial susceptibility guidelines as well as doses for patients are presented in table formats on pages 346–350. Drugs used in cardiopulmonary resuscitation are presented in table format on pages 341–345.

Doses listed are for adult patients with normal renal and hepatic function.

ACETAMINOPHEN (Tylenol, Paracetamol) Analgesic– antipyretic

Indications:	Pain, fever.
Actions:	Raises the pain threshold; acts directly on the hypothalamic heat regulating center.
Side effects:	Uncommon—rash, drug fever, mucosal ulcerations, leukopenia, and pancytopenia.
Comments:	Unlike aspirin, acetaminophen has no anti-inflammatory action, does not irritate the stomach, does not affect the aggregation of platelets, and does not interact with oral anticoagulants.
Dose:	325–1000 mg PO q4–6h PRN, up to 4000 mg/24 h.

ACETYLSALICYLIC ACID (see Aspirin)
ADALAT (see Nifedipine)

ALLOPURINOL (Zyloprim, Lopurin) Xanthine oxidase inhibitor

Indications:	Gout, uric acid nephropathy, tumor lysis syndrome.
Actions:	Inhibits the formation of uric acid.
Side effects:	Rash, fever, gastrointestinal upset, and hepatotoxicity.
Comments:	Reduce the dose in renal or hepatic insufficiency. Aminophylline, mercaptopurine, and azathioprine levels may be increased by allopurinol. Attacks of acute gout may occur shortly after starting allopurinol.
Dose:	100–300 mg PO once daily after meals. Doses up to 800 mg per day may be required in severe cases.

ALUMINUM HYDROXIDE (Amphogel, Basaljel) Antacid

Indications:	Pain due to peptic ulcer disease, reflux esophagitis, prophylaxis for stress ulcers, reduction of urinary

	phosphate in patients with phosphate-containing renal calculi.
Actions:	Buffers gastric acidity, binds phosphate in the intestine.
Side effects:	Constipation, anorexia, nausea, hypophosphatemia, aluminum toxicity in patients in renal failure.
Comments:	May bind and reduce intestinal absorption of tetracycline, thyroxine, and other medications.
Dose:	30–60 ml PO q1–2h during the acute phase. 30–60 ml PO q1 and 3h PC meals and QHS for chronic therapy.

AMICAR (see Aminocaproic Acid)

AMINOCAPROIC ACID (Amicar)   Plasminogen activator inhibitor

Indications:	Excessive bleeding due to fibrinolysis.
Actions:	Inhibits plasminogen activator, also has antiplasmin activity.
Side effects:	Increases the risk of DVT, pulmonary embolism, and cerebral vasospasm. Also, nausea, abdominal cramps, dizziness, rash, and headache.
Dose:	4–5 g IV over 1 h, followed by a maintenance infusion of 1–1.25 g/h to achieve plasma levels of 0.130 mg/ml or until bleeding has stopped.

AMINOPHYLLINE (Phyllocontin, Theophylline) Bronchodilator

Indications:	Bronchospasm.
Actions:	Phosphodiesterase inhibitor resulting in smooth muscle relaxation and bronchodilation. Also stimulates the respiratory center.
Side effects:	Tachycardia, ventricular ectopy, nausea, vomiting, headaches, seizures, insomnia, and nightmares.
Comments:	Theophylline clearance is decreased by the addition of erythromycin, cimetidine, propranolol, allopurinol, and a number of other drugs.
Dose:	Aminophylline loading dose is 6 mg/kg IV followed by 0.6 mg/kg/h maintenance. Maintenance doses for patients in CHF, those with liver disease, and the elderly should be reduced to 0.3 mg/kg/h, and smokers require a larger dose of 0.9 mg/kg/h.

AMOXICILLIN (see p. 348)
AMPHOGEL (see Aluminum Hydroxide)
AMPHOTERICIN B   Antifungal

Indications:	Systemic fungal infections.
Actions:	A polyene antibiotic that disrupts fungal cell membranes.
Side effects:	Fever, chills, nausea, vomiting, diarrhea, hypotension, nephrotoxicity, hypokalemia, hypomagnesemia, and thrombophlebitis.
Comments:	Premedication with antipyretics, antihistamines, antiemetics, and corticosteroids may reduce some of the side effects.

Dose: Patients should receive a test dose of 1 mg in 100 ml D5W over 2 h. If the test dose is tolerated, a further dose of 10 mg can be given on the first day. The dose can then be increased by 5 mg every day until the desired dose of 0.5 mg/kg/day is reached. Infusion time should be 4–6 h.

AMPICILLIN (see p. 348)
APRESOLINE (see Hydralazine)

ASPIRIN (Acetylsalicylic Acid)   Analgesic, antipyretic, anti-inflammatory

Indications: Pain due to inflammation, fever, antiplatelet agent in coronary syndromes.
Actions: Acts peripherally by interfering with the production of prostaglandins, thus reducing pain and inflammation, and acts centrally to reduce pain perception and reduce temperature by increasing heat loss.
Side effects: Gastric erosion and bleeding, tinnitus, fever, thirst, diaphoresis. Severe allergic reactions can occur, including asthma.
Dose: 325–650 mg PO q4–6h for mild pain or fever. 650 mg PO QID for chest pain due to pericarditis. 30–325 mg daily for angina and antiplatelet effects.
2.6–5.2 g per day in divided doses for rheumatoid arthritis.

ATIVAN (see Lorazepam)
ATROPINE (see p. 343)
AZT (see Zidovudine)
BASALJEL (see Aluminum Hydroxide)

BECLOMETHASONE (Beclovent, Vanceril)   Corticosteroid

Indications: Bronchial asthma long-term treatment.
Actions: Topical anti-inflammatory.
Side effects: Oral and pharyngeal candidiasis, laryngeal myopathy.
Comments: Has no role in the treatment of the acute asthma attack.
Dose: 2 inhalations BID to QID, may be more effective if administered 3–5 min after inhaled bronchodilator.

BECLOVENT (see Beclomethasone)
BENADRYL (see Diphenhydramine)

BISACODYL (Dulcolax)   Laxative

Indications: Constipation.
Actions: Stimulates peristalsis.
Side effects: Abdominal cramps, rectal bleeding.
Comments: Onset PO in 6–10 h; onset PR 15–60 min. Avoid in pregnancy, MI. May worsen orthostatic hypotension, weakness, and incoordination in the elderly.
Dose: 10–15 mg PO QHS PRN. 10 mg suppository PR PRN.

BRETYLIUM TOSYLATE (see p. 344)

BUMETANIDE (Bumex)   Loop diuretic

Indications: CHF.
Actions: Inhibits the reabsorption of Na and Cl in the ascending
                limb of the loop of Henle.
Side effects: Electrolyte depletion, rash, hyperuricemia, reversible
                deafness.
Comments: 1 mg bumetanide = 40 mg furosemide.
Dose: 0.5–1 mg PO or IV. If necessary repeat dose every 20
                min to a total dose of 3 mg.

BUMEX (see Bumetanide)
CALAN (see Verapamil)

CALCIUM GLUCONATE   Calcium supplement

Indications: Symptomatic hypocalcemia, hyperkalemia; adjunct in
                CPR protocol (see p. 345).
Actions: Replacment, decreases cardiac automaticity, raises
                cardiac cells resting potential.
Side effects: Administration of Ca to patients on digoxin may pre-
                cipitate ventricular dysrhythmias due to the combined
                effects of digoxin and Ca.
Comments: 500 mg of calcium gluconate = 2.3 mmol Ca^{2+}. 10%
                solution contains 0.45 mmol Ca^{2+}/ml.
Dose: 1–15 g PO daily for control of hypocalcemia. 5–10 ml
                of 10% solution IV for more rapid effects.

CANESTEN (see Clotrimazole)
CAPOTEN (see Captopril)

CAPTOPRIL (Capoten)   Angiotensin converting enzyme
                                                      inhibitor

Indications: Hypertension, CHF.
Actions: Inhibits the enzyme responsible for conversion of an-
                giotensin I to angiotensin II.
Side effects: Hypotension, dysgeusia, cough, rash, angioedema,
                neutropenia, proteinuria, and renal insufficiency.
Comments: May cause hyperkalemia if used in patients receiving
                potassium-sparing diuretics or potassium supple-
                ments.
Dose: Begin with a test dose of 6.25 mg PO and monitor BP
                for 4 h. For hypertension, titrate up to 25–50 mg PO
                BID and for CHF to 25–50 mg PO TID.

CEFAZOLIN (see p. 348)
CEFOXITIN (see p. 348)
CEFTAZIDIME (see p. 348)
CEFTRIAXONE (see p. 348)
CEFUROXIME (see p. 348)

CHLORAL HYDRATE (Noctec and others)   Hypnotic

Indications: Insomnia.
Actions: Hypnotic.

Side effects:	Gastric irritation, rash.
Comments:	Do not use in patients with liver or kidney disease.
Dose:	0.5–1.0 g PO/PR.

CHLORAMPHENICOL (see p. 348)
CHLORONASE (see Chlorpropamide)

CHLORDIAZEPOXIDE (Librium and others)   Benzodiazepine

Indications:	Anxiety, alcohol withdrawal.
Actions:	Benzodiazepine sedative–antianxiety agent.
Side effects:	CNS depression.
Comments:	Unpredictable absorption after IM injection.
Dose:	5–25 mg PO TID for anxiety. 50–100 mg IV q2h–6h PRN (maximum dose 500 mg for first 24 h) for alcohol withdrawal.

CHLORPROMAZINE (Largactil, Thorazine)   Antipyschotic phenothiazine

Indications:	Agitation, nausea, vomiting, hiccoughs.
Actions:	Dopamine, histamine$_1$, muscarine, and alpha$_1$-adrenergic antagonist.
Side effects:	CNS depression, hypotension, extrapyramidal effects, jaundice.
Comments:	In the acutely agitated patient, haloperidol may be a better choice because of its lesser effect on BP.
Dose:	25–75 mg for mild cases and 150 mg for severe cases daily PO. 25–50 mg IM repeated in q3–4h. 10–25 mg PO/IM q6–8h for hiccoughs.

CHLORPROPAMIDE (Diabinese, Chloronase)   Oral hypoglycemic

Indications:	NIDDM.
Actions:	Sulfonylurea, stimulates insulin secretion, increases the effect of insulin on the liver to increase gluconeogenesis and on muscle to increase glucose use.
Side effects:	Hypoglycemia, rash, blood dyscrasias, jaundice, hyponatremia, edema.
Comments:	Has a long duration of action (20–60h) and is cleared largely by the kidneys. Hypoglycemic reactions may be prolonged in the elderly and in patients with renal impairment.
Dose:	100–500 mg PO daily in one or two doses.

CIMETIDINE (Tagamet)   Histamine$_2$ antagonist

Indications:	Peptic ulcer disease, gastrointestinal reflux.
Actions:	Inhibits histamine-induced secretion of gastric acid.
Side effects:	Gynecomastia, impotence, confusion, diarrhea, leukopenia, thrombocytopenia, increase in serum creatinine.
Comments:	Reduces microsomal enzyme metabolism of drugs, including oral anticoagulants, phenytoin, and theophylline.

Dose: 300 mg PO/IV q6–8h. 800 mg PO QHS is effective in peptic ulcer disease and 400 mg PO BID in reflux.

CIPROFLOXACIN (p. 347)
CLINDAMYCIN (p. 349)
CLOXACILLIN (p. 349)

CODEINE   Narcotic analgesic

Indications: Pain, cough, diarrhea.
Actions: Narcotic analgesic, depresses the medullary cough center, decreases propulsive contractions of the small bowel.
Side effects: Dysphoria, agitation, pruritis, constipation, light-headedness, sedation.
Comments: Useful in mild to moderate pain.
Dose: 30–60 mg PO/SC/IM q4–6h for analgesia. 8–20 mg q4h for diarrhea and cough.

COLACE (see Docusate)

COTRIMAZOLE (Canesten and others)   Antifungal

Indications: Esophageal, vaginal, and intertrigonal candidiasis.
Actions: Damages fungal cell membranes.
Side effects: Local irritation, although generally well tolerated.
Dose: 10 mg troche PO QID for esophageal candidiasis, 100 mg intravaginally QHS × 7 nights for vaginal candidiasis, 1% cream or solution BID for intertrigonal candidiasis.

COUMADIN (see Warfarin)

ddC (dideoxycytidine, Hivid)   Nucleoside analog

Indications: Advanced HIV disease.
Actions: Inhibition of reverse transcriptase, thus inhibiting retrovirus replication. Cytidine analog.
Side effects: Mucosal ulcers and rash, peripheral neuropathy.
Comments: Used in combination therapy with AZT.
Dose: 0.01 mg/kg PO q8h.

ddI (dideoxyinosine, didanosine, Videx)   Nucleoside analog

Indications: Advanced HIV disease.
Actions: Inhibition of reverse transciptase, thus inhibiting retrovirus replication. Purine analog.
Side effects: Headache, insomnia, increase in uric acid, pancreatitis, increase in triglycerides, peripheral neuropathy.
Dose: 167–325 mg PO BID.

DEMEROL (see Meperidine)
DIABINESE (see Chlorpropamide)

DIAZEPAM (Valium)   Benzodiazepine

Indications: Anxiety, seizure disorders, alcohol withdrawal.
Actions: Benzodiazepine sedative–antianxiety agent.

Side effects:	Sedation, hypotension, respiratory depression, paradoxical agitation.
Comments:	IM administration is not recommended because of unpredictable absorption. Patients have a wide variability in tolerance to the benzodiazepines. Always start with a conservative dose in patients who have not previously received them.
Dose:	For anxiety, 2–10 mg PO BID to QID. For status epilepticus, 2 mg/min IV until the seizures stop or to a total dose of 20 mg. For acute alcohol withdrawal or delirium tremens, 5–10 mg IV at a rate of 2–5 mg/min q30–60 min until the patient is sedated, then follow with a maintenance dose of 10–20 mg PO QID.

DIFLUCAN (see Fluconazole)

DIGOXIN (Lanoxin)   Digitalis glycoside

Indications:	Supraventricular tachycardia, CHF.
Actions:	Slows AV conduction, increases the force of cardiac contraction, Na-K-ATPase inhibitor.
Side effects:	Dysrhythmias, nausea, vomiting, neuropsychiatric disturbances.
Comments:	80% renally excreted. Dose must be reduced in patients with renal impairment and the elderly. Avoid hypokalemia, which can predispose to digitalis-induced arrhythmias.
Dose:	IV 0.125–0.5 mg q6h to a total of 1 mg, then 0.125–0.25 mg daily. Oral 0.125–0.5 mg q6h to a total of 1.5 mg, then 0.125–0.25 mg daily. Higher doses may be required to control some supraventricular tachycardias.

DILANTIN (see Phenytoin)

DIMENHYDRINATE (Dramamine, Gravol)   Antihistamine

Indications:	Nausea, vomiting, labyrinthine and vestibular disturbances.
Actions:	Antihistamine and anticholinergic.
Side effects:	Drowsiness, dizziness, dry mouth, urinary retention.
Comments:	Anticholinergic effect is additive to that of other drugs, such as the tricyclic antidepressants.
Dose:	50 mg PO or 25 mg IM/IV q4–6h PRN.

DIPHENHYDRAMINE (Benadryl)   Antihistamine

Indications:	Allergic reactions.
Actions:	Antihistamine and anticholinergic.
Side effects:	Drowsiness, dizziness, dry mouth, urinary retention.
Comments:	Anticholinergic effect is additive to that of other drugs, such as the tricyclic antidepressants.
Dose:	25–50 mg PO/IM/IV q6–8h PRN.

DOCUSATE (Colace, dioctyl sodium sulfosuccinate)   Laxative

Indications:	Prevention of constipation.
Actions:	Stool softener, lowers surface tension.

Side effects: Nausea, bitter taste.
Dose: 100 mg PO TID.

DOPAMINE HYDROCHLORIDE (p. 341)
DRAMAMINE (see Dimenhydrinate)
DULCOLAX (see Bisacodyl)
EDECRIN (see Ethacrynic Acid)

ENALAPRIL (Vasotec) Angiotensin converting enzyme inhibitor

Indications: Hypertension, CHF.
Actions: Inhibits the enzyme responsible for conversion of angiotensin I to angiotensin II.
Side effects: Hypotension, headache, nausea, diarrhea.
Comments: May cause hyperkalemia if used in patients receiving
                 potassium-sparing diuretics or potassium supplements.
Dose: Begin with a test dose of 2.5 mg PO and monitor BP
                 for 4 h. For hypertension, titrate up to 2.5–40 mg PO
                 daily and for CHF to 10–25 mg PO BID.

EPINEPHRINE (see p. 341)
ERYTHROMYCIN (see p. 349)
ESIDRIX (see Hydrochlorothiazide)

ETHACRYNIC ACID (Edecrin)   Loop diuretic

Indications: CHF, edema.
Actions: Inhibition of the reabsorption of Na and Cl in the
                 ascending limb of the loop of Henle.
Side effects: Electrolyte depletion, hyperuricemia, hyperglycemia,
                 anorexia, nausea, vomiting, diarrhea, sensorineural
                 hearing loss.
Comments: Associated with more side effects than other loop diuretics.
Dose: 50 mg IV × one or two doses.

FAMOTIDINE (Pepcid)   Histamine$_2$ antagonist

Indications: Peptic ulcer disease, gastrointestinal reflux.
Actions: Inhibits histamine-induced secretion of gastric acid.
Side effects: Headache, dizziness, constipation, diarrhea.
Comments: Generally well tolerated. Does not have the same effects as cimetidine on microsomal enzymes or androgen blocking.
Dose: 40 mg PO QHS or 20 mg IV BID for acute conditions.
                 20 mg PO QHS for maintenance.

FERROUS SULFATE   Iron supplement

Indications: Iron deficiency.
Actions: Replaces iron stores.
Side effects: Constipation, nausea, diarrhea, abdominal cramps.
Comments: Stools may turn black but do not have the typical tarry
                 appearance of melena.
Dose: 325 mg PO TID.

FLUCONAZOLE (Diflucan)   Antifungal

Indications:	Oropharyngeal, esophageal, and systemic candidiasis, cryptococcal meningitis.
Actions:	Inhibition of cell membranes of yeasts and fungi.
Side effects:	Nausea, vomiting, headache, rash, abdominal pain, diarrhea, hepatic necrosis.
Comments:	Many drug interactions due to microsomal enzyme inhibition—sulfonylureas, phenytoin, warfarin, cyclophosphamide.
Dose:	200 mg PO followed by 100 mg PO daily. For systemic candidiasis and cryptococcal meningitis, 200–400 mg once daily. Reduce doses in patients with renal impairment.

FUROSEMIDE (Lasix)   Loop diuretic

Indications:	CHF, edema, hyperkalemia, hypercalcemia.
Actions:	Inhibition of the reabsorption of Na and Cl in the ascending limb of the loop of Henle.
Side effects:	Electrolyte depletion, hyperuricemia, hyperglycemia, reversible deafness.
Comments:	Loop diuretics are well absorbed orally, with a prompt onset of action.
Dose:	For acute pulmonary edema, 40 mg PO or IV repeated in 60–90 min if required. Higher doses may be required in patients with life-threatening pulmonary edema or renal impairment.

GELUSIL (aluminum hydroxide–magnesium hydroxide)
Antacid

Indications:	Pain due to peptic ulcer disease, reflux esophagitis, prophylaxis of stress ulcers.
Actions:	Buffers gastric acidity.
Side effects:	Diarrhea, hypermagnesemia in renal failure.
Comments:	Aluminum salts cause constipation, and magnesium salts cause diarrhea. The mixture attempts to balance these effects. May bind and reduce absorption of tetracycline, thyroxine, and other medications.
Dose:	30–60 ml PO q1–2h during the acute phase. 30–60 ml PO q1 and 3h PC meals and QHS for chronic therapy.

GENTAMICIN (see p. 349)
GRAVOL (see Dimenhydrinate)
HALDOL (see Haloperidol)

HALOPERIDOL (Haldol)   Antipsychotic

Indications:	Psychotic disorders, acute agitation.
Actions:	Antipsychotic neuroleptic butyrophenone.
Side effects:	Extrapyramidal reactions, postural hypotension, sedation, galactorrhea, jaundice, blurred vision, bronchospasm, neuroleptic malignant syndrome.
Comments:	Extrapyramidal effects are more pronounced but hypotension is less frequent than with phenothiazines.

Dose:	0.5–2 mg PO TID. 2–10 mg IM as frequently as q1h, if necessary, to control acute psychotic crises.

HEPARIN   Anticoagulant

Indications:	Prophylaxis and treatment of DVT, pulmonary embolism, embolic CVA; adjunct in treatment of unstable angina, thrombolytic therapy.
Actions:	Acts in conjunction with antithrombin III, which neutralizes several activated clotting factors—antithrombin effect.
Side effects:	Hemorrhage, thrombocytopenia.
Comment:	Monitor aPTT closely when using IV.
Dose:	For treatment of DVT or pulmonary embolism, 5000–10,000 units IV bolus, followed by 1000–2000 unit/h maintenance, according to desired aPTT.

HYDRALAZINE (Apresoline)   Arteriolar vasodilator

Indications:	Hypertension.
Actions:	Arteriolar vasodilator.
Side effects:	Tachycardia, SLE reaction at higher doses (>200 mg/day.)
Comments:	Very limited effect on veins, so little postural hypotension.
Dose:	10–25 mg PO q6h.

HYDROCHLOROTHIAZIDE (Hydrodiuril, Esidrix)   Thiazide diuretic

Indications:	Hypertension, CHF, edema.
Actions:	Blocks Na and Cl reabsorption in the cortical diluting segment of the loop of Henle.
Side effects:	Electrolyte depletion, hyperuricemia, hyperglycemia, hypercalcemia, pancreatitis, jaundice.
Comments:	In spite of the long list of side effects, thiazides are generally well tolerated when used in appropriate doses.
Dose:	12.5–50 mg PO daily.

HYDROCORTISONE   Corticosteroid

Indications:	Severe bronchospasm, anaphylaxis, hypercalcemia.
Actions:	Anti-inflammatory.
Side effects:	Na retention, hyperglycemia, potassium loss.
Comments:	Side effects are few during short-term use.
Dose:	250 mg IV followed by 100 mg IV q6h.

HYDRODIURIL (see Hydrochlorothiazide)

IBUPROFEN (Motrin and others)   NSAID

Indications:	Inflammation due to arthritis, soft-tissue injuries; analgesia.
Actions:	Proprionic acid derivative. Interferes with the production of prostaglandins.

Side effects: Nausea, diarrhea. May compromise renal function in patients with renal impairment. Contraindicated in the syndrome of aspirin sensitivity, nasal polyps, and bronchospasm.

Comments: Available as an analgesic in many countries without prescription.

Dose: For analgesia, 200 mg PO TID to QID. For anti-inflammatory effects, 200–400 mg PO TID to QID.

IMIPENEM (see p. 349)
IMITREX (see Sumatriptan Succinate)
INDERAL (see Propranolol)
INDOCIN (see Indomethacin)

INDOMETHACIN (Indocin)   NSAID

Indications: Inflammation due to arthritis, soft-tissue injury, pericarditis.

Actions: Indole acetic acid derivative. Interferes with the production of prostaglandins.

Side effects: Headaches, dizziness and lightheadedness, epigastric pain. May compromise renal function in patients with renal impairment.

Comments: Contraindicated in the syndrome of aspirin sensitivity, nasal polyps, and bronchospasm. May increase the risk of GI bleeding if used in patients receiving oral anticoagulants.

Dose: 25–50 mg PO TID

INSULIN   Hypoglycemic

Indications: Diabetes mellitus.

Actions: Enhances hepatic glycogen storage, enhances the entry of glucose into cells, inhibits the breakdown of protein and fat, enhances the entry of K into cells.

Side effects: Hypoglycemia, local skin reactions, lipohypertrophy.

Comments: Less immunogenicity seen with human insulin than with insulin from natural sources.

Dose: Extremely variable.

Insulin	Example	Onset	Peak	Duration
Regular	Humulin R	15–60 min	2–4 h	5–7 h
NPH	Humulin N	1.5–4 h	6–16 h	12–28 h
Lente	Humulin L	1–4 h	6–16 h	14–28 h

ISOPROTERENOL (see p. 343)
ISOPTIN (see Verapamil)
ISORDIL (see Isosorbide Dinitrate)

ISOSORBIDE DINITRATE (Isordil, Sorbitrate)   Vasodilator

Indications: Angina pectoris, CHF.

Actions: Venous, coronary, and arteriolar vasodilator.

Side effects: Headache, hypotension, flushing.

Comments: Nitrate tolerance may develop with prolonged continuous administration.

Dose: 5–30 mg PO QID.

KAYEXALATE (see Sodium Polystyrene Sulfonate)

KETOCONAZOLE (Nizoral)   Antifungal

Indications:	Esophageal candidiasis, pulmonary histoplasmosis.
Actions:	Inhibition of yeast and fungal cell growth.
Side effects:	Nausea, anorexia, vomiting, rash, pruritis. Inhibits microsomal enzymes. Gynecomastia, impotence. Interacts with warfarin and cyclophosphamide.
Comments:	Absorption is impaired in patients receiving drugs reducing gastric acidity.
Dose:	200–400 mg PO daily.

LABETALOL (Trandate)   Alpha$_1$ and beta blocker

Indications:	Hypertensive emergencies.
Actions:	Alpha$_1$ blocking action is predominant in acute use but is accompanied by nonspecific beta blockade.
Side effects:	Postural hypotension, bronchospasm, jaundice, bradycardia, negative inotropic effect.
Comments:	Effect is largely due to alpha-$_1$-adrenergic blocking activity. Contraindicated in conditions where beta blockers are contraindicated.
Dose:	20 mg IV q10–15 min in incremental doses (e.g., 20 mg, 20 mg, 40 mg, 40 mg). Alternatively, an infusion beginning at 2 mg/min and titrating to BP response may be given, with a maximum daily dose of 2400 mg.

LANOXIN (see Digoxin)
LARGACTIL (see Chlorpromazine)
LASIX (see Furosemide)
LEVARTERENOL (see p. 342)

LEVODOPA-CARBIDOPA (Sinemet)   Dopamine agonist

Indications:	Parkinson's disease.
Actions:	Levodopa is converted to dopamine in the basal ganglia. Carbidopa inhibits the peripheral destruction of levodopa.
Side effects:	Anorexia, nausea, vomiting, abdominal pain, dysrhythmias, behavioral changes, orthostatic hypotension, involuntary movements.
Comments:	Side effects are common.
Dose:	Begin with one tablet 100 mg/10 mg PO BID, increasing the dose until desired response is obtained, with a maximum dose of 8 tablets (800 mg/80 mg) per day.

LIBRIUM (see Chlordiazepoxide)

LIDOCAINE (Xylocaine)   Class IB antiarrhythmic

Indications:	Prophylaxis and treatment of ventricular tachycardia.
Actions:	Lengthens the effective refractory period in ventricular conducting system. Decreases ventricular automaticity.
Side effects:	Nausea, vomiting, hypotension, confusion, seizures, perioral paresthesias.

Comments:	Lower maintenance doses are required in the elderly and in patients with CHF, liver disease, and hypotension.
Dose:	I mg/kg IV loading dose in 2–3 min. A further dose of 50 mg may be given at 5–10 min intervals to a total dose of 300 mg, followed by a maintenance dose of 1–4 mg/min IV. For prophylaxis, a loading dose of 200 mg given as 50 mg q5min, followed by a maintenance infusion of 3 mg/min IV.

LOPURIN (see Allopurinol)

LORAZEPAM (Ativan)   Benzodiazepine

Indications:	Insomnia, anxiety.
Actions:	Benzodiazepine sedative–hypnotic.
Side effects:	Sedation, respiratory depression.
Comments:	Peak effect in 1–6 h
Dose:	0.5–1.0 mg PO QHS for sleep. 1.0 mg PO TID for anxiety.

MAALOX (aluminum hydroxide–magnesium hydroxide)
                                                         Antacid

Indications:	Pain due to peptic ulcer disease, reflux esophagitis, prophylaxis of stress ulcer.
Actions:	Buffers gastric acidity.
Side effects:	Diarrhea, hypermagnesemia in renal failure.
Comments:	Aluminum salts cause constipation, and magnesium salts cause diarrhea. The mixture attempts to balance these effects. May bind and reduce absorption of tetracycline, thyroxine, and other medications.
Dose:	30–60 ml PO q1–2h during the acute phase. 30–60 ml PO q1 and 3h PC meals and QHS for chronic therapy.

MANNITOL   Osmotic diuretic

Indications:	Cerebral edema, hemolytic transfusion reactions.
Actions:	Osmotic diuretic.
Side effects:	Volume overload, hyperosmolality, hyponatremia.
Comments:	Contraindicated in renal failure.
Dose:	25 g IV over 15–30 min q2–3h PRN.

MEPERIDINE (Demerol)   Narcotic analgesic

Indications:	Moderate to severe pain.
Actions:	Narcotic analgesic.
Side effects:	Respiratory depression, hypotension, nausea, vomiting, constipation, agitation, rash.
Comments:	100 mg meperidine SC/IV = 10 mg morphine SC/IV. Antidote is naloxone.
Dose:	50–150 mg SC/IM q4h.

METOLAZONE (Zaroxolyn)   Thiazide diuretic

Indications:	Hypertension, CHF, edema, some forms of renal failure.

Actions:	Blocks Na and Cl reabsorption in the cortical diluting segment of the loop of Henle.
Side effects:	Electrolyte depletion, hyperuricemia, hyperglycemia, hypomagnesemia.
Comments:	Only difference from hydrochlorothiazide is the longer duration of effect.
Dose:	2.5–10 mg PO daily.

METRONIDAZOLE (see p. 349)

MIDAZOLAM (Versed)   Benzodiazepine

Indications:	Premedication before surgery or diagnostic procedure.
Action:	Benzodiazepine sedative–hypnotic.
Side effects:	Sedation, paradoxical agitation, respiratory depression.
Comments:	Should be used only in the presence of individuals equipped to provide resuscitation. Benzodiazepine effects can be reversed with the antagonist flumazenil.
Dose:	0.20–0.35 mg/kg IV PRN in 20–30 sec as an induction dose in the unpremedicated healthy adult. Smaller doses in the elderly, the debilitated, and in the premedicated patient. Always inject IV slowly to avoid respiratory depression and hypotension.

MORPHINE SULFATE   Narcotic analgesic

Indications:	Moderate to severe pain, pulmonary edema.
Actions:	Narcotic analgesic, splanchnic venodilation.
Side effects:	Respiratory depression, hypotension, nausea, vomiting.
Comments:	10 mg morphine IM/SC = 100 mg meperidine IM/SC.
Dose:	For pulmonary edema or chest pain due to coronary ischemia, 2–4 mg IV q5–10min to a maximum dose of 10–12 mg. For pain, 2–15 mg IV/IM/SC q4h PRN.

MOTRIN (see Ibuprofen)
MYCOSTATIN (see Nystatin)

MYLANTA (aluminum hydroxide–magnesium hydroxide)
        Antacid

Indications:	Pain due to peptic ulcer disease, reflux esophagitis, prophylaxis of stress ulcer.
Actions:	Buffers gastric acidity.
Side effects:	Diarrhea, hypermagnesemia in renal failure.
Comments:	Aluminum salts may cause constipation, and magnesium salts may cause diarrhea. The mixture attempts to balance these effects. May bind and reduce absorption of tetracycline, thyroxine, and other medications.
Dose:	30–60 ml PO q1–2h during the acute phase. 30–60 ml PO q1 and 3h PC meals and QHS for chronic therapy.

NALOXONE HYDROCHLORIDE (Narcan) Narcotic antagonist

Indications:	Narcotic antagonism.
Actions:	Competitive antagonist of narcotics.
Side effects:	Nausea, vomiting, may precipitate withdrawal in narcotic addicts.
Comments:	Effect is shorter than that of many narcotics.
Dose:	0.2–2.0 mg IV/IM/SC q5min to a maximum dose of 10 mg.

NAPROXEN (Naprosyn) NSAID

Indications:	Inflammation due to arthritis, soft-tissue injury, pericarditis.
Actions:	Proprionic acid derivative. Interferes with production of prostaglandins.
Side effects:	Headaches, dizziness and lightheadedness, epigastric pain. May compromise renal function in patients with renal impairment.
Comments:	Should be used with caution in anticoagulated patients, contraindicated in the syndrome of aspirin sensitivity, nasal polyps, and bronchospasm.
Dose:	250 mg PO BID.

NARCAN (see Naloxone Hydrochloride)

NIFEDIPINE (Adalat, Procardia) Calcium channel blocker

Indications:	Angina pectoris, coronary spasm, hypertension.
Actions:	Calcium channel blocker, arterial vasodilator.
Side effects:	Hypotension, flushing, dizziness, headache, peripheral edema.
Comments:	The edema is due to vasodilation and does not respond to diuretics. Nifedipine has a greater effect than verapamil and diltiazem on peripheral vasculature.
Dose:	10–30 mg PO TID.

NITROGLYCERIN Vasodilator

Indications:	Angina pectoris, CHF.
Actions:	Venous, coronary, and arteriolar vasodilator.
Side effects:	Headache, hypotension, flushing.
Comments:	Nitrate tolerance may develop with prolonged continuous administration.

Dose:		
	Sublingual	0.15–0.6 mg
	Lingual aerosol	One or two doses sprayed on or under the tongue q3–5min to a maximum of 3 times/15 min
	Transdermal patch	0.2 mg/h, increasing to 0.4 mg/h. Patch should be left on 10–12 h, then off for 12–14 h to avoid tolerance.
	Transdermal ointment	0.5–4 inches q4–8h. Rotate sites
	Oral sustained release	2–9 mg BID to TID

NIZORAL (see Ketoconazole)
NOCTEC (see Chloral Hydrate)
NOREPINEPHRINE (see p. 342)

NYSTATIN (Mycostatin)   Antifungal

Indications:	Oral and esophageal candidiasis.
Actions:	Disruption of fungal cell membranes.
Side effects:	Nausea, vomiting.
Comments:	Not absorbed orally.
Dose:	400,000–600,000 units PO (swish and swallow) QID.

OXAZEPAM (Serax)   Benzodiazepine

Indications:	Insomnia, anxiety.
Actions:	Benzodiazepine sedative–hypnotic.
Side effects:	Sedation, respiratory depression, confusion.
Comments:	Peak effect in 1–4 h and relatively short duration.
Dose:	10–30 mg PO QHS PRN for sleep. 30–100 mg/day in divided doses for anxiety.

PARACETAMOL (see Acetaminophen)
PENICILLIN (see p. 349)
PENTACARINATE (see Pentamidine Isoethionate)

PENTAMIDINE ISOETHIONATE (Pentacarinate)   Anti-PCP
agent

Indications:	*Pneumocystic carinii* pneumonia (PCP).
Action:	Unknown.
Side effects:	Hypotension, renal failure, cardiac arrythmia, hypoglycemia, pancreatitis.
Comments:	Reduce dose in renal impaired patients.
Dose:	4 mg/kg in 50–250 ml D5W IV given over 2 h daily.

PHENAZOPYRIDINE (Pyridium)   Urinary analgesic

Indications:	Urethritis, cystitis.
Actions:	Analgesic effect on inflamed urinary tract mucosa.
Side effects:	Orange discoloration of urine, nausea.
Comments:	Has no antibacterial effect.
Dose:	200 mg PO TID after meals.

PHENYLEPHRINE (see p. 342)

PHENYTOIN (Dilantin)   Anticonvulsant, antiepileptic

Indications:	Seizure disorders.
Actions:	Anticonvulsant, reduces Na transport across cerebral cell membranes.
Side effects:	Hypotension, cardiac dysrhythmias, ataxia, nystagmus, dysarthria, hepatotoxicity, gingival hypertrophy, hirsutism, megaloblastic anemia, lymphadenopathy, fever, rash.
Comments:	At therapeutic doses, the drug is metabolized in the liver at zero order (a fixed absolute amount per unit time). Relatively small changes in dose can cause ma-

> jor changes in serum concentrations over the long term.

Dose: For status epilepticus, 18 mg/kg loading dose IV in NS at a rate of ≤25–50 mg/min. For epilepsy, 300 mg PO–IV daily.

PHYTONADIONE (Vitamin K$_1$)   Vitamin K

Indications: Vitamin K deficiency, reversal of warfarin effect.
Actions: Essential for hepatic synthesis of factors II, VII, IX, X.
Side effects: Hematoma formation with SC/IM administration.
Comment: Avoid IV administration because of hypotension and anaphylaxis. Serious hemorrhage due to excessive warfarin is better treated with fresh frozen plasma.
Dose: 2.5–5.0 mg PO/SC/IM.

PIPERACILLIN (see p. 349)

POTASSIUM   Potassium supplements

Indications: Hypokalemia.
Actions: Potassium supplement.
Side effects: Nausea, vomiting, diarrhea, abdominal discomfort, hyperkalemia.
Comments: Danger of hyperkalemia in patients with renal impairment, patients receiving potassium-sparing diuretics, and those on angiotensin-converting enzyme inhibitors.
Dose:

Micro-K Extencaps	= 8 mmol K$^+$
Micro-K-10 Extencaps	= 10 mmol K$^+$
Slow-K	= 8 mmol K$^+$
Kay Ciel Elixir	= 20 mmol/15 ml
Prevention	24–40 mmol per day
Treatment	60–120 mmol per day or more

PROCAINAMIDE (Pronestyl, Procan) Class IA antiarrhythmic

Indications: Atrial and ventricular tachyarrhythmias.
Actions: Reduces the maximum rate of depolarization in atrial and ventricular conducting tissue. Class IA antiarrhythmic.
Side effects: Hypotension, anorexia, nausea, vomiting, heart block, proarrhythmia, rash, fever, SLE-like syndrome, arthralgias.
Comments: Similar to quinidine except that it does not have an atropinic effect. Cross allergy to procaine.
Dose: 1 g load PO followed by 250–500 mg PO q3h. Delayed release preparations may be given q6h. For life-threatening tachydysrhythmias, 100 mg IV over 2 min repeatedly until the arrhythmia has abated or until a total dose of 1 g has been given. If successful, follow with a maintenance dose of 2–4 mg/min IV.

PROCAN (see Procainamide)
PROCARDIA (see Nifedipine)

PROMETHAZINE (Phenergan)   Antihistamine

Indications:	Sedation, nausea, vomiting.
Actions:	Antihistamine and anticholinergic.
Side effects:	Drowsiness, dizziness, constipation, dry mouth, urinary retention.
Comments:	Anticholinergic effects are additive with those of other drugs, such as the tricyclic antidepressants.
Dose:	25–50 mg PO/PR/IM q4–6h PRN or 12.5–25 mg IV q4–6h PRN.

PRONESTYL (see Procainamide)

PROPRANOLOL (Inderal)   Nonspecific beta blocker

Indications:	Angina pectoris; post-MI treatment of SVT, hypertension; thyrotoxicosis.
Actions:	Nonspecific beta-adrenergic blockade.
Side effects:	Hypotension, bradycardia, bronchospasm, CHF, nausea, vomiting, fatigue, nightmares, may mask symptoms of hypoglycemia.
Comments:	Abrupt withdrawal may precipitate angina in patients with coronary heart disease.
Dose:	10–80 mg PO BID to QID. Begin with a low dose and adjust to desired effect.

PROTAMINE SULFATE   Heparin antagonist

Indications:	Reversal of heparin anticoagulation.
Actions:	Binds to and inactivates heparin.
Side effects:	Hypotension, bradycardia, flushing.
Comments:	Overdosage may paradoxically result in worsening hemorrhage, since protamine possesses anticoagulant activity.
Dose:	1 mg/100 units of heparin, IV slowly, based on an estimation of the circulating heparin. Do not give more than 50 mg in a 10 min period.

PROVENTYL (see Salbutamol)
PYRIDIUM (see Phenazopyridine)

QUININE SULFATE   Antimalarial

Indications:	Nocturnal leg cramps.
Actions:	Unknown.
Side effects:	Nausea, visual disturbances, hemolytic anemia, thrombocytopenia.
Comments:	Side effects are unusual at this dose, which is 1/10 that used in malaria.
Dose:	300 mg PO QHS PRN.

RANITIDINE (Zantac)   Histamine$_2$ antagonist

Indications:	Peptic ulcer disease, gastrointestinal reflux.
Actions:	Inhibits histamine-induced secretion of gastric acid.
Side effects:	Jaundice, gynecomastia, headache, confusion, leukopenia.

Comments:	Generally well tolerated. Does not have the same effect as cimetidine on microsomal enzymes or androgen blocking.
Dose:	50 mg IV q8h or 150 mg PO BID or 300 mg PO once daily. Maintenance therapy 150 mg PO QHS.

SALBUTAMOL (Ventolin, Proventyl) Beta$_2$ antagonist

Indications:	Bronchospasm.
Actions:	Beta$_2$-adrenergic antagonist.
Side effects:	Headache, dizziness, nausea, tremor, palpitations.
Comments:	Larger doses cause tachycardia.
Dose:	2.5–5 mg in 3 ml NS by nebulizer q4h PRN. In severe bronchospasm, may be required q3–5min initially.

SERAX (see Oxazepam)
SINEMET (see Levodopa-Carbidopa)
SODIUM BICARBONATE (see p. 345)

SODIUM POLYSTYRENE SULFONATE (Kayexalate) Cation exchange resin

Indications:	Hyperkalemia.
Actions:	Nonabsorbable cation exchange resin.
Side effects:	Nausea, vomiting, gastric irritation, sodium retention.
Comments:	20 mmol of Na are exchanged for 20 mmol of K for each 15 g given orally. Mg and Ca also may be exchanged.
Dose:	15–30 g in 50–100 ml of 20% sorbitol PO q3–4h or 50 g in 200 ml 20% sorbitol or D20W PR by retention enema for 30–60 min q6h PRN.

SORBITRATE (see Isosorbide Dinitrate)

SPIRONOLACTONE (Aldactone) Diuretic, aldosterone antagonist

Indications:	Ascites, edema, hypertension, hyperaldosteronism.
Actions:	Aldosterone antagonist.
Side effects:	Hyponatremia, gynecomastia, confusion, headache.
Comments:	Most effective in states of hyperaldosteronism; however, equipotent to thiazides in hypertension.
Dose:	50–100 mg PO once daily. Higher doses are required in states of hyperaldosteronism.

SUMATRIPTAN SUCCINATE (Imitrex)

Indications:	Intermittent treatment of migraine.
Actions:	Selective 5-hydroxytryptamine-like receptor agonist. Causes vasoconstriction particularly of the dilated carotid arterial circulation in migraine.
Side effects:	Can cause coronary artery spasm. Contraindicated in coronary artery disease, concomitant use of ergot alkaloids, uncontrolled hypertension, use of MAOs, and hemiplegic migraine. Flushing, dizziness, feelings of heat, pressure, malaise, fatigue, drowsiness, nausea, vomiting.

Comments:	SC injection accompanied by local pain. Peak effects after SC in 15 min, after PO 0.5–5 h.
Dose:	100 mg PO or 6 mg SC. Do not repeat if first dose has not had an effect. If successful, recrudescences can be treated with further doses not to exceed 300 mg PO in 24 h.

TAGAMET (see Cimetidine)
TETRACYCLINE (see p. 349)
THEOPHYLLINE (see Aminophylline)

THIAMINE (Vitamin B_1)   Vitamin B_1

Indications:	Thiamine deficiency, prophylaxis of Wernicke's encephalopathy.
Action:	Vitamin B_1 replacment.
Side effects:	IV administration may result in hypotension or, rarely, anaphylactic shock. Well absorbed orally.
Comments:	Consider the oral route even in emergencies.
Dose:	100 mg PO/IM/IV daily for 3 days. If given IV, give slowly over 5 min.

THORAZINE (see Chlorpromazine)
TOBRAMYCIN (see p. 349)
TRANDATE (see Labetalol)
TYLENOL (see Acetaminophen)
VALIUM (see Diazepam)
VANCERIL (see Beclomethasone)
VANCOMYCIN (see p. 349)
VASOTEC (see Enalapril)
VENTOLIN (see Salbutamol)

VERAPAMIL (Isoptin, Calan)   Calcium channel blocker

Indications:	Angina pectoris, treatment of SVTs, hypertension, left ventricular diastolic dysfunction.
Actions:	Calcium channel blocker, depresses AV conduction.
Side effects:	CHF, bradycardias, hypotension, headaches, dizziness, constipation.
Comments:	Calcium gluconate 1–2 g IV may reverse the negative inotropic and hypotensive effects but not the AV block.
Dose:	80–120 mg PO TID. IV administration should take place only in monitored patients: 5–10 mg IV may be given for rate control to break an SVT.

VERSED (see Midazolam)
VITAMIN B_1 (see Thiamine)
VITAMIN K_1 (see Phytonadione)

WARFARIN (Coumadin)   Oral anticoagulant

Indications:	Prophylaxis and treatment of DVT, pulmonary embolism, embolic CVA.
Actions:	Inhibits vitamin K-dependent clotting factors.

Side effects:	Hemorrhage, nausea, vomiting, skin necrosis, fever, rash.
Comments:	Individualize dosage to maintain PT in the desired range. Many drugs interact to increase or decrease the effect of warfarin. Always look up new medications before starting them in patients on warfarin to see whether they interact. Fresh frozen plasma is the treatment of choice to rapidly reverse warfarin's effect. An alternative is vitamin K_1.
Dose:	10 mg PO daily for 2 days, then estimated maintenance dose of 5–7.5 mg PO daily modified according to PT.

XYLOCAINE (see Lidocaine)
ZANTAC (see Ranitidine)
ZAROXOLYN (see Metolazone)
ZIDOVUDINE (AZT, azidothymidine, Retrovir) Nucleoside analog

Indications:	Advanced HIV disease.
Actions:	Inhibition of reverse transcriptase, thus inhibiting virus replication, thymidine analog.
Side effects:	Headache, anorexia, nausea, vomiting, myalgias, anemia, leukopenia.
Comments:	Mild anemia (macrocytic and megaloblastic) is common but readily reversible on stopping the drug.
Dose:	100 mg PO q4h or 200 mg PO q8h.

ZYLOPRIM (see Allopurinol)

INDEX

Note: Page numbers in *italics* refer to illustrations; page numbers followed by t refer to tables